THE AGING LUNGS

MECHANISMS AND CLINICAL SEQUELAE

THE AGING LUNGS

MECHANISMS AND CLINICAL SEQUELAE

Editors

Richard Bucala

Patty J Lee

Yale University

World Scientific

NEW JERSEY • LONDON • SINGAPORE • BEIJING • SHANGHAI • HONG KONG • TAIPEI • CHENNAI • TOKYO

Published by

World Scientific Publishing Co. Pte. Ltd.
5 Toh Tuck Link, Singapore 596224
USA office: 27 Warren Street, Suite 401-402, Hackensack, NJ 07601
UK office: 57 Shelton Street, Covent Garden, London WC2H 9HE

British Library Cataloguing-in-Publication Data
A catalogue record for this book is available from the British Library.

Accelerated lung aging in a MIF deficient mouse. Photo credit: Maur Sauler, MD.

THE AGING LUNGS
Mechanisms and Clinical Sequelae

ISBN 978-981-4635-00-4

Typeset by Stallion Press
Email: enquiries@stallionpress.com

Printed in Singapore

Preface

Patty J. Lee and Richard Bucala

> I'm the same person I was back then, A little less hair, a little less chin, A lot less lungs, much less wind. But ain't I lucky I can still breathe in.
>
> *Excerpt from Maya Angelou's 'On Aging'*

The lungs represent the largest interface between the host and the external environment. As a result they have the capacity to mount diverse, complex stress responses but eventually exhibit the cumulative effects of inhaled as well as circulating toxins, antigens and pathogenic microbes. Aging reduces ventilatory capacity and increases vulnerability to stressors, which manifest as increased rates of pulmonary infections, acute respiratory failure and a variety of chronic lung diseases. As the number of Americans over age 65 is estimated to reach 19% of the population, or over 72 million, by 2030, there is urgency in better understanding fundamental mechanisms of lung aging and their clinical manifestations. Dysregulated inflammation, immunosenescence, genomic instability and mitochondrial dysfunction are a few of the emerging theories that link aging and lung disease. This volume will provide a comprehensive overview of the state-of-the-art paradigms in aging lung by leaders in the field.

Contents

Chapter 1

Normal Development, Anatomy, Histology and Aging of the Lung

Xuchen Zhang*,‡ and Robert J. Homer†

1. Introduction

The primary function of the lungs is to exchange gas between air in the external environment and blood in the cardiovascular system. Although this process sounds straightforward, it is fraught with multiple barriers to its success.[1] The entire airway is constantly exposed to the external environment and must cope with challenges including temperature, particles and allergens, toxicants and pathogens. Terrestrial life has adapted to these and other challenges through the evolution of a complex respiratory system consisting of more than 40 different cell lineages.[2,3] The lung's major anatomic components are the airway, including the conducting airways and

*Assistant Professor of Pathology, Yale University School of Medicine, New Haven, CT 06510; Pathology and Laboratory Medicine Service, VA CT Healthcare System, West Haven, CT 06516, USA, E-mail: Xuchen.Zhang@yale.edu

†Professor of Pathology, Yale University School of Medicine, New Haven, CT 06510; Pathology and Laboratory Medicine Service, VA CT Healthcare System, West Haven, CT 06516, E-mail: Robert.Homer@yale.edu

‡Corresponding Author.

the alveoli; the vasculature, including both pulmonary and systemic circulation; the interstitium, including all supporting tissue, smooth muscle and nerves; the hematopoietic and lymphoid tissues that provide host defense; and finally the poorly understood cells, such as stem (progenitor) cells, perivascular epithelioid cells, meningothelioid cells and others.[2]

The lung is extremely complex not only in structure, with its abundant, diverse cell types in distinct locations, but also in the comprehensive mechanisms of development, maturation, repair and aging processes. The complex nature of lung impacts its normal function, ability to respond to injury and age-associated structural and physiological changes.

2. Lung Development

Mammalian lung development encompasses both prenatal and postnatal life.[4,5] During early embryonic life, the foregut endoderm is specified into domains that will give rise to organs, such as the thyroid, lung, liver and pancreas. Once respiratory cell fate has been established, the tracheal and lung primordial form, which subsequently develops into a tree-like system of epithelial tubules and vascular structures that ultimately becomes the airways and the alveoli. During development the endoderm differentiates into the multiple resident epithelial cell lineages, while the mesoderm will give rise to structures such as the vascular components of the lung, airway smooth muscle, lymphatics, tracheal cartilage, and pleura. Lung development has been extensively studied in recent years, generating new insights into the origins of the different cell lineages that exist in the lung as well as the molecular pathways that regulate these lineages. This has led to novel insights into congenital lung diseases, lung abnormalities and acquired lung diseases, including asthma and chronic obstructive pulmonary disease (COPD), and the lung's response to acute injuries.[1]

2.1. *Lung morphogenesis*

Lung development is essential for terrestrial life and follows a stereotypic program orchestrated by interactions among epithelial

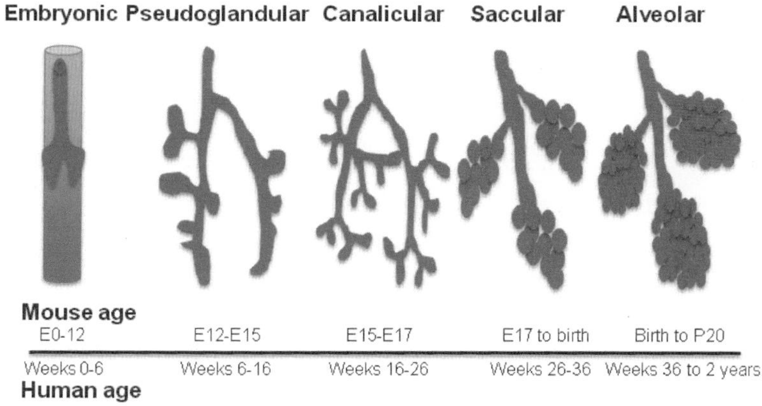

Fig 1. Lung Development. Lung Development in both Mouse and Human Progresses through Five Overlapping Phases: Embryonic, Pseudoglandular, Canalicular, Saccular and Alveolar. E–Embryonic Days, P–Postnatal Days.

and mesenchymal tissues. Lung morphogenesis, together with the trachea, arises from the anterior foregut endoderm, a tissue that generates multiple organs, including the respiratory system, esophagus, thyroid and liver. Typically, lung morphogenesis is divided into five phases (Fig. 1) with some overlap of the beginning and end of each of these phases.[5] It is generally accepted in humans that weeks 0 to 6 of gestation comprise the embryonic phase, weeks 6 to 16 the pseudoglandular phase, weeks 16 to 24 the canalicular phase, weeks 24 to term (40 weeks) the saccular phase, and weeks 36 to 2 years postnatal life the alveolar phase.

2.1.1. *Embryonic phase (Weeks 0 to 6)*

The initiation of lung formation as a bud off the lateral foregut endoderm occurs in the 4th week in humans post conception. During this stage, the trachea completes its separation from the esophagus and branches into the right and left main bronchi and subsequently into lobar and segmental bronchi. Lobar and segmental bronchi appear at about the 5th week and by the end of this stage, 18 major lobules are recognizable. Meanwhile, the bud protrudes into the mesenchyme, which gives rise to the fibroblasts and vascular cells of the lung as well as to the cartilage and smooth muscle of the airways.

2.1.2. *Pseudoglandular phase (Weeks 6 to 16)*

Pseudoglandular stage is characterized by further branching of airway and vascular network and progressive differentiation of epithelial cells to form adult structures of cartilage, submucosal gland, bronchial smooth muscle and epithelial cell types.[6] By the 7th week, the trachea and the segmental and subsegmental bronchi are evident. By the end of the 16th week, all bronchial divisions are completed. Of note, although the conducting airways will continually enlarge as the fetus and newborn grow (airway diameter and length increase 2–3 folds between birth and adulthood), large airway branching ceases by the end of this phase. Thus, during pseudoglandular phase, all pre-acinar structures, including pre-acinar airway, pulmonary arteries and veins are formed.

2.1.3. *Canalicular phase (Weeks 16 to 26)*

The canalicular phase is marked by completion of the conducting airways through the level of the terminal bronchioles, and the development of the rudimentary gas exchange unit of the lung acinus. The acinus is comprised of a respiratory bronchiole, its associated alveolar ducts and primitive alveoli. Differentiation of type I and type II alveolar cells and formation of the alveolar capillary barrier are established in this canalicular phase. Surfactant protein is detectable by weeks 24 and only by the end of this phase is the fetus able to survive outside the uterus.

2.1.4. *Saccular phase (Weeks 26 to 36)*

By this stage, division of the airways is almost complete and further growth and development of lung structures comprise of enlargement of the peripheral airways with dilatation of acinar tubules forming “saccules” and thinning of the primary septa between saccules that contain two layers of capillaries from the neighboring saccules. This ensures increased surface area for gas exchange. There is also further differentiation of type II alveolar cells to type I cells, increment in surfactant containing laminar bodies in type II alveolar cells and lung maturation can be measured by surfactant from amniotic fluid. By the end of this phase (at birth), one third of alveoli are developed. Therefore, the human lung is not fully mature structurally, even at term delivery.

2.1.5. *Alveolar phase (36 weeks to 2 years)*

The alveolar phase is characterized by the presence of secondary septa and the formation of definitive alveoli. Alveoli are formed by septation of the terminal sacs to create more numerous, smaller airspaces in a process termed secondary septation. Alveolar walls are formed by the secondary crests that protrude from the walls of the terminal sacs (primary crests). These secondary septa contain fibroblasts, connective tissue, and two layers of capillaries, and they are covered on either side by epithelium. As with all earlier events in lung development, signaling between the epithelium and mesenchyme is key to coordinating this morphogenesis. As the wall matures, the double layer of capillaries interconnects and eventually fuses to form the single layer present in the adult lung. There are about 50 million alveoli in the lungs of the full-term infant, which provide sufficient gas exchange for the beginning of extra-uterine life. Postnatal, alveoli continue to grow in size and number by septation, until the child reaches 2–3 years of age. Some alveoli may continue to be developed up to 8–10 years of age. The final numbers of alveoli in the fully developed lung range from 300–600 million with a total surface area of about 70 m^2, which is approximately 1000 alveoli per acinus.

3. Mechanisms of Lung Development

During the lung morphogenesis, separation of the tracheal tube from the esophagus and formation of the branching lung are the two major developmental processes. The understanding of these basic lung developmental processes has significantly improved through extensive studies in mouse molecular genetics and genomics. It is well recognized that these developmental processes are regulated by diverse signaling crosstalk between the epithelial cells and surrounding mesenchyme, which are highly coordinated by growth factors, transcriptional factors, and extracellular matrix residing in the lung microenvironment. In addition, a number of epigenetic regulators and non-coding RNAs have been identified as key regulators of lung development.[4,7] A full review of signaling pathways involved in lung morphogenesis is beyond the scope of this chapter, but the best-established pathways will be briefly discussed.

3.1. *Specification of the lung endoderm from the anterior foregut*

The first and most important transcription factor in the lung specification from the anterior foregut endoderm is thyroid transcription factor-1 (TTF-1), a product of the *NKX2.1* gene. Expression of the transcription factor TTF-1 occurs at about embroyal (E) day 9.0 in the mouse and 4 weeks gestation in the human. TTF-1 is considered a master regulator of specification of the lung endoderm in the anterior foregut, as *NKX2.1* null mice exhibit absence of lung specification by showing markedly foreshortened trachea that remains fused to the esophagus, resembling a relatively rare anatomical deformity in humans, known as 'complete tracheo-esophageal cleft'. Studies have shown that Wnt signaling pathway plays a crucial role in specifying *NKX2*.1+ respiratory endoderm progenitors during development. Wnt2 and Wnt2b are expressed in the ventral anterior mesoderm surrounding the region of the anterior foregut endoderm where *NKX2*.1+ respiratory endoderm progenitors are located.[8] In Wnt2/2b combined null mutants, embryos lacking Wnt2/2b expression exhibit complete lung agenesis and do not express *NKX2*.1.[8] This phenotype is recapitulated by an endoderm-restricted deletion of β-catenin.[8,9] On the contrary, conditional expression of an activated form of β-catenin leads to an expansion of *NKX2.1*+ progenitors in the posterior gut, including the stomach, suggesting that Wnt is not only necessary but also sufficient to drive lung progenitor identity in foregut endoderm.[8,9] Wnt signaling does not act alone in specifying lung fate; the ability of Wnt/β-catenin signaling to promote *NKX2.1*+ respiratory endoderm progenitor fate is dependent upon other associated signaling pathways, such as active bone morphogenetic protein (BMP) signaling.[10] Bmp4 is expressed in the ventral mesenchyme surrounding the anterior foregut, and loss of Bmp signaling in the foregut endoderm through inactivation of the BMP receptors Bmpr1a and Bmpr1b leads to tracheal agenesis with retention of the branching region of the lungs. Bmp signaling appears to act by repressing the transcription factor SRY-box containing gene 2 (SOX2), which allows for expression of *NKX2.1* in the presumptive lung endoderm.[10,11] Thus, both Wnt and Bmp signaling appear to modulate early lung specification and development.

3.2. *Branching morphogenesis and epithelial differentiation of the lung*

After the early budding of the main bronchi or airways, the lung buds extend into the surrounding mesenchyme and develop rapidly through a process called branching morphogenesis. Branching morphogenesis is essential for forming both the structural airways as well as the terminal alveolar compartments in which gas exchange occurs.[1] Although the exact mechanisms are still unclear, several pathways have been found to be involved in the branching morphogenesis process. Fibroblast growth factor (FGF) signaling, in particular FGF10 signaling to its cognate receptor FGFr2 in the developing endoderm, is essential for branching morphogenesis, and loss of this pathway leads to complete abrogation of branching.[12,13] FGF10 is one of the most-studied family members during lung development. FGF10-null mice lack distal lung despite formation of larynx and trachea is normal.[14] FGF10 is expressed focally in E11–E12 mouse peripheral lung mesenchyme and signals through adjacent distal epithelial FGFr2. These sites of expression change dynamically, compatible with the sites of lung bud formation. Several key regulatory molecules such as Wnt, sonic hedgehog (Shh), BMPs, and TGF-β crosstalk with FGF10 during embryonic lung branching morphogenesis, suggesting a complex interplay of signaling molecules.[15–17]

During branching morphogenesis, the lung endoderm also begins to develop distinct cell lineages along its proximal-distal axis. SOX2 expression marks the proximal endoderm progenitor lineage whereas the combined expression of Sox9 and the transcriptional regulator inhibitor of DNA binding 2 (ID2) marks the distal endoderm progenitor lineage. Importantly, these two populations have distinct fates: The proximal progenitors give rise to airway neuroendocrine cells, secretory cells, ciliated cells and mucosal cells, whereas the distal progenitors give rise to type 1 and type 2 alveolar epithelial cells.[1] Studies have shown that SOX2 is necessary for the differentiation of proximal progenitors into their various progeny; loss of SOX2 expression leads to loss of the mature secretory and ciliated lineages in the lung airways.[18,19] The precise molecular pathways required for the formation and differentiation of distal SOX9/Id2 progenitors are poorly understood. Inhibition of both Wnt/β-catenin signaling and BMP signaling results in a loss of distal lung epithelial lineages.[20–22] In addition, transcription factors, such as NKX2.1 and forkhead box (Foxp1/2), appear to play important roles in the differentiation of distal endoderm progenitors.[23,24]

TTF-1, regulator of lung specification from the anterior foregut, also has a prominent role in establishing cell fate along the proximal to distal lung epithelium. TTF-1 expression continues to be expressed by epithelial cells at the distal tips of the branching lung epithelium, ultimately becoming more restricted to Clara cells and alveolar type 2 cells. TTF-1 is critical for the expression of genes that are unique to differentiated epithelium, such as CC10 expression in Clara cells and sftp in alveolar type 2 cells. DNA binding sites for TTF-1 are found in the promoter regions of all four surfactant proteins (sftp a-d), CC10, and *NKX2.1* itself, creating a positive feedback loop for sustained TTF-1 expression. Furthermore, *NKX2.1* expression can itself interact with additional transcriptional regulators such as Gata-6 and Foxa2.[25,26] Gata-6 is a member of the Gata family of zinc finger proteins and is expressed in endodermally derived tissues including the lung.[27] GATA-6 and NKX2.1 directly interact and regulate sftp-C gene expression.[27] Mice heterozygous for both Gata-6 and *NKX2*.1 have defects in lung epithelial cell differentiation.[28] The Fox family proteins, Foxa1 (also known as hepatocyte nuclear factor-3, Hnf-3α) and Foxa2 (also known as Hnf-3β), are key regulators of endoderm identity and development. The combined loss of Foxa1 and Foxa2 leads to severe defects in lung epithelial cell differentiation, including loss of the alveolar type 2 cell markers (Sftpc and Sftpb) and the airway epithelial markers for the secretory (secretoglobin 1A member 1, Scgb1a1) and ciliated (Foxj1) epithelial lineages.[29] Both Foxa1 and Foxa2 regulate the expression of *NKX2*.1, which in turn regulates transcription of the sftp genes in lung epithelial cells.[26,30] Other Fox transcription factors, such as Foxj1, which is required for differentiation of proximal SOX2+ progenitors into ciliated epithelium, and overexpression of Foxj1 throughout the developing lung epithelium leads to ectopic formation of ciliated epithelium.[31–33] Foxp1, Foxp2 and Foxp4 are highly expressed in the developing and postnatal lung; Foxp1 and Foxp4 are expressed in both proximal and distal epithelial lineages while Foxp2 is expressed primarily in distal epithelium. Loss of Foxp2 in mouse leads to defective postnatal lung alveolarization and death, 3 weeks after birth.[24] When the lung alveolus is formed, Foxp2 modulates the *NKX2*.1-mediated sftp C expression in type II alveolar cells.[34]

4. Lung Anatomy and Histology

The lungs are paired intrathoracic organs that are divided into 5 lobes (3 on the right-upper, middle and lower lobes; two on the left-upper and lower lobes), and the lobes are further divided into bronchopulmonary segments. The segmental anatomy of the lung is important for radiologists, bronchoscopists, pathologists and thoracic surgeons in accurately defining the location of lesions and performing the segmentectomy procedures.[35] The lingula is a rudimentary appendage arising from the left upper lobe and is analogous to the middle lobe on the right. The right lung usually weighs about 625 gm and the left 567 gm, but much variation is met with according to the amount of blood or serous fluid they may contain. The lungs are heavier in the male than in the female. Increased lung weight can be an indication of congestion, edema, or inflammatory conditions. The right main bronchus is more vertical and more directly in line with the trachea than is the left. Consequently, aspirated foreign material, such as vomitus, blood and foreign bodies, tend to enter the right lung rather than the left.

The lung and all surfaces connected to the lung including diaphragm, mediastinum and inner chest wall are covered by a serosal surface lined by mesothelial cells. The visceral and parietal pleurae are continuous with each other around the hilar structures. The potential space between them is the pleural cavity, which is maintained at a negative pressure by the inward elastic recoil of the lung and the outward pull of the chest wall. It contains a small amount of fluid that allows for smooth, friction free movement of the lung. However, the entry of air or the accumulation of fluid in the pleural cavity may lead to mechanical dysfunction of breathing.[36] Thoracoscopy allows the direct inspection of both the parietal and visceral surfaces. The parietal pleura is translucent and at thoracoscopy the underlying muscles and blood vessels are visible. The visceral pleura is also translucent and has a grey variegated appearance due to the underlying lung and the vascular network in the subpleural layer.

The muscles of respiration and the diaphragm, acting together, create a negative pressure within the pleural space. The resultant reduction in intra-alveolar pressure prompts the conduction of air through the upper respiratory tract into the trachea and airways and then into the alveoli, where gaseous exchange occurs. The respiratory muscles are skeletal muscles similar to the skeletal muscles of the limbs. However, certain functions of respiratory muscles are distinct. They must work without sustained rest throughout life and as a result have high oxidative capacity with increased numbers of mitochondria, high capillary density and greater maximal blood flow than other skeletal muscles. The fiber type distribution in respiratory muscles is consistent with this profile.[37,38] Aging and a number of respiratory diseases e.g. emphysema, have dramatic effects on the function and composition of respiratory muscles and ultimately lead to improper function of respiratory muscles.[38–40]

Within the lung, the airway can be subdivided into a conducting zone and a gas exchange zone. The conducting zone contains the trachea, the bronchi, terminal bronchioles, respiratory bronchioles and alveolar ducts. The respiratory zone, where gas exchange occurs, contains the respiratory bronchioles, the alveolar ducts, and the alveoli. The alveolar ducts are lined entirely by alveoli but are architecturally more like airways. The conducting zone humidifies and warms the air to body temperature. It also cleanses the air by removing particles via cilia and mucus located on the walls of the passageways.[41]

4.1. *Structure of conducting airways*

The airway forms the connection between the atmosphere and the terminal respiratory units. The conducting airways are lined internally by a mucosa, and the epithelium lies on a thin connective tissue lamina propria. External to this is a submucosa, also composed of connective tissue, in which are embedded airway smooth muscle, glands, cartilage plates (depending on the level of the respiratory tree), vessels, lymphoid tissue and nerves. Cartilage is present from the trachea to the smallest bronchi, but is absent from bronchioles. The most proximal bronchioles are referred to as membranous bronchioles (Fig. 2(a)) while the most distal bronchioles without gas exchange are called terminal bronchioles. Terminal and respiratory bronchioles are distinguished in that only the lining of the respiratory bronchioles includes alveoli (Fig. 2(b)). In the trachea and extrapulmonary bronchi, the smooth muscle is mainly confined to the posterior, non-cartilaginous part of the tracheal tube. Along the entire intrapulmonary bronchial tree, smooth muscle forms two opposed helical tracts, which become thinner and finally disappear at the level of the alveoli. Airway smooth muscle regulates airway flow in both large and small airways in response to a variety of stimuli.

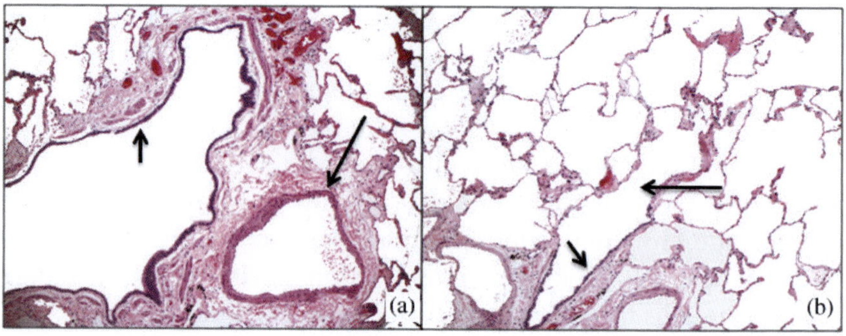

Fig 2. Bronchioles. (a) Normal Bronchioles with Low Columnar Mucosa, Circumferential Smooth Muscle and is Surrounded by an Adventitial Layer (Short Arrow). A Companying Pulmonary Artery is also Present (Long Arrow). **(b)** A Terminal Bronchiole is Continuous with the Respiratory Bronchiole (Short Arrow), which Extends into the Alveolar Ducts (Long Arrow) and Ultimately the Alveoli.

Abnormal contraction may be caused by circulating smooth muscle stimulants or by local release of excitants such as serotonin, histamine, leukotrienes or other inflammatory mediators, which produces bronchospasm. Airway smooth muscle plays a role in inflammation through production of inflammatory mediators and expression of receptors that promote cell adhesion and leukocyte activation. Airway smooth muscle cells also are a key contributor to extracellular matrix composition and amount by production of extracellular matrix, growth factors and matrix modifying enzymes such as matrix metalloproteinases (MMPs) and their inhibitors such as the tissue inhibitors of matrix MMPs (TIMMPs). The altered matrix in turn regulates airway smooth muscle cell function and growth. Numerous mast cells are present in the connective tissue of the respiratory tree, especially towards the bronchioles.

The components of the epithelium lined the mucosa are highly heterogeneous from the larger to smaller airways. The extrapulmonary and larger intrapulmonary airways are lined with respiratory epithelium, which is pseudostratified, predominantly ciliated, and contains interspersed mucus-secreting goblet cells (Fig. 3(a)). There are fewer cilia in terminal and respiratory bronchioles, and the cells

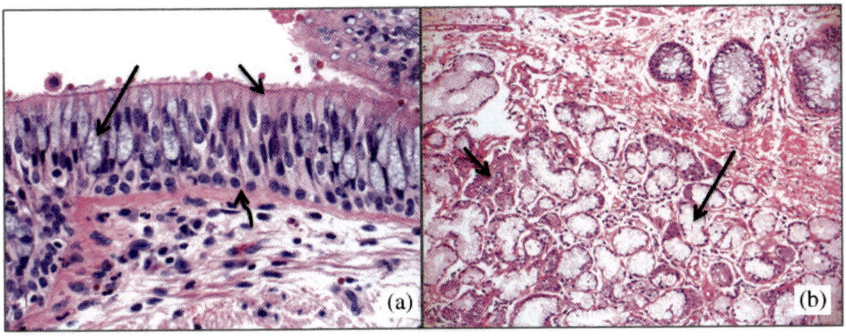

Fig 3. Bronchial Epithelium and Submucosal Glands. (a) Normal Bronchial Epithelium is Pseudostratified and Columnar with Numerous Ciliated Cells (Short Straight Arrow), Scattered Basophilic and Flocculent-Appearing Goblet Cells (Long Straight Arrow) and Basal Cell (Black Curved Arrow). **(b)** The Bronchial Submucosal Glands Contain Mixed Seromucinous Glands (Short Arrow-Serous Cells and Long Arrow-Mucinous Cells) with Ducts Leading to the Bronchial Mucosa.

are reduced in height to low columnar or cuboidal. The epithelium in the respiratory bronchioles progressively reduces in height towards the alveoli, and is eventually composed of cuboidal, non-ciliated cells. Six types of epithelial cell have been described in the conducting airways: Ciliated columnar, goblet, Clara, basal, brush and neuroendocrine cells. Lymphocytes and mast cells migrate into the epithelium from the underlying connective tissue. It is generally thought that pulmonary epithelial cells, including those in the conducting airways and the respiratory alveoli, share a common lineage, distinguished by expression of the transcription factor *NKX2*.1 (TTF-1) during development. In the adult lung, *NKX2*.1 (TTF-1) expression is limited to Clara cells and type II alveolar epithelial cells.

Ciliated columnar cells are the most common epithelial cell of the airway accounting for over 50% of all epithelial cells within the human airways.[42] They vary from low to tall columnar, and each has roughly 200–300 cilia projecting from the apical surface. The cilia extend into a watery fluid secreted by serous cells of the submucosal glands, but their tips are in contact with a more superficial layer of thicker mucus secreted by surface goblet cells and mucous cells in the submucosal glands. The rate of ciliary beating is usually 20 times per second. In addition to tight junctions which seal the apical intercellular space from the airway lumen, the ciliated columnar cells are coupled by gap junctions which allow the cilia beating in a coordinated fashion. The beating is spontaneous and independent of nervous control. The role of the cilia is to move the mucus blanket layer which coats the conducting airway epithelium up to the pharynx where it is either swallowed or expectorated. The mucus layer provides both direct protection against particulates and microbes and allows trapped dust and microbes to be eliminated.[41]

The goblet cells, also called mucus cells, of the surface epithelium in humans are present from the trachea (6000–7000 per mm^2) down to the smaller bronchi, but are normally absent from bronchioles. The ratio of ciliated columnar to mucus cells in humans is estimated to be between 7:1 and 25:1 in the large bronchi. Goblet cells contain an apical region full of large secretory vacuoles filled with mucinogen. When the epithelium is irritated, e.g. by tobacco smoke, goblet cell hyperplasia and metaplasia occur, and they may also extend into the bronchioles, which lead to excessive sputum production.[42] While mucus is produced by the goblet cells in the surface epithelium, in humans the submucosal glands are the main source of bronchial fluid secretion. These glands are mixed seromucinous glands with a narrow duct lined by ciliated epithelium in continuity with the surface epithelium (Fig. 3(b)). The secretory acini are either serous cells or mucus producing cells. In older individuals, oncocytic metaplasia can be seen in these glands. The submucosal glands produce fluid and electrolytes that contribute to the periciliary fluid layer and hydration of mucus and the production of mucus and proteins that contribute to host defense. Serous cells produce various antimicrobial products including lysozyme, lactoferrin, beta defensins, proline rich proteins and secretory leukocyte proteinase inhibitor (SLPI) among other products. The serous cells also are a major site for transport of IgA. Glandular secretion is assisted by myoepithelial cells which are situated between the surface epithelial cells (ductal and secretory) and the basement membrane.

The other major non-ciliated secretory cell of the airway is the Clara cell which was named after the Austrian histologist Max Clara in 1937.[43] Clara cells are cuboidal non-ciliated cells with apices which bulge into the lumen. They contain numerous electron-dense secretory granules and many lysosomes. Clara cells have at least four functions in the lung.[43,44] One function is as progenitor cells for themselves and for ciliated epithelial cells. Another function is detoxification of xenobiotics via cytochrome p450 dependent mixed function oxidase activity. The third function is secretion. Clara cells are a source of some of the sftp (sftpa, sftpb and sftpd). They also are a source of lipids, proteins (such as Clara cell 10kDa protein), glycoproteins, and modulators of inflammation (such as leukocyte protease inhibitor and trypsin-like protease). The fourth function is fluid balance by influencing ion channels.

Basal cells are found predominantly in the larger airways. The basal cell containing pseudostratified airway epithelium extends distally to terminal bronchioles and only the respiratory bronchioles are lined by a simple cuboidal epithelium lacking basal cells. They are relatively undifferentiated and characteristically express transcription factor Trp-63 (p63) and cytokeratins 5 and 14. The development of basal cells, which is completed postnatally, is dependent on the transcription factor p63 such that p63-null mice lack basal cells in the tracheal epithelium.[45] Basal cells have only sparse electron-dense cytoplasm and often contain bundles of cytokeratin tonofilaments, which lead to formation hemidesmosomes firmly attaching to the basement membrane. Basal cells have also been demonstrated to possess stem cell-like properties in that they can self-renew and give rise to secretory and ciliated epithelial cells in response to epithelial injury.[46,47] In addition to their structural and progenitor roles, basal cells have been shown to produce a variety of bioactive molecules including neutral endopeptidase, 15-lipoxygenase products and cytokines.[48]

Neuroendocrine cells, also known as Kulchitsky cells, constitute about 1 to 2% of bronchial epithelial cells in neonates and 0.5% in adults. They are found both in the basal layer of the surface epithelium and in the bronchial glands. Aggregates of neuroendocrine cells are called neuroepithelial bodies; they tend to occur at airway bifurcations. The cells are characterized by cytoplasmic 70–150 nm granules, with a dense central core separated from an outer membrane by a clear halo. During lung development, neuroendocrine cells are the first cell type to form and differentiate within the airway epithelium, increase in number at birth and peak during the neonatal period.[42] The cells contain L-amino acid decarboxylase and 5-hydroxytrptamine, general neuroendocrine markers such as neuron specific enolase, chromogranin A, synaptophysin and Neural Cell Adhesion Molecule (NCAM, CD56), and neuroendocrine peptides such as gastrin-releasing peptide (bombesin), calcitonin, substance P, endothelin, and enkephalin. Neuroendocrine cells are typically tall and pyramidal in shape, extend from the basal lamina of the epithelium and possess apical microvilli. The cells are located within the epithelium lining the larynx, trachea, bronchi and down to the bronchiole-alveolar junctions. They integrate signaling from the environment and from neural input and release their mediators into the surrounding tissue and blood. These cells are thought to be important in regulating airway epithelial regeneration and in responding to a variety of different physiological or pathological stimuli.[49,50]

Brush cells, also termed tuft, caveolated, multivesicular, fibrillovesicular cells or cholinergic chemosensory cells, are characterized by the presence of a tuft of blunt, squat microvilli (approximately 120–140/cell) on the cell surface. The microvilli contain filaments that stretch into the underlying cytoplasm. They have a distinctive pear shape with a wide base and a narrow microvillous apex.[51,52] The function of the brush cells is still obscure although secretory, absorptive and receptive functions have been proposed.[53]

The bronchial basement membrane on which the epithelium sits is a thin layer of extracellular matrix that provides support for the epithelium. Ultra structurally, a basement membrane consists of the basal lamina (true basement membrane) and the deeper lamina reticularis. The major molecular constituent of the basal lamina is collagen IV and laminin synthesized predominantly by epithelial cells; while the lamina reticularis consists of collagens III and IV and fibronectin synthesized by subepithelial fibroblasts. The dense basement membrane beneath the airway epithelium has several important roles in maintaining epithelial integrity: Acting as an anchor facilitating adhesion of epithelial cells, establishing and maintaining correct cellular polarity, providing a barrier between the surface epithelium and the underlying connective tissue and delivering essential survival signals to the epithelium.[42] Studies have demonstrated that the basement membrane contains pores, which can be used as conduits for immune cells to traffic between the epithelial and mesenchymal compartments without perturbing the basement extracellular matrix.[54,55]

Airway-associated lymphoid tissue may be present in the normal lung, but it is very sparse and typically occurs at the bifurcation points of the airways. This lung lymphoid tissue is generally referred to as bronchus-associated lymphoid tissue (BALT), and is felt to be analogous to the mucosa-associated lymphoid tissue of the gastrointestinal tract, such as Peyer's patches and appendiceal lymphoid tissue.[56] The strategic location of BALT at airway divisions may be a consequence to which to inhaled antigens and other particles that are likely to impact these areas. BALT foci are associated with specialized epithelial cells in the mucosa and the constituent lymphoid cells (mainly *B* lymphocytes) are admixed with macrophages and dendritic cells. The epithelial and dendritic cells of the BALT presumably play a role in the detection of inhaled allergens, viruses and bacteria, such that BALT is considered to be a critical component of the lung's immune defense system. The bronchial BALT may become hyperplastic, with follicular germinal center formation. BALT may also be important in diseases of immunologic origin that produce bronchiolitis, such as connective tissue disease (e.g. Sjogren's syndrome and rheumatoid arthritis), as well as graft-versus-host disease in organ transplantation, immunoglobulin deficiency states and even inflammatory bowel disease.

4.2. *Structure of the alveoli*

Gas exchange occurs in the alveolus based on a very thin barrier of very large surface area between air and blood. Alveolar walls comprise greater than 99% of the internal surface area of the mammalian

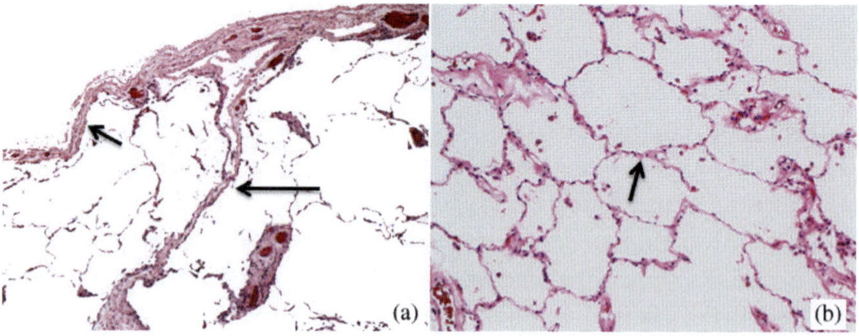

Fig 4. Distal Lung Parenchyma and Visceral Pleura. (a) An Interlobular Septum (Long Arrow) and the Visceral Pleura (Short Arrow) are Present. **(b)** Lung Parenchyma Showing Alveoli are Demarcated by Septa Composed of a Continuous Layer of Alveolar Epithelial Cells Overlying a Thin Interstitium (Arrow).

lung.[57] Alveoli are demarcated by septa composed of a continuous layer of epithelial cells overlying a thin interstitium (Figs. 4(a) and (b)). The former consists principally of two morphologically distinct cells, type I and type II alveolar epithelial cells; the interstitium contains capillaries involved in gas exchange, as well as connective tissue and a variety of cells responsible for maintaining alveolar shape and defense.

Type I alveolar cells cover approximately 95% of the alveolar surface while comprising only 8% of the total cells in the normal adult human lung.[58] The nucleus of this cell type is small and covered by a thin rim of cytoplasm containing few organelles. The rest of the cytoplasm extends as a broad sheet. Adjacent type I cells are joined to one another by tight junctions that provide a complete barrier to the diffusion of fluid and water soluble substances into the alveolar airspace. The cell cytoplasm contains pinocytotic vesicles that can theoretically transport material in either direction across the air–blood barrier. In addition to providing a mechanical barrier that allows gas exchange, fluid and ion transport is a major function of type I cells in order to keep the alveolus functional. In fact, type I alveolar epithelial cells are in rich with solute active transport proteins, water channels and impermeable tight junctions between cells, such as caveolae, amiloride-sensitive epithelial sodium channels (ENaC), cystic fibrosis transmembrane conductance regulator (CFTR) chloride channels and aquaporin 5 (AQP-5).[59–61] Furthermore, type I cells are part of the innate immune system, capable of producing pro-inflammatory mediators, which could contribute to the increase in inflammation seen in early Bronchopulmonary dysplasia or LPS-induced lung injury.[61,62]

Type II alveolar cells are cuboidal in shape and account for approximately 15% of total cells but only about 5% of the alveolar surface area in the healthy human lung.[63] Mainly located in the corner of the mammalian alveolus, type II cells are characterized by their distinctive secretory granules called lamellar bodies, intracellular storage organelles for pulmonary surfactants.[57] Lamellar bodies are among the largest secretory organelles of all cells in the body. Owing to their content of lysosomal enzymes (e.g. acid phosphatase and cathepsins) and proteins (members of the LAMP protein family) and their acid pH of about 5.5, lamellar bodies are regarded as secretory lysosome related organelles. Type II cells are commonly known for the synthesis, secretion and re-uptake of pulmonary surfactants. In addition, type II cells can also regulate alveolar fluid balance and act as progenitor cells following injury to the alveolar epithelium.[64,65]

The evolution of mammalian lungs was closely linked with the parallel development of surfactant. Alveolar surfactant is a complex mixture of approximately 90% phospholipids and 10% protein that is synthesized and recycled by type II cells. This mixture of lipids and proteins reduces the surface tension of the air–fluid interfaces of the lung. The major surfactant proteins are surfactant protein (sftp a, b, c and d). Surfactant facilitates distention of air spaces and also inhibits the tendency of small units to empty into larger units. This tendency is related to Laplace's law that the surface tension of a bubble is inversely proportionate to its radius. Because surfactant is more active in smaller than larger alveoli, it serves to make surface tension of the alveoli more uniform. Overall respiratory compliance is therefore highly dependent on presence of surfactant. States in which surfactant function is reduced including ALI can therefore be expected to have reduced compliance and more alveolar collapse.

A surfactant film is also present in smaller airways where it also prevents airway collapse, promotes mucociliary transport and interacts with pathogens and particles. Sftpa, b and d are synthesized by rodent Clara cells while human Clara cells produce little sftpa or sftpd. Unlike type II alveolar epithelial cells, Clara cells are not involved in re-uptake or recycling of surfactant components.

Alveoli are surrounded and separated from one another by an exceedingly thin connective tissue layer that contains blood capillaries. The tissue between adjacent alveolar air spaces is called the alveolar septum. The alveolar epithelium lies on a basal lamina, which, in the thin portions of a septum, is fused with the basal lamina surrounding the adjacent capillaries. The total barrier to diffusion between air and blood in the thin portions of a septum may be as thin as 0.2 μm. The thick portions of a septum contain connective tissue elements, including elastic and collagen fibers, migratory cells and resident cells. The principal resident cell present is fibroblast (mesenchymal contractile interstitial cell), which has ultra-structural features suggestive of both fibroblast and muscle differentiation. These cells have long slender projections of cytoplasm that extend into the interstitial space. They are closely associated with collagen and elastin fibers of which they are the most likely source. Functions of these cells include local regulation of alveolar gas exchange (their contraction resulting in a reduction in capillary blood flow), regulation of the fluid content of the alveolar interstitium and production of connective tissue, such as collagen and elastin fibers. Loss of elastic fibers in the alveolar interstitium plays an important role in the failure of the lungs to contract adequately in patients who have emphysema. The capillary endothelial cells are non-fenestrated and form a continuous lining. The individual cells are joined by tight junctions, which are more permeable than are the junctions between epithelial cells. On the other hand, overgrowth of fibrous tissues in the lungs in patients with pulmonary fibrosis is responsible for the difficulty that they experience during inhalation. There are also small pores (interalveolar pores of Kohn) lined by epithelium (usually type II alveolar cells), which cross interalveolar septa to link adjacent alveolar airspaces. Humans have up to 7 pores per alveolus, ranging in size from 2 to 13 μm. These small passages may sustain the flow of air in the event of blockage of one of the alveolar ducts and also provide routes of migration for alveolar macrophages(AM) and spread inflammation between alveoli.

AMs, located in the alveolus, provide the first line of phagocytic defense against microbial or toxic invasion in the lower respiratory tract. Besides their phagocytic and microbicidal functions, AMs also secrete numerous chemical mediators upon stimulation, thereby playing a role in regulating inflammatory reactions in the lung.[66] AMs are terminally differentiated cells of the myeloid lineage which are derived from circulating and resident monocytes. They are long-lived cells with life spans of many months up to several years and the turnover rate is only approximately 40% in 1 year.[67,68] However, studies also showed that AMs have a marked capacity for self-renewal and that this is the main means by which these cells are replenished throughout life.[69] Several macrophage subsets with distinct functions have been described. Classically activated macrophages (M1 macrophages) mediate defence of the host from a variety of bacteria, protozoa and viruses and have roles in antitumor immunity. Alternatively activated macrophages (M2 macrophages) have anti-inflammatory and immune regulation functions and regulate wound healing.[70] Similarly, a transcriptional analysis of human AMs that were polarized *ex vivo* using interferon-γ (IFNγ), or with interleukin-4 (IL-4) and IL-13, subgrouped human AMs into M1 and M2 macrophages, respectively.[71] Genes associated with M1 AMs include those encoding CD69, Toll-like receptor 2 (TLR2), TLR4, CXC-chemokine ligand 9 (CXCL9), CXCL10, CXCL11 and CC-chemokine ligand 5 (CCL5); whereas genes associated with M2 AMs include those encoding the mannose receptor (also known as CD206), matrix MMP2, MMP7, MMP9, the tyrosine protein kinase MER, growth arrest-specific protein 7 (GAS7), CD163, stabilin 1 (STAB1), arginase and the adenosine A3 receptor.[71] In humans, there is no general consensus yet about whether AMs in the healthy state are M1 or M2 in nature.[72] Studies have shown that AMs in the healthy lungs are predominantly M1 phenotype.[71,73] However, other studies have shown that up to 50% of macrophages in human bronchoalveolar lavage fluid(BAL) are M2 macrophages.[74,75]

An increase in M2 AMs seems to be a feature of many inflammatory lung diseases in humans including allergic asthma, idiopathic pulmonary fibrosis and COPD.[76–78]

4.3. *Pulmonary vasculature*

The lungs have two functionally distinct vascular systems: Bronchial (systemic) arteries and veins and pulmonary arteries and veins. The latter is a low-pressure high-capacity system which is structurally organized to allow a large change of volume with a minimal change in pressure; they convey deoxygenated blood to the alveolar walls and drain oxygenated blood back to the left side of the heart. The former, the bronchial arteries, provides oxygenated blood to lung tissues that do not have close access to atmospheric oxygen, e.g. those of the bronchi and larger bronchioles.

The bronchial arteries in the walls of bronchi are part of the systemic circulation and have pressures similar to systemic arterial pressures. Most individuals have 2 to 4 bronchial arteries, a relatively common pattern being one on the right (originating from the third intercostal artery) and two on the left (arising directly from the aorta). As part of the systemic circulation, the bronchial arterial system delivers blood at high pressure and high arterial oxygen content. The bronchial arteries accompany the bronchial tree and supply bronchial glands, the walls of the bronchial tubes and larger pulmonary vessels. The bronchial branches form a capillary plexus in the muscular tunic of the air passages which supports a second, mucosal plexus that communicates with branches of the pulmonary artery and drains into the pulmonary veins. Other arterial branches ramify in interlobular loose connective tissue and most end in either deep or superficial bronchial veins; some also ramify on the surface of the lung, forming subpleural capillary plexuses. Bronchial arteries supply the bronchial wall as far as the respiratory bronchioles and anastomose with branches of the pulmonary arteries in the walls of the smaller bronchi and in the visceral pleura. In addition to the main bronchial arteries, smaller bronchial branches exist arising from the descending thoracic aorta.

Pulmonary arteries are intimately related to the airways and divide with them, a branch accompanying the adjacent airway to the level of the respiratory bronchioles. The endothelial cells of pulmonary arteries and veins are similar to that of capillaries, but with more organelles. They are rich in Weibel–Palade bodies which contain von Willibrand factor, *p*-selectin, tissue type plasminogen activator, endothelin-1, various adhesion molecules and other factors involved in hemostasis, inflammation and vasoactivity.[79] A classic example is the conversion of angiotensin I to angiotensin II and the inactivation of bradykinin by angiotensin-converting enzyme. Accumulating evidence has demonstrated a physiological and pathological role of angiotensin-converting enzyme in lungs with COPD and SARS coronavirus or influenza H5N1 virus-mediated ALIs.[80–82] Large (elastic) pulmonary arteries in infants are similar to the aorta structurally; the elastic fiber lamellae become more irregular, fragmented and less compact in adulthood. Elastic tissue remains relatively prominent in the pulmonary arterial tree including the main pulmonary artery and its lobar, segmental and subsegmental branches extending approximately to the point where bronchi become bronchioles. At this juncture, the pulmonary arteries become primarily muscular arteries. The muscular pulmonary arteries and arterioles have an internal and external elastic membrane. Arterioles continue to divide within the acinus, some accompanying bronchioles and alveolar ducts to the level of the alveolar sacs and others penetrating the adjacent parenchyma directly. The smaller branches ramify to form the capillary network of the alveoli. Unlike pulmonary arteries, pulmonary veins and venules are not associated with airways instead in the parenchyma or in the connective tissue septa. Pulmonary veins have only a lamellated single (outer) elastica. Small intra-acinar pulmonary veins merge into larger veins in the interlobular septa. It may be difficult to separate small pulmonary arterioles from venules, since both of them contain a single elastic lamina. In pathologic states, the veins may develop muscular hypertrophy with increased mural thickness (arterialization), making the distinction of arteries from veins even more difficult. The location of the vessel, particularly if it is in a septum or accompanied by an airway, is extremely helpful when separating pulmonary veins from pulmonary arteries.

The lung has a highly developed lymphatic network, which are divided into the subpleural, or superficial, plexus that drains the outer parts of the lung via the visceral pleural lymphatics and the deep, or peribronchovascular, plexus that drains in the bronchovascular connective tissue toward the hilar lymph nodes. Anastomotic channels between these two lymphatic systems can be seen at the boundaries of their distribution and between lobes or lobules and the pleura near the hilum. Alveolar walls do not have lymphatic spaces, but some lymphatics are located immediately adjacent to alveolar airspaces in the interlobular, peribronchial and perivascular connective tissue. These channels have been termed juxta-alveolar lymphatics because of their close topographic and possible functional relationship with the alveolar airspaces.

4.4. *Incidental findings of the lung*

A variety of structures may be incidentally observed in lung tissue samples. They can be endogenous or exogenous materials in both pathologic and non-pathologic conditions of the lungs.

Minute pulmonary meningothelial-like nodules(MPMN) (formerly called pulmonary chemodectomas) were originally thought to represent an intrapulmonary proliferation of perivenular chemoreceptor cells. However, the accumulated evidence suggests that the cells resemble meningothelial cells, hence the present nomenclature. MPMN are composed of interstitial clusters of fusiform cells with pale eosinophilic cytoplasm, forming small stellate nodules near small veins (Fig. 5(a)). MPMN can be seen in all lobes and the incidence is not different between lobes or between age groups.[83,84] The clinic-pathologic significance of the presence of MPMN remains unclear.

Corpora amylacea are 30–200μm round to oval eosinophilic endogenous concretions arranged in concentric layers (Fig 5. (b)); they are more common in the alveoli and alveolar walls of older individuals. Sometimes they may have a black or birefringent central

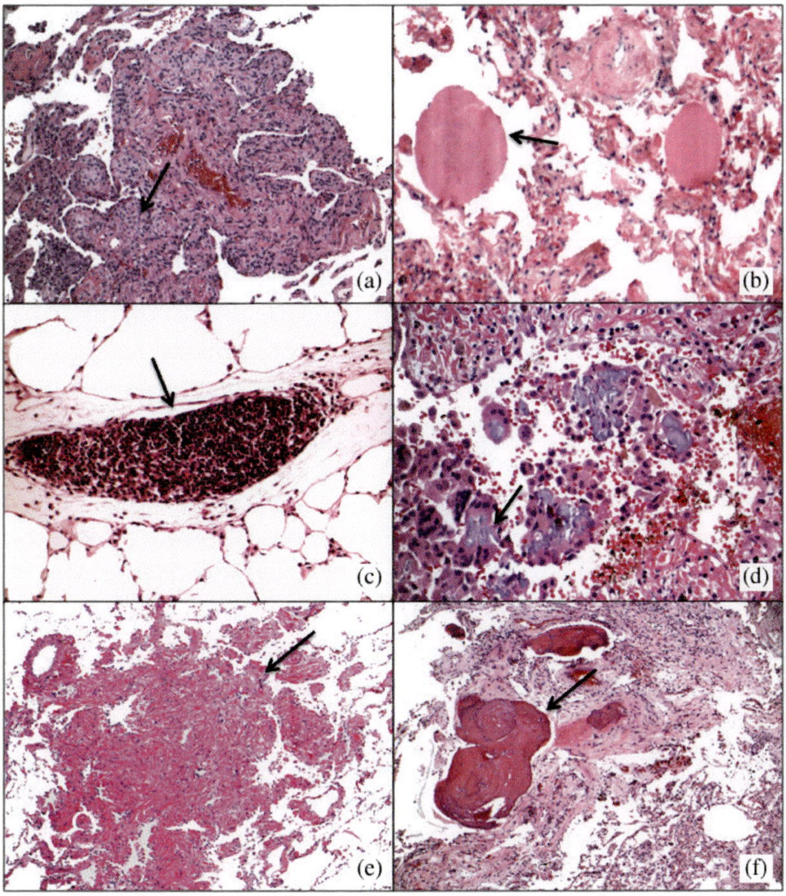

Fig 5. Incidental Findings of the Lung. (a) MPMN. MPMN is Composed of Interstitial Clusters of Fusiform Cells with Pale Eosinophilic Cytoplasm (Arrows), Forming Small Stellate Nodules Near Small Veins. **(b)** Corpora Amylacea. Round to Oval Eosinophilic Concretions Arranged in Concentric Layers in the Alveoli. **(c)** Intraulmonary Lymph Node. Lymph Node within the Lung Parenchyma (Arrow). **(d)** Blue Bodies. Blue Bodies are Gray or Blue, Intra-Alveolar, Calcified, Lamellated Structures Often Associated with Clusters of Macrophages, Including Giant Cells. **(e)** Incidental Parenchymal Scar. These Scars are Typically Seen in Subpleural Parenchyma and Appear to Center on Alveolar Ducts (arrow) and Commonly Have Fascicles of Normal Appearing Smooth Muscle. **(f)** Osseous Metaplasia. A Focus of Pulmonary Osseous Metaplasia (Arrow) is Present in the Lung Parenchyma.

core surrounded by a rim of macrophages. The exact nature and cause of corpora amylacea are still unclear, but they are of no clinical significance.

Pulmonary lymph nodes are usually found at the bifurcation of the bronchi, where they are referred to as peribronchial lymph nodes. Occasionally, lymph nodes can exist within the lung parenchyma, which are designated as intrapulmonary lymph nodes. They vary from loosely organized microscopic foci of lymphoid tissue to fully developed lymph nodes (Fig. 5(c)). Diseases occurring in other lymph nodes can also be seen in intrapulmonary lymph nodes. Although they are not of direct clinical relevance, they are becoming more important in relation to the differential diagnosis of peripheral nodules, especially in relation to computed tomography screening for lung carcinoma.

Blue bodies are intra-alveolar, lamellated, round to oval, basophilic, calcified structures found in airspaces associated with AMs and giant cells (Fig. 5(d)). They should not be mistaken as exogenous foreign material. They are a non-specific finding in variety of lung diseases related to accumulation of macrophages and are of no diagnostic significance.

Focal scars are among other incidental nodular lesions occasionally encountered in the lung. One form of the scars is frequently seen in (ex)smokers and located in the periphery of the lung. They are round or somewhat stellate in shape and have numerous fascicles of smooth muscle (Fig. 5(e)).

Osseous metaplasia is an aging change that is occasionally seen in bronchial cartilages and sometimes seen in lung parenchyma (Fig. 5(f)). In lung parenchyma, osseous metaplasia is commonly seen in lungs with fibrous process, such as that in interstitial pneumonia, lung scarring, or pleural plaques, although it can also be seen in normal lung parenchyma. Rarely osseous metaplasia can be seen in malignant lung tissue. There is no clinical significance by itself, but it may be mistaken as neoplasm radiologically.

Occasionally, megakaryocytes can present in the pulmonary circulation especially alveolar wall capillaries. Megakaryocytes are produced in the bone marrow and some are evidently released intact into circulation. Because of their massive size, megakaryocytes are lodged in the capillary bed of the lung where they released platelets. They generally appear as irregular hematoxyphilic clumps representing only the condensed nuclei. They are devoid of cytoplasm and have evidently discharged their platelets in the lung. Lung may be a site of platelet production and the platelet levels in the pulmonary veins are higher compared to that of pulmonary artery. There is also evidence that platelets regulate pulmonary vascular permeability and the barrier function of the alveolar capillaries and influence pulmonary vasoreactivity. Platelets likely have specialized activities in lung repair.[85] Megakaryocytes are particularly easy to find in pulmonary capillaries in conditions such as ALI/acute respiratory distress syndrome, burns, disseminated intravascular coagulation, thrombosis, shock and carcinomatosis, which lead to increased platelet consumption.

5. Structural Aspects of Aging of the Lung

The lung constantly interacts with the environment through thousands of liters of air containing toxic chemicals and particles or pathogenic microorganisms that are inhaled daily. This poses a challenge to lung structure and function and contributes to the aging process of lungs. Increasing age is associated with failing pulmonary health that includes the development of COPD/emphysema[86] and an increased susceptibility to numerous pulmonary infections, e.g. influenza, pneumococcal pneumonia, tuberculosis.[87–89] Age-related cellular, histologic and structural changes in the lung are linked to these disease states.

5.1. *Cellular changes*

AM is the major cellular components in BAL fluid. Studies have demonstrated that age-related differences in the cell populations of BAL fluid. The older subjects (mean age, 74 years; range, 70–80 years) had a higher percentage of neutrophils (40% versus 10%, $p < 0.005$) and a lower percentage of macrophages (32% versus 67%,

$p < 0.0001$) as compared with the younger group (mean age, 27 years; range, 19–34 years).[90] Similar to age-associated increases in neutrophils in BAL samples, higher levels of IL-8 and neutrophil elastase were seen in older subjects.[91] Induced sputum cell counts provide a relatively non-invasive method to evaluate the presence, type, and degree of inflammation in the airways of the lungs. Similar to BAL, sputum cell distribution of healthy subjects aged ≥50 years was mainly composed of neutrophils; however, macrophage counts showed a proportionate, inverse correlation with increasing age.[92,93] The mechanism by which neutrophils are recruited into the airways of older healthy subjects is still unclear. However, the accumulation of neutrophils in the lungs of older people could create a favorable microenvironment for the development of diseases associated with chronic airway inflammation.

5.2. *Tissue composition changes*

Age-related changes in tissue composition that may have a significant effect on lung mechanics (e.g. compliance) and lung repair. Collagen and elastin are the main proteins in the extracellular matrix that make up the framework of the alveolar structure and are the most important components in determining the mechanical properties of lung parenchyma. Changes of lung mechanics are closely associated with alterations of the stromal components of the lung parenchyma. A study of normal lung parenchyma obtained at autopsy from the elderly (mean age 76 years, range 67–88 years) and the young controls (mean age 45 years, range 28–58 years) demonstrated that the elastic fibers were thin and fragmented, while the type III collagen strands were thick in the alveolar wall. Furthermore, the type III collagen was also observed at the alveolar-capillary membrane with thickening of basement membrane in the elderly versus the young controls.[94] However, early studies showed that the reduced elastic recoil of the aging lungs is not related to changes in the amount of elastin and collagen in the lung parenchyma.[95] It is suggested that the loss of lung elasticity may be due to alterations in cross-linkage and/or configuration of elastin and/or collagen.[96] Interestingly, age-related alteration of extracellular matrix collagen have the capacity to diminish the invasive behavior of lung carcinoma cells and may deter the development of invasive lung tumors in the elderly compared with their younger counterparts.[97]

In addition to the alterations of collagen and/or elastin in lung parenchyma, other tissue composition changes outside of the lung including calcification of the cartilaginous articulations of the spine, ribs and sternum; Calcification and ossification of cartilages in the large airways; hyalinized and sclerotic intimal thickening of pulmonary arteries and veins; mural hyalinization of small arterioles; oncocytic changes of the bronchial seromucinous glands; disproportionate degeneration of large myelinated phrenic nerve fibers of diaphragm; and atrophy and loss of fast twitch diaphragmatic muscle fibers also contribute to the impaired lung function in the elderly.[40]

Alveolar lining fluid is generated, secreted and recycled by alveolar epithelial cells and is essential for maintaining lung function. Components of alveolar lining fluid, such as sftp (especially sftpa and sftpd), complement protein C3 and alveolar hydrolases, play a significant innate immune role in controlling microbial infections in the lung. It has been shown that pro-inflammatory cytokines (increased IL-6), sftps (higher levels of sftpa and sftpd), complement components (decreased complement C2), antimicrobial enzymes (decreased hydrolases activity) and oxidized components (increased levels of myeloperoxidase and carbonyl and nitrotyrosine residues) are significantly altered in the aged lung in both mice and humans.[98] These data indicate that the molecular composition of the alveolar lining fluid in the aging lung can potentially modify lung immune responses, thereby impacting pulmonary infection susceptibility and other pulmonary diseases in the elderly population.

5.3. *Structural changes*

The combination of loss of lung elasticity, alteration of extracellular matrix elastin and/or collagen, increases stiffness of the chest wall and reduces respiratory muscle strength which eventually results in a homogeneous increase in distal airspace (alveolar ducts and alveoli) (Fig. (6)) along with a loss of alveolar gas exchange surface area

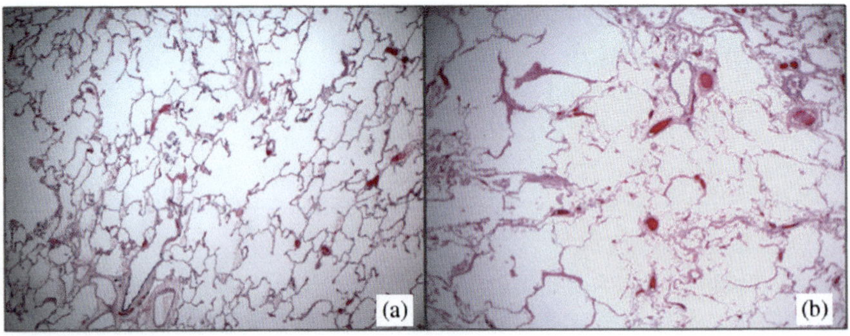

Fig 6. Lung Parenchyma of Normal and Aging (senile) Lungs. (a) Lung Parenchyma of a 42-Year-Old Subject. **(b)** Lung Parenchyma of an 80-Year-Old Subject with Remarkable Dilatation of the Distal Airspace.

and a decline in the number of capillaries per alveolus. All these are consistent with changes seen in emphysema or small airways disease. The descriptive term "senile emphysema" has been used to describe this finding. Aging lung was suggested as an alternative term to acknowledge that "senile emphysema" might be misleading since it lacks alveolar wall destruction, a pathologic hallmark of emphysema. In this context, it is proposed that the term "senile lung" seems more appropriate to describe these structural changes associated with normal aging.[99–101] These changes are responsible for the decrease in expiratory flow rates and an increase in residual volume at the expense of vital capacity.

References

1. Herriges M, Morrisey EE. (2014) Lung development: Orchestrating the generation and regeneration of a complex organ. *Development* **141**: 502–513.
2. Cardoso W V, Whitsett J A. (2008) Resident cellular components of the lung: Developmental aspects. *Proc Am Thorac Soc* **5**: 767–771.
3. Franks TJ, Colby TV, Travis WD *et al.* (2008) Resident cellular components of the human lung: Current knowledge and goals for research on cell phenotyping and function. *Proc Am Thorac Soc* **5**: 763–766.
4. Morrisey EE, Cardoso WV, Lane RH *et al.* (2013) Molecular determinants of lung development. *Ann Am Thorac Soc* **10**: S12–S16.

5. Burri PH. (2006) Structural aspects of postnatal lung development — alveolar formation and growth. *Biol Neonate* **89**: 313–322.
6. Joshi S, Kotecha S. (2007) Lung growth and development. *Early Hum Dev* **83**: 789–794.
7. Hagood JS. (2014) Beyond the genome: Epigenetic mechanisms in lung remodeling. *Physiol* **29**: 177–185.
8. Goss AM, Tian Y, Tsukiyama T *et al.* (2009) Wnt2/2b and beta-catenin signaling are necessary and sufficient to specify lung progenitors in the foregut. *Dev Cell* **17**: 290–298.
9. Harris-Johnson KS, Domyan ET, Vezina CM *et al*. (2009) beta-Catenin promotes respiratory progenitor identity in mouse foregut. *Proc Natl Acad Sci U S A* **106**: 16287–16292.
10. Domyan ET, Ferretti E, Throckmorton K *et al.* (2011) Signaling through BMP receptors promotes respiratory identity in the foregut via repression of Sox2. *Dev* **138**: 971–981.
11. Ferri A, Favaro R, Beccari L *et al.* (2013) Sox2 is required for embryonic development of the ventral telencephalon through the activation of the ventral determinants Nkx2.1 and Shh. *Dev* **140**: 1250–1261.
12. Sekine K, Ohuchi H, Fujiwara M *et al.*(1999) Fgf10 is essential for limb and lung formation. *Nat Genet* **21**: 138–141.
13. Ohuchi H, Hori Y, Yamasaki M *et al.*(2000) FGF10 acts as a major ligand for FGF receptor 2 IIIb in mouse multi-organ development. *Biochem Bioph Res Co* **277**: 643–649.
14. Min HS, Danilenko DM, Scully SA *et al.* (1998) Fgf-10 is required for both limb and lung development and exhibits striking functional similarity to Drosophila branchless. *Gene Dev* **12**: 3156–3161.
15. Bellusci S, Grindley J, Emoto H *et al.* (1997) Fibroblast growth factor 10 (FGF10) and branching morphogenesis in the embryonic mouse lung. *Development* **124**: 4867–4878.
16. Pepicelli CV, Lewis PM, McMahon AP. (1998) Sonic hedgehog regulates branching morphogenesis in the mammalian lung. *Curr Biol : CB* **8**: 1083–1086.
17. Weaver M, Dunn NR, Hogan BL. (2000) Bmp4 and Fgf10 play opposing roles during lung bud morphogenesis. *Dev* **127**: 2695–2704.
18. Que J, Luo X, Schwartz RJ *et al.* (2009) Multiple roles for Sox2 in the developing and adult mouse trachea. *Dev* **136**: 1899–1907.
19. Tompkins DH, Besnard V, Lange AW *et al.* (2011) Sox2 activates cell proliferation and differentiation in the respiratory epithelium. *Am J Respir Cell Mol Biol* **45**: 101–110.

20. Weaver M, Yingling JM, Dunn NR *et al.* (1999) Bmp signaling regulates proximal-distal differentiation of endoderm in mouse lung development. *Dev* **126**: 4005–4015.
21. Lu MM, Yang H, Zhang L *et al.* (2001) The bone morphogenic protein antagonist gremlin regulates proximal-distal patterning of the lung. *Dev Dynam : An official publication of the American Association of Anatomists* **222**: 667–680.
22. Mucenski, ML, Wert SE, Nation JM *et al.* (2003) beta-catenin is required for specification of proximal/distal cell fate during lung morphogenesis. *J Biol Chem* **278**: 40231–40238.
23. Okubo T, Knoepfler PS, Eisenman RN *et al.* (2005) Nmyc plays an essential role during lung development as a dosage-sensitive regulator of progenitor cell proliferation and differentiation. *Dev* **132**: 1363–1374.
24. Shu W, Lu MM, Zhang Y *et al*. (2007) Foxp2 and Foxp1 cooperatively regulate lung and esophagus development. *Dev* **134**: 1991–2000.
25. Shaw-White, JR, Bruno MD, Whitsett JA. (1999) GATA-6 activates transcription of thyroid transcription factor-1. *J Biol Chem* **274**: 2658–2664.
26. Ikeda K, Shaw-White JR, Wert SE *et al.*(1996) Hepatocyte nuclear factor 3 activates transcription of thyroid transcription factor 1 in respiratory epithelial cells. *Mol Cell Biol* **16**: 3626–3636.
27. Liu C, Glasser SW, Wan H *et al*. (2002) GATA-6 and thyroid transcription factor-1 directly interact and regulate surfactant protein-C gene expression. *J Biol Chem* **277**: 4519–4525.
28. Zhang Y, Rath N, Hannenhalli S *et al.* (2007) GATA and Nkx factors synergistically regulate tissue-specific gene expression and development *in vivo. Dev* **134**: 189–198.
29. Wan H, Dingle S, Xu Y *et al.* (2005) Compensatory roles of Foxa1 and Foxa2 during lung morphogenesis.*J Biol Chem* **280**: 13809–13816.
30. Minoo P, Hu LY, Xing YM *et al.* (2007) Physical and functional interactions between homeodomain NKX2.1 and winged helix/forkhead FOXA1 in lung epithelial cells. *Mol Cell Biol* **27**: 2155–2165.
31. Chen J, Knowles HJ, Hebert JL *et al.* (1998) Mutation of the mouse hepatocyte nuclear factor/forkhead homologue 4 gene results in an absence of cilia and random left-right asymmetry. *J Clin Invest* **102**: 1077–1082.
32. Tichelaar JW, Lim L, Costa RH *et al.* (1999) HNF-3/forkhead homologue-4 influences lung morphogenesis and respiratory epithelial cell differentiation *in vivo. Dev Biol* **213**: 405–417.

33. Whitsett JA, Tichelaar JW. (1999) Forkhead transcription factor HFH-4 and respiratory epithelial cell differentiation. *Am J Respir Cell Mol Biol* **21**: 153–154.
34. Yang Z, Hikosaka K, Sharkar MT *et al.* (2010) The mouse forkhead gene Foxp2 modulates expression of the lung genes. *Life Sci* **87**: 17–25.
35. Oizumi H, Kato H, Endoh M *et al.* (2014) Techniques to define segmental anatomy during segmentectomy. *Ann Cardiothorac Surg* **3**: 170–175.
36. Yalcin NG, Choong CK, Eizenberg N. (2013) Anatomy and pathophysiology of the pleura and pleural space. *Thorac Surg Clin* **23**: 1–10.
37. Polla B, D'Antona G, Bottinelli R *et al.* (2004) Respiratory muscle fibres: Specialisation and plasticity. *Thorax* **59**: 808–817.
38. McKenzie DK, Butler JE,Gandevia SC. (2009) Respiratory muscle function and activation in chronic obstructive pulmonary disease. *J Appl Physiol* **107**: 621–629.
39. Sharma G, Goodwin J. (2006) Effect of aging on respiratory system physiology and immunology. *Clin Interv Aging* **1**: 253–260.
40. Lalley PM. (2013) The aging respiratory system–pulmonary structure, function and neural control. *Respir Physiol Neurobiol* **187**: 199–210.
41. Brand-Saberi BE, Schafer T. (2014) Trachea: Anatomy and physiology. *Thorac Surg Clin* **24**: 1–5.
42. Tam A, Wadsworth S, Dorscheid D *et al.* (2011) The airway epithelium: More than just a structural barrier. *Ther Adv Respir Dis* **5**: 255–273.
43. Reynolds SD,Malkinson AM. (2010) Clara cell: Progenitor for the bronchiolar epithelium. *Intl J Biochem Cell Biol* **42**: 1–4.
44. Wang H, Liu Y, Liu Z. (2013) Clara cell 10-kD protein in inflammatory upper airway diseases. *Curr Opin Allergy Clin Immunol* **13**: 25–30.
45. Arason AJ, Jonsdottir HR, Halldorsson S *et al.* (2014) deltaNp63 has a role in maintaining epithelial integrity in airway epithelium. *PloS one* **9**: e88683.
46. Rock JR, Gao X, Xue Y *et al.* (2011) Notch-dependent differentiation of adult airway basal stem cells. *Cell Stem Cell* **8**: 639–648.
47. Lynch TJ, Engelhardt JF. (2014) Progenitor Cells in Proximal Airway Epithelial Development and Regeneration. *J Cell Biochem*
48. Nadel JA, Borson DB. (1991) Modulation of neurogenic inflammation by neutral endopeptidase. *Am Rev Respir Dis* **143**: S33–S36.
49. Lembrechts R, Brouns I, Schnorbusch K *et al.* (2013) Functional expression of the multimodal extracellular calcium-sensing receptor in pulmonary neuroendocrine cells. *J Cell Sci* **126**: 4490–4501.

50. Gu X, Karp PH, Brody SL *et al.* (2014) Chemosensory functions for pulmonary neuroendocrine cells. *Am J Respir Cell Mol Biol* **50**: 637–646.
51. Reid L, Meyrick B, Antony, VB *et al.* (2005) The mysterious pulmonary brush cell: A cell in search of a function. *Am J Respir Critic Care Med* **172**: 136–139.
52. Krasteva G, Canning BJ, Hartmann P *et al.* (2011) Cholinergic chemosensory cells in the trachea regulate breathing. *Proc Natl Acad Sci USA* **108**: 9478–9483.
53. Sato A. (2007) Tuft cells. *Anat Sci Intl* **82**: 187–199.
54. Howat WJ, Holmes JA, Holgate ST *et al.* (2001) Basement membrane pores in human bronchial epithelium: A conduit for infiltrating cells? *Am J Pathol* **158**, 673–680
55. Mestres P, Gomez LL, Lopez TN *et al.* (2014) The basement membrane of the isolated rat colonic mucosa. A light, electron and atomic force microscopy study. *Annals Anat = Anatomischer Anzeiger: Official organ of the Anatomische Gesellschaft* **196**: 108–118.
56. Randall TD. (2010) Bronchus-associated lymphoid tissue (BALT) structure and function. *Adv Immunol* **107**: 187–241.
57. Dobbs LG, Johnson MD. (2007) Alveolar epithelial transport in the adult lung. *Respir Physiol Neurobiol* **159**: 283–300.
58. Herzog EL, Brody AR, Colby TV, *et al.* (2008) Knowns and unknowns of the alveolus. *Proc Am Thorac Soc* **5**: 778–782.
59. Maniatis NA, Chernaya O, Shinin V *et al.* (2012) Caveolins and lung function. *Adv Ex Med Biol* **729**: 157–179.
60. Matsuzaki T, Hata H, Ozawa, H, *et al.* (2009) Immunohistochemical localization of the aquaporins AQP1, AQP3, AQP4, and AQP5 in the mouse respiratory system. *Acta Histochem Cytoc* **42**: 159–169.
61. Rozycki HJ. (2014) Potential Contribution of Type I Alveolar Epithelial Cells to Chronic Neonatal Lung Disease. *Frontiers in pediatrics* **2**: 45.
62. Wong MH, Chapin OC, Johnson MD. (2012) LPS-stimulated cytokine production in type I cells is modulated by the renin-angiotensin system. *Am J Respir Cell Mol Biol* **46**: 641–650.
63. Crapo JD, Barry BE, Gehr P *et al.* (1982) Cell number and cell characteristics of the normal human lung. *Am Rev Respir Dis* **126**: 332–337.
64. Bove PF, Dang H, Cheluvaraju C *et al.* (2014) Breaking the *in vitro* alveolar type II cell proliferation barrier while retaining ion transport properties. *Am J Respir Cell Mol Biol* **50**: 767–776.

65. Barkauskas CE, Cronce MJ, Rackley CR *et al.* (2013) Type 2 alveolar cells are stem cells in adult lung. *J Clin Invest* **123**: 3025–3036.
66. Cheung DO, Halsey K, Speert DP. (2000) Role of pulmonary alveolar macrophages in defense of the lung against Pseudomonas aeruginosa. *Infect Immun* **68**: 4585–4592.
67. Maus UA, Janzen S, Wall G *et al.* (2006) Resident alveolar macrophages are replaced by recruited monocytes in response to endotoxin-induced lung inflammation. *Am J Respir Cell Mol Biol* **35**: 227–235.
68. Janssen WJ, Barthel L, Muldrow A *et al.* (2011) Fas determines differential fates of resident and recruited macrophages during resolution of acute lung injury. *Am J Respir Critic Care Med* **184**: 547–560.
69. Hashimoto D, Chow A, Noizat C *et al.* (2013) Tissue-resident macrophages self-maintain locally throughout adult life with minimal contribution from circulating monocytes. *Immunity* **38**: 792–804.
70. Murray PJ, Wynn TA. (2011) Protective and pathogenic functions of macrophage subsets. *Nat Rev. Immunol* **11**: 723–737.
71. Shaykhiev R, Krause A, Salit J ,*et al.* (2009) Smoking-dependent reprogramming of alveolar macrophage polarization: Implication for pathogenesis of chronic obstructive pulmonary disease. *J Immunol* **183**: 2867–2883.
72. Hussell T, Bell TJ. (2014) Alveolar macrophages: Plasticity in a tissue-specific context. *Nat Rev. Immunol* **14**: 81–93.
73. Kim EY, Battaile JT, Patel AC. (2008) Persistent activation of an innate immune response translates respiratory viral infection into chronic lung disease. *Nat Med* **14**, 633–640.
74. Pechkovsky DV, Prasse A, Kollert F *et al.* (2010) Alternatively activated alveolar macrophages in pulmonary fibrosis-mediator production and intracellular signal transduction. *Clin Immunol* **137**: 89–101.
75. Melgert BN, ten Hacken NH, Rutgers B *et al.* (2011) More alternative activation of macrophages in lungs of asthmatic patients. *J Allergy Clin Immunol* **127**: 831–833.
76. Dasgupta P, Keegan AD. (2012) Contribution of alternatively activated macrophages to allergic lung inflammation: A tale of mice and men. *J Innate Immun* **4**: 478–488.
77. Stahl M, Schupp J, Jager B *et al.* (2013) Lung collagens perpetuate pulmonary fibrosis via CD204 and M2 macrophage activation. *PloS one* **8**: e81382.

78. Kaku Y, Imaoka H, Morimatsu Y *et al.* (2014) Overexpression of CD163, CD204 and CD206 on alveolar macrophages in the lungs of patients with severe chronic obstructive pulmonary disease. *PloS one* **9**: e87400.
79. Ochoa CD, Wu S,Stevens T. (2010) New developments in lung endothelial heterogeneity: Von Willebrand factor, P-selectin, and the Weibel-Palade body. *Semin Thromb Hemost* **36**: 301–308.
80. Xue T, Wei N, Xin Z *et al.* (2014) Angiotensin-converting enzyme-2 overexpression attenuates inflammation in rat model of chronic obstructive pulmonary disease. *Inhal Toxicol* **26**: 14–22.
81. Imai Y, Kuba K, Rao S *et al.* (2005) Angiotensin-converting enzyme 2 protects from severe acute lung failure. *Nature* **436**: 112–116.
82. Zou Z, Yan Y, Shu Y, *et al.* (2014) Angiotensin-converting enzyme 2 protects from lethal avian influenza A H5N1 infections. *Nat Commun* **5**: 3594.
83. Mizutani E, Tsuta K, Maeshima AM *et al.* (2009) Minute pulmonary meningothelial-like nodules: Clinicopathologic analysis of 121 patients. *Human Pathol* **40**: 678–682.
84. Mukhopadhyay S, El-Zammar OA, Katzenstein ALA. (2009) Pulmonary Meningothelial-like Nodules New Insights Into a Common but Poorly Understood Entity. *Am J Surg Pathol* **33**: 487–495.
85. Weyrich AS, Zimmerman GA. (2013) Platelets in lung biology. *Ann Rev Physiol* **75**: 569–591.
86. Ito K, Barnes PJ. (2009) COPD as a disease of accelerated lung aging. *Chest* **135**: 173–180.
87. Wroe PC, Finkelstein JA, Ray GT *et al.* (2012) Aging population and future burden of pneumococcal pneumonia in the United States. *J Infect Dis* **205**: 1589–1592.
88. Cruz-Hervert LP, Garcia-Garcia L, Ferreyra-Reyes L *et al.* (2012) Tuberculosis in ageing: High rates, complex diagnosis and poor clinical outcomes. *Age and ageing* **41**: 488–495.
89. Hernandez-Vargas EA, Wilk E, Canini L *et al.* (2014) Effects of aging on influenza virus infection dynamics. *J Virol* **88**: 4123–4131.
90. Thompson AB, Scholer SG, Daughton DM, *et al.* (1992) Altered epithelial lining fluid parameters in old normal individuals. *J Gerontol* **47**: M171–176.
91. Meyer KC, Rosenthal NS, Soergel P *et al.* (1998) Neutrophils and low-grade inflammation in the seemingly normal aging human lung. *Mec Ageing Dev* **104**: 169–181.

92. Pignatti P, Ragnoli B, Radaeli A *et al.* (2011) Age-related increase of airway neutrophils in older healthy nonsmoking subjects. *Rejuvenation Res* **14**: 365–370.
93. Thomas RA, Green RH, Brightling CE *et al.* (2004) The influence of age on induced sputum differential cell counts in normal subjects. *Chest* **126**: 1811–1814.
94. D'Errico A, Scarani P, Colosimo E *et al.* (1989) Changes in the alveolar connective tissue of the ageing lung. An immunohistochemical study. *Virchows Archiv. A, Patholl Anat Histopathol* **415**: 137–144.
95. Pierce JA. (1965) Tensile strength of human lung. *J Lab Clin Med* **66**: 652–658.
96. Dyer C. (2012) The interaction of ageing and lung disease. *Chronic Respir Dis* **9**: 63–67.
97. Bartling B Desole M, Rohrbach S, *et al.* (2009) Age-associated changes of extracellular matrix collagen impair lung cancer cell migration. *FASEB J : Official publication of the Federation of American Societies for Experimental Biology* **23**: 1510–1520.
98. Moliva JI, Rajaram MV, Sidiki S, *et al.* (2014) Molecular composition of the alveolar lining fluid in the aging lung. *Age*
99. Fukuchi Y. (2009) The aging lung and chronic obstructive pulmonary disease: similarity and difference. *Proc Am Thorac Soc* **6**: 570–572.
100. Teramoto S, Ishii M. (2007) Aging, the aging lung, and senile emphysema are different. *Am J Respir Critic Care Med* **175**: 197–198.
101. Verbeken EK, Cauberghs M, Mertens I *et al.* (1992) The senile lung. Comparison with normal and emphysematous lungs. 1. Structural aspects. *Chest* **101**: 793–799.

Chapter 2

Physiology of the Aging Lung

Brienne Miner*,†, Thomas M. Gill†, and Carlos A. Vaz Fragoso†,‡

1. Introduction

Across the adult lifespan, there is a decline in respiratory physiology. This is a consequence of age-related changes, termed normal aging, and of an increased vulnerability for having respiratory disease.[1–4] Hence, normal aging must be taken into account when establishing a diagnosis of respiratory disease, especially if based on pulmonary function testing (physiologic criteria) as is commonly employed in clinical practice and research settings. This chapter provides an updated and expanded review of the aging lung, [4] focusing on the physiology of normal aging, risk factors for respiratory disease, and diagnostic use of pulmonary function tests.

2. Normal Aging

As shown in Table 1, normal aging of the respiratory system is associated with impairments in multiple physiologic domains, including

* Corresponding author.
†Yale School of Medicine, Department of Internal Medicine, 333 Cedar Street, New Haven, CT, 06520, USA.
‡Veterans Affairs Clinical Epidemiology Research Center, 950 Campbell Avenue, West Haven, CT, 06516, USA.

Table 1. Age-related changes in respiratory physiology (normal aging as measured across the adult lifespan).

Domain	Impairment	Mechanism
Ventilatory Control	• Equivocal response to hypoxemia and hypercapnia (see text) • Increased prevalence of central sleep apnea • Decreased symptom awareness (bronchoconstriction)	• Decreased cerebrovascular response to CO_2 • Decreased number of medullary ventral respiratory neurons • Decreased peripheral chemoreflex CO_2 sensitivity • Decreased feedback from peripheral mechanoreceptors
Respiratory Muscles	• Decreased inspiratory (MIP) and expiratory (MEP) strength	• Impaired respiratory mechanics and sarcopenia
Respiratory Mechanics	• Airflow-limitation (decreased FEV1, FVC, FEV1/FVC) • Air trapping (increased RV) • Hyperinflation (increased FRC, unchanged TLC) • Increased closing volume	• Increased rigidity of the chest wall and decreased elastic recoil of the lung
Gas Exchange	• Increased ventilation-perfusion mismatch, with heterogeneous distribution of lung units having high and low V_A/Q ratios, increased V_D, increased PA systolic pressure, decreased DLCO, decreased PaO_2, unchanged $PaCO_2$	• Increased closing volume • Decreased alveolar surface area and density of lung capillaries • Increased pulmonary vascular resistance • Decreased cardiac output response to exercise
Exercise	• Low breathing reserve $([V_{Emax}/MBC] - 1) \times 100\%$ • Flow limitation (expiratory flow rates approach the maximal predicted flow-rate) and dynamic hyperinflation	• Impaired respiratory mechanics • Impaired respiratory muscles • Impaired gas exchange

Abbreviations: CO_2, carbon dioxide; FEV1, forced expiratory volume in 1 second; FVC, forced vital capacity; FRC, functional residual capacity; MBC, maximum breathing capacity; MIP, maximal inspiratory pressure; MEP, maximal expiratory pressure, RV, residual volume; TLC, total lung capacity; V_A/Q, ventilation to perfusion ratio; V_D, dead space ventilation; V_{Emax}, ventilation at maximal exercise.

ventilatory control, respiratory muscle strength, respiratory mechanics and gas exchange, and these are most evident during exercise.

2.1. *Ventilatory control*

Studies involving healthy older persons have evaluated age-related changes in ventilatory control, based on the P100 and minute ventilation (V_E) response to hypoxemia and hypercapnia. The P100 is defined as the inspiratory pressure that is generated at the mouth 100 ms after airway occlusion and is considered a validated index of central respiratory drive.[5] Based on the P100, prior work has shown that healthy persons aged 65–79 years had an approximate 50% reduction in their response to hypoxemia and hypercapnia, relative to those aged 22–29 years.[6] Similarly, prior work based on V_E has shown that healthy men aged 64–73 years had a 51% and 41% reduction in their response to hypoxemia and hypercapnia, respectively, as compared to those aged 22–30 years.[7] In another study, healthy persons aged 67–79 years had a one-third reduction in the V_E response to hypercapnia, relative to those aged 22–37 years.[8] As a potential explanation for the age-related reduction in ventilatory control, a decrease in peripheral chemoreflex CO_2 sensitivity in older persons has been demonstrated in a subsequent study.[9] Other studies, however, have not confirmed these age-related changes in ventilatory control, including changes in peripheral chemoreflex CO_2 sensitivity.[10–14] Reconciling these conflicting results is difficult because of differences in techniques used to evaluate ventilatory control, as well as limitations imposed by the distinct characteristics of the different study populations. For example, the hypoxic and hypercapneic challenges varied across studies, having included the use of progressive, steady-state and dynamic end-tidal forcing techniques, respectively. Furthermore, study populations were small in size, ranging from only 5 to 14 older persons and with none older than 80 years (age range of 61–80 years),[6–14] and one study selectively enrolled older persons from a health and fitness center.[14]

Some investigators have posited that the increased prevalence of central sleep apnea among older persons suggests an age-related adverse effect on ventilatory control.[15–18] Based on a frequency of ≥2.5 central apneic events per hour of sleep, the prevalence of central sleep apnea is 12.1% for persons aged 65–100 years, but only 1.7% for those aged 45–64 years.[15] The age-related increase in central sleep apnea, including its potential role as a sleep-related cause of death, may be due to a reduction in the number of medullary ventral respiratory neurons.[16–18] Preliminary work shows that aging is associated with loss of gray matter volume in brain regions that involve breathing function.[16–18] Nonetheless, a more likely mechanism for the age-related increase in central sleep apnea is a decreased cerebrovascular response to CO_2 that, in turn, leads to breathing instability (cerebrovascular and ventilatory responses to $PaCO_2$ are tightly linked).[19–23]

Finally, prior research comparing persons aged 60–80 years with those 20–46 years has shown an age-related reduction in awareness of methacholine-induced bronchoconstriction, characterized by older persons having less severe respiratory symptoms despite having greater reductions in lung function (a lower forced expiratory volume in 1-s (FEV1)).[24, 25] The mechanisms underlying the reduced awareness are unknown, but could involve diminished feedback from peripheral mechanoreceptors.[24,25]

2.2. *Respiratory muscles*

Several large studies have shown that advancing age is associated with a reduction in both the maximal inspiratory pressure (MIP), a measure of inspiratory muscle strength, and the maximal expiratory pressure (MEP), a measure of expiratory muscle strength.[26–28] For example, for a man of average height and weight, the MIP at age 50 and 80 years are 111 and 70 cm H_2O, respectively.[28] The age-related reductions in MIP and MEP are likely a consequence of impaired respiratory mechanics (discussed below) and an age-related increase in the prevalence of sarcopenia (loss of muscle mass and function).[1,29–31]

2.3. *Respiratory mechanics*

Age-related reductions are especially pronounced in respiratory mechanics. Over the course of the adult lifespan, there is an increase in the rigidity of the chest wall and a decrease in the elastic recoil of the lung.[1,2,29,32] These age-related changes in respiratory mechanics lead to airflow-limitation, defined by a decreased FEV1 and a decrease in the ratio of FEV1 to forced vital capacity (FVC), along with worsening air trapping and hyperinflation, defined by an increase in residual volume (RV) and functional residual capacity (FRC), respectively.[1,2,29,32] In addition, because of a loss in supporting elastic tissue, there is an increase in the "closing volume", defined as the lung volume above which there is premature collapse of small airways, a phenomenon that is most evident in the gravity-dependent regions of the lung.[29,33] The net effects of these age-related changes include a decline in FEV1 of up to 30 mL/year, an increase in RV of about 50% between ages 20 and 70 years and an increase in the closing volume, which approaches the FRC (including during normal tidal breathing) by age 65 years.[2,29,32,33]

The noted age-related changes in respiratory mechanics lead to considerable physiologic limitations, even in healthy older adults. As the FEV1 declines, the tidal breathing response during exercise is reduced because of expiratory flow limitation and dynamic hyperinflation.[29,34] As the RV increases, the curvature of the diaphragm is reduced, shifting the length-tension relationship to a shorter length and, in turn, decreasing the force generating capacity of the muscle.[1,29,31] As the closing volume increases, the small airways are more likely to collapse prematurely, leading to a reduced ratio of alveolar ventilation to lung perfusion (V_A/Q) and, in turn, decreased oxygenation.[29,33,35,36]

2.4. *Gas exchange*

Gas exchange is dependent on the matching of ventilation with lung perfusion.[37] Prior work has shown that normal aging is associated with increased ventilation-perfusion mismatch, characterized by heterogeneous distribution of lung units that have high and low V_A/Q ratios.[38–42] As discussed earlier, the age-related increase in closing volume can lead a low V_A/Q ratio and, in turn, reduced oxygenation.[29,33,35,36] In addition, age-related changes in the pulmonary circulation may further exacerbate ventilation-perfusion mismatch.[43–45] In a study involving 3,790 participants aged 1–89 years with normal echocardiograms, the pulmonary arterial systolic pressure rose an average of 1 mmHg per decade of age, yielding an upper limit of 40 mmHg in those older than 50 years.[44] This rise in pulmonary arterial systolic pressure has been attributed to an increase in pulmonary vascular resistance, possibly reflecting increased vascular stiffness.[44,46]

Gas exchange may also be impaired as a consequence of an age-related decrease in the diffusion capacity of the lung for carbon monoxide (DLCO), a measure of the transfer capacity of oxygen across the alveolar-capillary interface.[29,47,48] In a study involving 74 healthy participants aged 69–104 years and 55 healthy participants aged 20–40 years, there was a 50% reduction in the DLCO for the older age group.[47] The reduction in DLCO may be due to a decline in the alveolar surface area and, possibly, in the density of lung capillaries.[45,47,48]

Age-related impairments in gas exchange are also associated with a subtle but important change in the arterial tension for carbon dioxide (P_aCO_2).[35,36] P_aCO_2 is largely dependent on V_E, which is the sum of alveolar ventilation (V_A) and dead space ventilation (V_D).[37] In contrast to V_D, which does not participate in gas exchange and thus denotes wasted ventilation (ventilation without perfusion), V_A includes areas of the lung that are both ventilated and perfused and is thus critical for CO_2 elimination. Because of an age-related increase in ventilation-perfusion mismatch, normal aging leads to an increase in V_D, thus requiring an increase in V_E to maintain V_A and, in turn, also maintain a normal P_aCO_2.[37–45] This compensatory increase in V_E is most evident during maximal exercise.[34]

Subtle changes in the arterial tension for oxygen (P_aO_2) also occur across the lifespan.[35,36] In the setting of age-related increases in ventilation-perfusion mismatch, the PaO_2 declines from an average of 100 mmHg in young adults (18–24 years) to 89 mmHg in older adults (≥65 years).[33,36] Moreover, the age-related decline in DLCO also reduces the PaO_2, but this effect is minimal and only when oxygen consumption is substantially elevated, as during maximal exercise in a highly fit individual (discussed below).[34,47] Nonetheless, because the reduced PaO_2 levels remain on the flat portion of the O_2 dissociation curve, the O_2 saturation remains normal with advancing age.[37]

Although the above noted age-related changes in gas exchange confer only mild physiologic impairments, they increase the risk of exercise intolerance and respiratory failure among older persons who have respiratory disease or experience an episode of acute lung injury such as pneumonia.

2.5. *Exercise*

The metabolic requirements of maximal exercise present a substantial challenge to the gas exchange capacity of the respiratory system. In a physically fit older person, for example, maximal exercise can lead to a 14-fold increase in O_2 consumption (VO_2) and CO_2 production (VCO_2).[34] To achieve such a high level of VO_2, the delivery of oxygen to the exercising muscle must be increased, concurrent with increased oxygen extraction at the tissue-capillary interface of the exercising muscle. VCO_2 is a byproduct of metabolic activity within the exercising muscle, but at heavier exercise workloads, is also due to bicarbonate buffering of lactic acid. Specifically, at workloads beyond the anaerobic threshold, the exercising muscle shifts to glycolysis as its energy source, thereby increasing lactic acid production. The lactic acid is then released into the circulation and buffered by sodium bicarbonate, further increasing VCO_2. The net effect of these exercise-induced metabolic changes is that the venous blood returning to the lung is acidotic, including a high CO_2 tension (rising to 60 mmHg) and a low O_2 saturation (declining to 40%).[49] In response, the respiratory system must increase its gas exchange capacity to reverse the acidosis and to restore an adequate arterial oxygen content.

A major determinant of the gas exchange capacity of the respiratory system during exercise is the "*breathing reserve*", defined as a ratio of the minute ventilation that is required at maximal exercise (V_{Emax}) relative to an individual's maximum breathing capacity (MBC).[34] The formula to calculate the breathing reserve is[34]: $([V_{Emax}/MBC] - 1) \times 100\%$, where the MBC (in liters/m) is 35 times the FEV1 in females and 40 times the FEV1 in males. A low breathing reserve (<15%) leads to a diminished capacity for exercise and, as discussed below, may occur as a consequence of normal aging, through an increase in V_{Emax} and a decrease in MBC.

The age-related increase in V_{Emax} is due to ventilation-perfusion mismatch. In particular, the increase in lung perfusion that normally occurs in response to exercise is attenuated in older persons, due to an age-related reduction in cardiac output and pulmonary capillary density, as well as an increase in pulmonary vascular resistance.[34,38,39,43–46] The reduced lung perfusion increases V_D and the dead space fraction of the tidal volume (termed the dead space ratio $[V_d/V_t]$). As a result, V_{Emax} needs to increase to maintain adequate levels of alveolar ventilation (V_A) and, in turn, CO_2 elimination ($V_A = V_{Emax} - V_D$).

The MBC component of the breathing reserve declines across the adult lifespan, largely due to age-related changes in respiratory mechanics. To illustrate, a healthy 30-year-old male of average height who has an FEV_1 of 4.5 L will have an MBC of 180 L/m. At age 70 years, however, his FEV_1 will have decreased to 3.3 L, thus yielding an MBC of only 132 L/m. At peak exercise, this age-related reduction in MBC is accompanied by a reduction in tidal volume, a consequence of expiratory flow limitation (expiratory flow rates approach the maximal predicted flow-rate) and dynamic hyperinflation.[29,34,50,51]

The MBC may also be diminished in the setting of age-related reductions in respiratory muscle strength, which often coexist with impairments in the muscles of ambulation.[26–28,34,52,53] Prior work, for example, has shown that a reduced MIP is associated with moderate-to-severe mobility impairment, defined by a Short Physical

Performance Battery score <8,[52] while another study has shown that higher MIP levels are associated with a slower rate of mobility decline over time.[53] Age-related increases in the prevalence of sarcopenia, therefore, may have an important adverse affect on both the muscles of respiration and muscles of ambulation.[30,52,53]

Another potential contributor to reduced gas exchange capacity during exercise is a decrease in oxygenation. As noted earlier, age-related changes in respiratory mechanics can lead to lung regions having a low V_A/Q ratio which, in turn, reduces oxygenation. In addition, aging is associated with impaired oxygen diffusion across the alveolar-capillary interface that is most evident during exercise. In particular, exercise-induced increases in cardiac output substantially shorten the transit time of the red blood cell in the pulmonary capillary bed, thus reducing the available time for diffusion of oxygen across the alveolar-capillary interface and decreasing oxygenation.[34,37,47,48] The noted adverse effects of a low V_A/Q ratio and a diffusion defect on oxygenation are further amplified during exercise by the returning venous blood having an extremely low oxygen saturation (40%).[34,37,49]

The age-related reduction in gas exchange capacity, particularly in breathing reserve, increases the risk of an exercise limitation in older persons, even among those who are physically fit.[34,50–54] To illustrate, as compared with a healthy but sedentary 30-year-old, a physically fit 70-year-old at a similar VO_{2max} (42–43 mL/kg/m) will have a substantially higher ventilatory requirement (V_{Emax} of 120 versus 100 L/m) but the same P_aCO_2 (34 mmHg).[34] This occurs as a consequence of higher dead space ventilation (V_D of 32 versus 14 L/m; V_d/V_t 0.28 versus 0.12).[34] Moreover, relative to a 30-year-old, the higher V_{Emax} in a 70-year-old is accompanied by a lower MBC (132 versus 180 L/m) and limitations in pulmonary mechanics at peak exercise (expiratory flow-limitation and dynamic hyperinflation). The net effect of these age-related differences is a substantially lower breathing reserve in a 70-year-old versus a 30-year-old (9% versus 44%), despite a comparable VO_{2max}. Because of the age-related increase in lung regions having a low V_A/Q ratio and the decrease in the diffusion of oxygen across the alveolar-capillary interface, a 70-year-old at peak exercise will also have a lower P_aO_2 (84 versus 92 mmHg) than a 30-year-old.[34]

Nonetheless, in the absence of respiratory disease, age-related changes in the cardiovascular and musculoskeletal systems are usually the limiting factor to maximal exercise in healthy but sedentary older persons, since the resulting workload does not lead to a respiratory limitation.[34] However, in the presence of respiratory disease, age-related reductions in respiratory physiology substantially increase the likelihood of exercise intolerance.

2.6. *Risk factors*

The most frequent risk factors that can lead to respiratory disease are exposures to environmental toxins, including tobacco smoke, respiratory infections, ambient indoor and outdoor air pollution and occupational dusts.[55–77] The respiratory system is especially vulnerable because it has a large interface with the environment — the alveolar surface area is 85 m^2 versus the skin at 1.8 m^2.[37]

Older persons have high cumulative rates of exposure to environmental toxins.[62–77] For example, the prevalence of smoking in the mid-1960s was about 50%, as compared with 9% in 2008.[68] In recent cohorts of older persons, the prevalence of ever-smokers and never-smokers was 56% and 44%, respectively.[65] Even among never-smokers, however, smoking exposure can be substantial. In 2008, among non-smoking Americans who were ≥60 years, 32% had documented exposure to second-hand smoke, also known as environmental tobacco smoke (ETS).[69]

Respiratory infections are also highly prevalent in older populations. In a large cohort of community-dwelling older persons, 27% reported a history of pneumonia.[67] From the period 1979 through 2001, persons aged ≥75 years had a 10-fold or greater increase in the rate of influenza-associated hospitalization, relative to any other age-group.[70] Outdoor air pollution is another common respiratory exposure.[71–74] In 2009, 34% of older Americans lived in a major city, a surrogate for outdoor air pollution.[71,74] Additional airway exposures include a prior high-risk occupation (freight, stock and material handlers and metal and wood workers) and the use of biomass fuel for indoor cooking or heating.[59,74,75] The prevalence rates for these exposures among older non-smokers are 12% and 18%, respectively.[74]

In susceptible persons, the above noted environmental exposures can lead to chronic lung inflammation and, in turn, reductions in respiratory physiology that are subsequently associated with adverse outcomes.[1,2,34,37,55–77] In aging populations, the most common forms of chronic lung inflammation relate to respiratory diseases such as chronic obstructive pulmonary disease (COPD) and idiopathic pulmonary fibrosis.[56,57,59]

3. Pulmonary Function

The predominant physiologic impairment in respiratory disease is in respiratory mechanics, which is most often evaluated by spirometric measures of pulmonary function and, in select cases, by a peak flow meter.[4] However, because respiratory diseases can also adversely affect ventilatory control, respiratory muscle strength and gas exchange, additional tests of pulmonary function may be required. To facilitate our discussion, common pulmonary function terminology is summarized in Table 2.

3.1. *Spirometry*

Spirometry may be conveniently performed using a portable, handheld device. In spirometric testing, the individual performs a series of forceful and complete exhalation maneuvers, starting from maximal inspiration.[78,79] Based on guidelines published by the American Thoracic and European Respiratory Societies (ATS/ERS), these breathing maneuvers generate several physiologic measures, of which the most important are the FEV1 (a timed lung volume) and FVC (an untimed lung volume).[78,79]

As shown in Tables 2 and 3, respiratory diseases that lead to a greater reduction in the timed lung volume than the untimed lung volume, resulting in a reduced FEV1/FVC, are characterized by airflow-limitation that is due to airways obstruction.[79,80] Conversely,

Table 2. Abbreviations and explanations of common tests of pulmonary function.

Spirometry	
FEV1	FEV in 1-second: The lung volume that is delivered in the first second of an FVC maneuver.
FVC	FVC: The lung volume that is delivered during a forceful and complete exhalation, starting from maximal inspiration.
FEV1/FVC	The ratio of FEV1 to FVC.
Normal spirometry	Defined by a normal FEV1/FVC and FVC.
Airflow-limitation	Defined by a reduced FEV1/FVC, with severity staged according to FEV1; includes respiratory diseases that lead to airways obstruction, most commonly chronic obstructive pulmonary disease (COPD), asthma, bronchiectasis, and cystic fibrosis.
Restrictive-pattern	Defined by a normal FEV1/FVC but reduced FVC; includes respiratory diseases that involve the chest wall (kyphosis, scoliosis, ankylosing spondylitis), respiratory muscles (sarcopenia, myasthenia gravis, diaphragmatic paralysis), pleura (effusions, fibrosis), and interstitium (edema, fibrosis) — among others.
Peak flow meter	
PEF	PEF: The maximal expiratory flow delivered with maximal force, starting from maximal inspiration. Reductions in PEF may indicate airways obstruction, respiratory muscle weakness, disorders that limit the expansion of the chest wall, or poor effort.
Static lung volumes (body plethysmography or helium dilution)	
TLC	TLC: The lung volume after a full inhalation. When reduced, it confirms restrictive lung disease; when increased, it establishes hyperinflation (most often due to airflow-limitation).
FRC	FRC: The lung volume after a normal (passive) exhalation. When increased, it indicates hyperinflation (most often due to airflow-limitation).
RV	RV: The lung volume after a full exhalation. When increased, it indicates air trapping (most often due to airflow-limitation).
DLCO	DLCO: Indicates oxygen transfer across the alveolar-capillary interface; is potentially reduced in interstitial lung disease, COPD, and pulmonary hypertension.
MIP	MIP: Reductions indicate respiratory muscle (diaphragmatic) weakness.

Table 3. Spirometric criteria for normal function and respiratory disease (airflow-limitation and restrictive-pattern).

	Spirometric Criteria				
		Airflow-limitation			
Method	**Normal**	**Mild**	**Moderate**	**Severe**	**Restrictive-Pattern**
GOLD					
FEV1/FVC	≥0.70		<0.70		≥0.70
FEV1	NA	≥80%Pred	50–79%Pred	<50%Pred	NA
FVC	≥80%Pred		NA		<80%Pred
ATS/ERS					
FEV1/FVC	≥ATS/ERS-LLN		<ATS/ERS-LLN		≥ATS/ERS-LLN
FEV1	NA	≥70%Pred	50–69%Pred	<50 %Pred	NA
FVC	≥ATS/ERS-LLN		NA		<ATS/ERS-LLN
LMS					
FEV1/FVC	≥5 LMS-tile		<5 LMS-tile		≥5 LMS-tile
FEV1	NA	≥5 LMS-tile	0.5 to 4.9 LMS-tile	<0.5 LMS-tile	NA
FVC	≥5 LMS-tile		NA		<5 LMS-tile

respiratory diseases that lead to comparable reductions in the timed and untimed lung volumes, resulting in a reduced FVC but normal FEV1/FVC, suggest a restrictive-pattern.[79,80] Otherwise, normal spirometry is defined by a normal FEV1/FVC and FVC.[79]

3.2. *Current practice*

Current practice establishes respiratory disease based on spirometric criteria from the Global Initiative for Obstructive Lung Disease (GOLD) and from a combined task force from the ATS/ERS.[55,79] As shown in Table 3, GOLD establishes respiratory disease using an FEV1/FVC threshold of 0.70 and FVC threshold of 80% predicted (%Pred), with airflow-limitation further staged according to FEV1 thresholds of 80, 50, and 30%Pred.[55] Alternatively, the ATS/ERS establishes respiratory disease based on thresholds for FEV1/FVC and FVC set at the lower limit of normal (LLN), with airflow-limitation further staged according to FEV1 thresholds of 70, 60, 50 and 35%Pred.[79] The LLN is calculated by the ATS/ERS as the 5th percentile distribution of reference values.[79,81] For both GOLD and ATS/ERS, the %Pred is calculated as ([measured/predicted] × 100).[55,79]

The GOLD and ATS/ERS spirometric thresholds for establishing respiratory disease may not be age-appropriate for three reasons.[2,4,64-67,82–84] First, because normal aging impairs respiratory mechanics, the FEV1/FVC is frequently <0.70 in otherwise healthy, asymptomatic never-smokers who are aged ≥65 years.[1,2,4,74,85] Second, because normal aging is associated with variability in spirometric performance, the use of %Pred thresholds for FEV1 and FVC incorrectly assumes that a given cut-point is equivalent for all persons, regardless of age, height, sex and ethnicity.[83,84] To illustrate the effect of age on spirometric performance, at the 5th percentile as calculated in a reference population of healthy never-smokers, a white male of average height has a value for FEV1 of 74%Pred at age 30 years but only 63%Pred at age 70 years.[83] Third, the calculation of the LLN as currently recommended by the ATS/ERS is based on multiple regression equations that incorrectly assume a linear relationship between the predictor variables (age and height) and spirometric measures, as well as incorrectly assume that reference values are distributed normally and have constant variability across the life-span.[2] In older populations, for example, multiple regression equations for FEV1/FVC have limited explanatory ability, with R-squared values ranging from only 0.01–0.15 (indicating that data points fit poorly in regression models).[86–88]

3.3. *Z scores*

To address limitations in current practice, investigators have suggested that spirometric thresholds be expressed as a Z score, which converts a raw measurement on a test to a standardized score in units of standard deviations.[83,84] More recently,[2] a novel method for calculating spirometric Z scores has been developed, termed Lambda–Mu–Sigma (LMS). This strategy uses all three elements of the distribution, including: The median (Mu) — representing how spirometric measures change based on predictor variables (age, height, sex and ethnicity); the coefficient-of-variation (Sigma) — representing the spread of reference values and adjusting for non-uniform dispersion; and skewness (Lambda) — representing the departure from normality.[2] The LMS-derived Z score is then calculated as follows[2]: $[(\text{measured/predicted median})^{\text{Lambda}}$ minus 1]/(Lambda x Sigma). Clinically, Z scores are also routinely used to diagnose osteopenia and osteoporosis based on bone mineral density testing and the LMS method is already widely applied to growth charts in children.[2,89]

We have proposed that respiratory disease should be defined by LMS-calculated spirometric Z scores, as shown in Table 3.[4] To assess the clinical validity of this approach, we evaluated the associations between LMS-defined respiratory disease and health outcomes, using data from the Cardiovascular Health Study (CHS), a longitudinal cohort of community-dwelling older persons aged 65–80 years.[65,66] As shown in Fig 1, the presence of LMS-defined restrictive-pattern and the presence and severity of LMS-defined airflow-limitation were

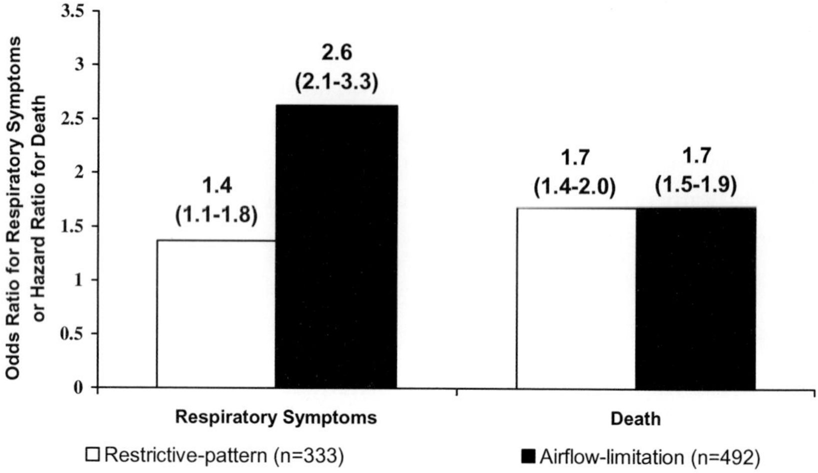

(a) LMS-defined restrictive-pattern and airflow-limitation, relative to normal spirometry

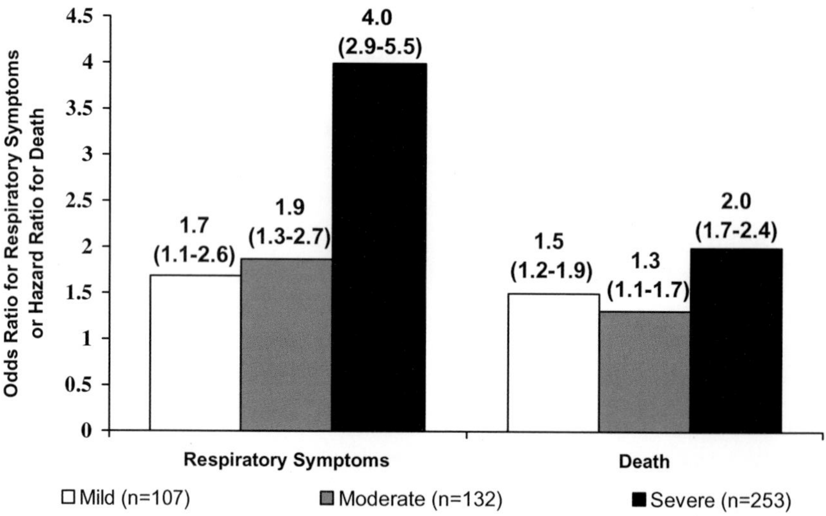

(b) LMS-staged severity of airflow-limitation, relative to normal spirometry

Fig 1. Adjusted Odds Ratios (95% Confidence Intervals) for Respiratory Symptoms and Adjusted Hazard Ratios (95% Confidence Intervals) for Death According to LMS Criteria among Community-dwelling Persons Aged 65–80. (Reproduced with Permission from Ref 4).

significantly associated with respiratory symptoms and mortality, respectively.[65,66] Similar associations have subsequently been found in other cohorts, including middle-aged persons and non-whites and for several other health outcomes, including frailty status (Fried-phenotype), COPD hospitalization and mobility disability.[65–67,90–92] Importantly, because participants in our analytical samples had high smoking rates and no history of asthma, our results for airflow-limitation are most directly applicable to COPD.

Among older persons, when the LMS approach is considered the reference standard, both airflow-limitation and restrictive-pattern are commonly misclassified by GOLD and the ATS/ERS.[65] As shown in Fig 2, using data from CHS, we found that false-positive and false-negative designations occur frequently in GOLD, with

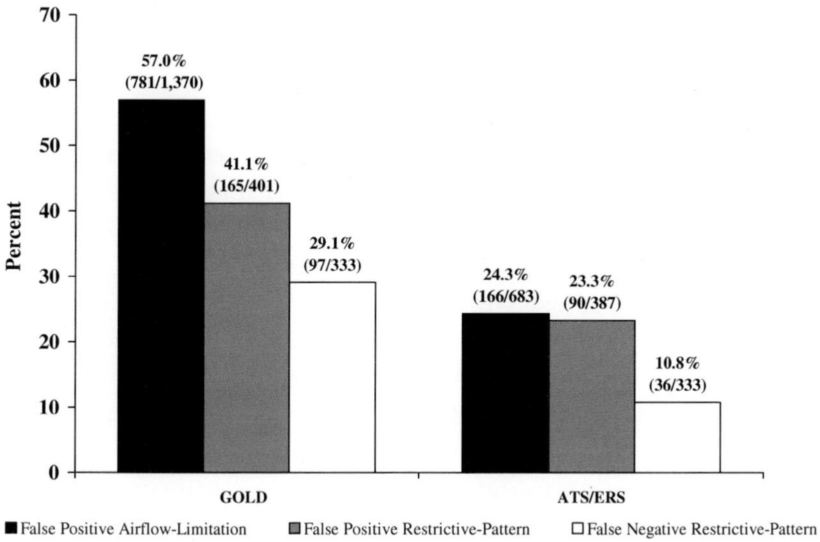

Fig 2. Prevalence of False-Positive and False-Negative Designations of GOLD- and ATS/ERS-Defined Airflow-Limitation and Restrictive-Pattern, Respectively, Relative to LMS Criteria, among Community-Dwelling Persons Aged 65–80 Years. There was no False-Negative Designation for Airflow-Limitation, because all Participants who had Airflow-Limitation by LMS also had Airflow-Limitation by GOLD and ATS/ERS, Respectively. (Reproduced with Permission from Ref 4).

more modest misclassifications seen in the ATS/ERS approach. Both GOLD and the ATS/ERS also misclassify the severity of airflow-limitation, as shown in Table 4.[66] For example, using data from CHS, we found that among the 576 participants classified as having moderate airflow-limitation by GOLD, 330 (57.3%) had normal spirometry by LMS, while 43 (7.5%) and 71 (12.3%) had mild and severe airflow-limitation.

In the absence of pathologic confirmation, it is difficult to directly compare the diagnostic accuracy for respiratory disease of current and alternative spirometric approaches, if the basis for direct comparisons is a reference group composed of persons having potentially misidentified normal spirometry.[93,94] In a prior study, for example, only 26% of community-dwelling older adults had normal spirometry as defined by GOLD.[93] This arguably represented a "super-normal" group that, in turn, misclassified the risk of adverse outcomes among elderly participants who had GOLD-defined respiratory disease. The latter study[93] also included an implausibly high rate of GOLD-defined respiratory disease (74%) and suggests that, if GOLD criteria are broadly applied to populations of older persons, it could lead to inappropriate and potentially harmful pharmacotherapy, as well as delays in considering other diagnoses.[3,85,95–98]

As an alternative approach, we have compared the prevalence rates of GOLD- and LMS-defined respiratory disease stratified according to respiratory symptoms and gait speed, as well as compared their cumulative incidence probabilities of developing mobility disability (characterized as "a lot of difficulty or unable to walk up 10 steps or walk a half-mile").[91] Using CHS data and defining respiratory disease as either spirometric airflow-limitation or restrictive-pattern, we found that the overall prevalence of respiratory disease was 49.7% when using GOLD and 23.2% when using LMS. Differences in the prevalence of respiratory disease were most evident, however, among participants who had no respiratory symptoms, with a value of 38.1% when classified by GOLD and 12.3% when classified by LMS. In addition, among those who had normal gait speed, the rate of respiratory disease more than doubled when

Table 4. Cross-tabulation of frequency distributions of normal spirometry and airflow-limitation (airway obstruction) according to GOLD and the ATS/ERS criteria, within strata of the LMS staging system, among community-dwelling persons aged 65–80 years. (Reproduced with permission from reference 4).

	GOLD Spirometric Category†			
		Airflow-limitation: FEV1 %Pred		
	Normal $N = 1,792$	***Mild:*** **≥ 80** $N = 680$	***Moderate:*** **50–79** $N = 576$	***Severe:*** **< 50** $N = 182$
LMS Spirometric Category‡			**No. (%)**§	
Normal	1,792(100)	**616(90.6)**	**330(57.3)**	0
Airflow-limitation: FEV1 LMS-tile				
Mild: ≥ 5	0	64(9.4)	**43(7.5)**	0
Moderate: 0.5–4.9	0	0	132(22.9)	0
Severe: < 0.5	0	0	**71(12.3)**	182(100)

	ATS/ERS Spirometric Category¶			
		Airflow-limitation: FEV1 %Pred		
	Normal $N = 2,482$	***Mild:*** **≥ 70** $N = 359$	***Moderate:*** **50–69** $N = 207$	***Severe:*** **< 50** $N = 182$
LMS Spirometric Category‡			**No. (%)**§	
Normal	2,482(100)	**214(59.6)**	**42(20.3)**	0
Airflow-limitation: FEV1 LMS-tile				
Mild: ≥ 5	0	107(29.8)	0	0
Moderate: 0.5–4.9	0	**38(10.6)**	94(45.4)	0
Severe: < 0.5	0	0	**71(34.3)**	182(100)

*Discordant spirometric designations are shown in bold.

†Normal spirometry was defined by FEV1/FVC ≥ 0.70 and FVC ≥ 80%Pred; airflow-limitation by an FEV1/FVC < 0.70.

‡Normal spirometry was defined by FEV1/FVC and FVC, both ≥ 5 LMS-tile; airflow-limitation by FEV1/FVC < 5 LMS-tile.

§Column percent.

¶Normal spirometry was defined by FEV1/FVC and FVC, both ≥ ATS/ERS-LLN; airflow-limitation by FEV1/FVC < ATS/ERS-LLN.

classified by GOLD (46.4%) versus LMS (19.3%). Conversely, the 5-year cumulative incidence probability of mobility disability was substantially higher for LMS-defined respiratory disease than for GOLD-defined respiratory disease (0.313 and 0.249 for never-smokers, and 0.352 and 0.289 for ever-smokers, respectively), but similar for LMS- and GOLD-defined normal spirometry (0.193 and 0.185 for never-smokers, and 0.219 and 0.216 for ever-smokers, respectively). These results suggest that the LMS approach (versus the GOLD approach) classifies respiratory disease less frequently in those who are asymptomatic and is more strongly associated with mobility disability.

In another study,[92] we found that the risk of COPD hospitalization over 5 years was increased more than 2-fold in older persons who had LMS-defined mild and moderate COPD and restrictive-pattern and more than 8-fold in those who had LMS-defined severe COPD. However, for the discordant designation of GOLD-defined respiratory disease (COPD or restrictive-pattern) but LMS-defined normal spirometry, the probability of COPD hospitalization was very low (0.04–0.06) and comparable to that in persons who had normal spirometry by either GOLD (0.03) or LMS (0.04).

Although the evidence supporting LMS-calculated Z-scores as a basis for establishing respiratory disease is strong and growing, the generalizability of LMS-calculated Z-scores has been limited because until recently reference equations were only available for whites aged ≤80 years.[2] In late 2012, the Global Lung Function Initiative (GLI) expanded the availability of LMS-calculated spirometric Z scores by publishing reference equations that include ages up to 95 years and multiple ethnicities.[99] Subsequent publications using the updated set of GLI equations have provided further clinical validation of LMS-calculated Z scores as a basis for establishing respiratory disease.[52,100,101]

3.4. *Peak expiratory flow (PEF)*

Because spirometry cannot be obtained in many older persons, especially those who are physically frail, and because primary care settings often lack access to high-quality spirometry, alternative strategies for establishing respiratory disease are needed.[102,103] One possible strategy is PEF, which is assessed by a simple and inexpensive peak flow meter. The PEF is defined as the maximum flow achieved during expiration delivered with maximal force, starting from maximal inspiration.[104] In prior work involving 754 community–dwelling older persons aged ≥70 years, 99.5% completed three PEF readings and variability in effort was minimal (intraclass correlation coefficient of 0.92).[62,63]

PEF is reduced most commonly in the setting of airflow-limitation, particularly asthma and COPD.[104] Other less common causes include extra-thoracic airway obstruction, respiratory muscle weakness and disorders of the chest wall.[104] Although PEF is an attractive alternative to spirometry, two limitations merit comment.[104,105] First, PEF is less sensitive than spirometry in establishing respiratory disease and cannot distinguish airflow-limitation from restrictive-pattern. Second, because it requires an explosive effort, PEF is more effort-dependent than spirometric measures such as the FEV1. Thus, PEF may be reduced simply because of poor effort.[104.105]

Despite these limitations, when spirometry is not available, PEF may be used as a screening tool to evaluate respiratory disease. Prior work has shown that PEF is cross-sectionally associated with health status and physical and cognitive function, and is longitudinally associated with cognitive decline, institutionalization and death.[106–112] Until recently, however, diagnostic thresholds for PEF could not be established because suitable reference values did not exist. To establish diagnostic thresholds, PEF can be expressed as a Z score, similar to that described for spirometry.[62,63] Because LMS and GLI equations are not yet available for PEF, we have instead used Z scores calculated as a standardized residual (SR)[62,63]: [(measured – predicted mean)/(standard deviation of the residuals)]. In this equation, the numerator is termed the "residual", whereas the denominator quantifies the spread of the reference data (accounting for variability in age, sex, height and ethnicity). Hence, an SR-derived Z score also converts a raw measurement on a test to a standardized score in units of standard deviations. Using data from a large cohort of community-dwelling persons aged ≥70 years, we have shown that the highest cut-point for PEF that conferred an increased risk of adverse outcomes occurred at the 10th SR-tile.[63] Specifically, a PEF <10th SR-tile, identifying nearly a quarter of the cohort, conferred an increased risk of disability in activities of daily living (adjusted HR [95% confidence interval]: 1.8 [1.2, 2.6]), mobility disability (1.9 [1.2, 3.1]) and death (2.3 [1.3, 4.1]).

3.5. *Diagnostic confirmation*

As shown in Fig 3, older persons who have respiratory symptoms may require several diagnostic tests to adequately evaluate respiratory disease. In particular, because its accuracy for identifying restrictive lung disease is limited, a spirometric restrictive-pattern will require diagnostic confirmation with static lung volumes as measured by

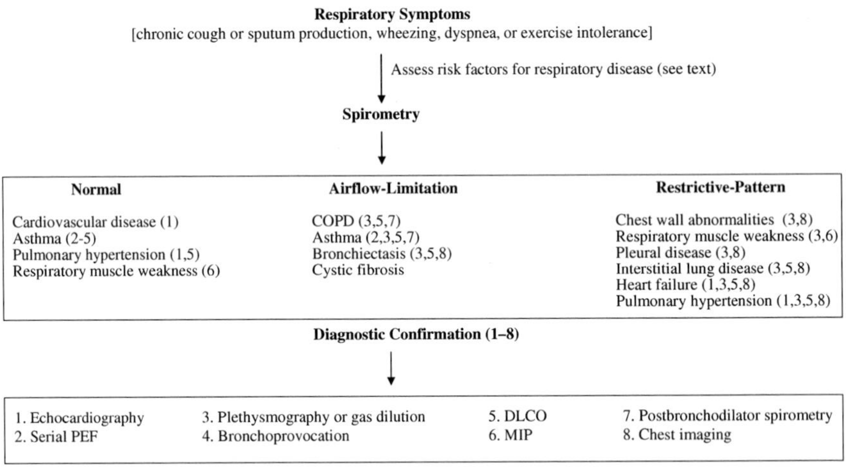

Fig 3. Evaluation of Respiratory Disease Based on Spirometry, Among Persons who have Respiratory Symptoms. Restrictive-Pattern Requires Body Plethysmography or Gas Dilution to Confirm Restrictive Lung Disease. Asthma may also Present with Normal Spirometry, because it is Reversible in its Physiologic Impairment or is Specific to Certain Settings or Symptoms (Exercise-Induced, Occupational, and Cough-Variant Forms of Asthma). (Reproduced with Permission from Ref 4).

Abbreviations: COPD, chronic obstructive pulmonary disease; DLCO, diffusion capacity for carbon monoxide; MIP, maximal inspiratory pressure; PEF, peak expiratory flow.

body plethysmography or gas dilution.[79,113] Older persons who have normal spirometry but are symptomatic may also require further evaluation, potentially including serial PEF measurements, bronchoprovocation, body plethysmography or gas dilution, DLCO, MIP, or echocardiography.[4,80] In the setting of multimorbidity, several tests may be jointly required to identify all the factors contributing to respiratory symptoms. For example, COPD and heart failure frequently coexist in older persons, potentially leading to multiple impairments in respiratory physiology that can contribute to respiratory symptoms.[80,114]

4. Conclusion

In healthy middle- and older-aged persons, normal aging leads to impairments in respiratory physiology, including ventilatory control, respiratory muscle strength, respiratory mechanics and gas exchange, and these are most evident during exercise. Middle- and older-aged persons also have high cumulative rates of exposure to environmental toxins, including tobacco smoke, respiratory infections, ambient air pollution and occupational dusts. In susceptible persons, these environmental exposures induce lung inflammation (respiratory disease) and, in turn, impairments in respiratory physiology, including ventilatory control, respiratory muscle strength and gas exchange but, most frequently, in respiratory mechanics.

Given the noted adverse effects on similar domains of respiratory physiology, normal aging must be taken into account when establishing a diagnosis of respiratory disease, especially if based on pulmonary function testing (physiologic criteria) as is commonly employed in clinical practice and research settings. In particular, because the most prominent physiologic impairment is in respiratory mechanics, the initial diagnostic approach will frequently include spirometric measures of pulmonary function, which are best expressed as Z-scores. The latter rigorously account for normal aging of the respiratory system. Further diagnostic testing may be required, however, depending on the clinical setting.

Acknowledgments

This work was supported by the Department of Veterans Affairs, the Yale Claude D. Pepper Older Americans Independence Center (P30AG021342) and an R03 award from the National Institute on Aging (R03AG037051 — Vaz Fragoso). Dr. Vaz Fragoso is the recipient of a Veterans Administration Merit Award. Dr. Gill is the recipient of an Academic Leadership Award [K07AG043587] from the National Institute on Aging. Dr. Miner is supported by T32AG1934 and the John A. Hartford Center of Excellence at Yale.

The authors report no conflict of interest.

References

1. Meyer KC. (2005) Aging. *Proc Am Thorac Soc* **2**: 433–439.
2. Stanojevic S, Wade A, Stocks J *et al.* (2008) Reference ranges for spirometry across all ages. *Am J Respir Crit Care Med* **177**: 253–260.
3. Qaseem A, Snow V, Shekelle P *et al.* (2007) Diagnosis and management of stable chronic obstructive pulmonary disease: A clinical practice guideline from the American College of Physicians. *Ann Intern Med* **147**: 633–638.
4. Vaz Fragoso CA, Gill T. (2012) Respiratory impairment and the aging lung: A novel paradigm for assessing pulmonary function. *J Gerontol Med Sci* **67**: 264–275.
5. Milic-Emili J, Whitelaw WA, Derenne JPh. (1975) Occlusion pressure — a simple measure of the respiratory center's output. *NEJM* 1029–1030.
6. Peterson DD, Pack AI, Silage DA *et al.* (1981) Effects of aging on ventilatory and occlusion pressure responses to hypoxia and hypercapnia. *Am Rev Respir Dis* **124**: 387–391.
7. Kronenberg RS, Drage CW. (1973) Attenuation of the ventilatory and heart rate responses to hypoxia and hypercapnia with aging in normal men. *J Clin Invest* **52**: 1812–1819.
8. Brischetto MJ, Millman RP, Peterson DD *et al.* (1984) Effect of aging on ventilatory response to exercise and CO_2. *J Appl Physiol Respir Environ Exerc Physiol* **56**: 1143–1150.
9. Poulin MJ, Cunninham DA, Paterson DH *et al.* (1993) Ventilatory sensitivity to CO2 in hyperoxia and hypoxia in older aged humans. *J Appl Physiol* **75**(5):2209–2216.

10. Rubin S, Tack M, Cherniack NS. (1982) Effect of aging on respiratory responses to CO_2 and inspiratory resistive loads. *J Gerontol* **37**: 306–312.
11. Pokorski VM, Marczak M. (2003) Ventilatory response to hypoxia in elderly women. *Ann Hum Biol* **30**: 53–64.
12. Smith WDF, Poulin M, Paterson DH *et al.* (2001) Dynamic ventilatory response to acute isocapnic hypoxia in septuagenarians. *Exp Physiol* **86**(1):117–126.
13. Vovk A, Smith WDF, Paterson ND *et al.* (2004) Peripheral chemoreceptor control of ventilation following sustained hypoxia in young and older adult humans. *Exp Physiol* **89**: 647–656.
14. Ahmed M, Giesbrecht GG, Serrette C *et al.* (1991) Ventilatory response to hypoxia in elderly humans. *Respir Physiol* **83**: 343–351.
15. Bixler EO, Vgontzas AN, Ten HT *et al.* (1998) Effects of age on sleep apnea in men: Prevalence and severity. *Am J Respir Crit Care Med* **157**: 144–148.
16. McKay LC, Janczewski WA, Feldman JL. (2005) Sleep-disordered breathing after targeted ablation of preBotzinger complex neurons. *Nat Neurosci* **8**: 1142–1144.
17. Celle S, Peyron R, Faillenot I *et al.* (2009) Undiagnosed sleep-related breathing disorders are associated with focal brainstem atrophy in the elderly. *Hum Brain Mapp* **30**: 2090–2097.
18. Feldman JL, Del Negro CA. (2006) Looking for inspiration: New perspectives on respiratory rhythm. *Nature Rev: Neurosci* **7**: 232–242.
19. Garcia-Touchard A, Somers VK, Olson LJ *et al.* (2008) Central sleep apnea: Implications for congestive heart failure. *Chest* **133**: 1495–1504.
20. Ainsliel PN, Duffin JD. (2009) Integration of cerebrovascular CO_2 reactivity and chemoreflex control of breathing: Mechanisms of regulation, measurement, and interpretation. *Am J Physiol Regul Integr Comp Physiol* **296**: R1473–R1495.
21. Flück DF, Beaudin AE2, Steinback GD *et al.* (2014) Effects of aging on the association between cerebrovascular responses to visual stimulation, hypercapnia and arterial stiffness. Available at *journal.frontiersin.org/Journal/10.3389/fphys.2014.00049/full.* Accessed April 14, 2014.
22. Fisher JP, Hartwich D, Seifert T *et al.* (2013) Cerebral perfusion, oxygenation and metabolism during exercise in young and elderly individuals. *J. Physiol* **591**: 1859–1870.

23. Nishiyama T, Sugai N, Hanaoka K. (1997). Cerebrovascular CO_2 reactivity in elderly and younger adult patients during sevoflurane anaesthesia. *Can J Anaesth* **44**: 160–164.
24. Connolly MJ, Crowley JJ, Charan NB *et al.* (1992) Reduced subjective awareness of bronchoconstriction provoked by methacholine in elderly asthmatic and normal subjects as measured on a simple awareness scale. *Thorax* **47**: 410–413.
25. Cuttitta G, Cibella F, Bellia V *et al.* (2001) Changes in FVC during methacholine-induced bronchoconstriction in elderly patients with asthma: Bronchial hyperresponsiveness and aging. *Chest* **119**: 1685–1690.
26. Chen H-I, Kuo C-S. (1989) Relationship between respiratory muscle function and age, sex, and other factors. *J Appl Physiol* **66**: 943–948.
27. Enright PL, Kronmal RA, Manolio TA *et al.* (1994) Respiratory muscle strength in the elderly; correlates and reference values. *Am J Respir Crit Care Med* **149**: 430–438.
28. Sachs MC, Enright PL, Stukovsky KDH *et al.* (2009) Performance of maximum inspiratory pressure tests and maximum inspiratory pressure reference equations for 4 race/ethnic groups. *Respir Care* **54**: 1321–1328.
29. Janssens J-P. (2005) Aging of the respiratory system: Impact on pulmonary function tests and adaptation to exertion. *Clin Chest Med* **26**: 469–484.
30. Cruz-Jentoft AJ, Baeyens JP, Bauer JM *et al.* (2010) Sarcopenia: European consensus on definition and diagnosis: Report of the European working group on sarcopenia in older people. *Age Ageing* **39**: 412–423.
31. Polkey MI, Hamnega C-H, Hughes PD *et al.* (1998) Influence of acute lung volume change on contractile properties of human diaphragm. *J Appl Physiol* **85**(4):1322–1328.
32. Fletcher C, Peto R. (1977) The natural history of chronic airflow obstruction. *BMJ* **1**: 1645–1648.
33. LeBlanc P, Ruff F, Milic-Emili J. (1970) Effects of age and body position on "airway closure" in man. *J Appl Physiol* **28**(4):448–451.
34. American Thoracic Society/American College of Chest Physicians (ATS/ACCP). (2003) Statement on Cardiopulmonary Exercise Testing. *Am J Respir Crit Care Med* **167**: 211–277.
35. Hardie JA, Vollmer WM, Buist AS *et al.* (2004) Reference values for arterial blood gases in the elderly. *Chest* **125**: 2053–2060.

36. Crapo RO, Jensen RL, Hegewald M *et al.* (1999) Arterial blood gas reference values for sea level and an altitude of 1,400 meters. *Am J Respir Crit Care Med* **160**: 1525–1531.
37. West, JB. (2008) *Respiratory physiology: The essentials.* 8th ed. Lippincott Williams and Wilkins, Baltimore.
38. Levin DL, Buxton RB, Spiess JP *et al.* (2007) Effects of age on pulmonary perfusion heterogeneity measured by magnetic resonance imaging. *J Appl Physiol* **102**: 2064–2070.
39. Ohlsson J, Middaugh M, Hlastala MP. (1989) Reduction of lung perfusion increases V_A/Q heterogeneity. *J Appl Physiol* **66**: 2423–2430.
40. Wagner P, Laravuso R, Uhl R *et al.* (1974) Continuous distribution of ventilation-perfusion ratios in normal subjects breathing air and 100 per cent O2. *J Clin Invest* **54**: 54–68.
41. Holland J, Milic-Emili J, Macklem PT *et al.* (1968) Regional distribution of pulmonary ventilation and perfusion in elderly subjects. *J Clin Invest* **47**: 81–92.
42. Cardus J, Burgos F, Diaz O *et al.* (1997) Increase in pulmonary ventilation–perfusion inequality with age in healthy individuals. *Am J Respir Crit Care Med* **156**: 648–653.
43. Ersham R, Perruchoud DA, Oberholzer M *et al.* (1983) Influence of age on pulmonary haemodynamics at rest and during supine exercise. *Clin Sci* **65**: 653–660.
44. McQuillan BM, Picard MH, Leavitt M *et al.* (2001) Clinical correlates and reference intervals for pulmonary artery systolic pressure among echocardiographically normal subjects. *Circulation* **104**: 2797–2802.
45. Butler C, Kleinerman J. (1970) Capillary density: Alveolar diameter, a morphometric approach to ventilation and perfusion. *Am Rev Respir Dis* **102**: 886–894.
46. Mackay EH, Banks J, Sykes B *et al.* (1978) Structural basis for the changing physical properties of human pulmonary vessels with age. *Thorax* **33**: 335–344.
47. Guénard H, Marthan R. (1996) Pulmonary gas exchange in elderly subjects. *Eur Respir J* **9**: 2573–2577.
48. Garcia-Rio F, Dorgham A, Galera R *et al.* (2012) Prediction equations for single-breath diffusing capacity in subjects aged 65 to 85 Years. *Chest* **142**: 175–184.
49. Casaburi R, Daly J, Hansen JE *et al.* (1989) Abrupt changes in mixed venous blood gas composition after the onset of exercise. *J Appl Physiol* **67**(3):1106–1112.

50. Johnson BD, Reddan WG, Pegelow DF *et al.*(1991). Flow limitation and regulation of functional residual capacity during exercise in a physically active aging population. *Am Rev Respir Dis* **143**: 960–967.
51. Johnson BD, Weisman IM, Zeballos RJ *et al.* (1999) Emerging concepts in the evaluation of ventilatory limitation during exercise; the exercise tidal flow-volume loop. *Chest* **116**: 488–503.
52. Vaz Fragoso CA, Beavers DP, Hankinson JL *et al.* (2014) Respiratory impairment and dyspnea and their associations with physical inactivity and mobility in sedentary community-dwelling older persons. *J Am Geriatr Soc.* In press
53. Buchman AS, Boyle PA, Wilson RS *et al.* (2008) Respiratory muscle strength predicts decline in mobility in older persons. *Neuroepidemiol* **31**: 174–180.
54. Johnson BD, Badr MS, Dempsey JA (1994) Impact of the aging pulmonary system on the response to exercise. *Clin Chest Med* **15**: 229–246.
55. GOLD executive summary. (2007) Global strategy for the diagnosis, management, and prevention of chronic obstructive pulmonary disease. *Am J Respir Crit Care Med* **176**: 532–555.
56. Raherison C, Girodet PO. (2009) Epidemiology of COPD. *Eur Respir Rev* **18**: 213–221.
57. Stockley RA, Mannino D, Barnes PJ. (2009) Burden and pathogenesis of chronic obstructive pulmonary disease. *Proc Am Thorac Soc* 6: 524–526.
58. Donaldson GC, Seemungal TA, Bhowmik A *et al.* (2002) Relationship between exacerbation frequency and lung function decline in chronic obstructive pulmonary disease. *Thorax* **57**: 847–852.
59. Raghu G, Collard HR, Egan JJ *et al.* (2011) An Official ATS/ERS/JRS/ALAT statement: Idiopathic pulmonary fibrosis: Evidence-based guidelines for diagnosis and management. *Am J Respir Crit Care Med* **183**: 788–824.
60. Chotirmall SH, Watts M, Branagan P *et al.* (2009) Diagnosis and management of asthma in older adults. *J Am Geriatr Soc* **57**: 901–909.
61. Gibson PG, McDonald VM, Marks GB. (2010) Asthma in older adults. *Lancet* **376**: 803–813.
62. Vaz Fragoso CA, Gahbauer E, Van Ness P *et al.* (2007) Reporting peak expiratory flow in older persons. *J Gerontol Med Sci* **62**A: 1147–1151.
63. Vaz Fragoso CA, Gahbauer E, Van Ness P *et al.* (2008) Peak expiratory flow as a predictor of subsequent disability and death in community-living older persons. *J Am Geriatr Soc* **56**: 1014–1020.

64. Vaz Fragoso CA, Concato J, McAvay G *et al.* (2010) The ratio of FEV1 to FVC as a basis for establishing chronic obstructive pulmonary disease. *Am J Respir Crit Care Med* **181**: 446–451.
65. Vaz Fragoso CA, Gill TM, McAvay G *et al.* (2011) Respiratory impairment and mortality in older persons: A novel spirometric method. *J Investig Med* 59(7):1089–1095.
66. Vaz Fragoso CA, Concato J, McAvay G *et al.* (2011) Staging the severity of chronic obstructive pulmonary disease in older persons based on spirometric Z-scores. *J Am Geriatr Soc* **59**: 1847–1854.
67. Vaz Fragoso CA, Enright P, McAvay G *et al.* (2012) Frailty and respiratory impairment in older persons. *Am J Med* **125**: 79–86.
68. Centers for Disease Control and Prevention. National Center for Health Statistics. National Health Interview Survey 1965–2008. Analysis for years 1997—2008 by the American Lung Association, Research and Program Services Division.
69. Kaufmann RB, Babb S, O'Halloran A *et al.* (2010) Vital Signs: Nonsmokers' exposure to secondhand smoke — United States, 1999–2008. *MMWR* **59**(35):1141–1146.
70. Thompson WW, Shay DK, Weintraub E *et al.* (2004) Influenza-associated hospitalizations in the United States. *JAMA* **292**: 1333–1340.
71. A Profile of Older Americans: 2013. U.S. Department of Health and Human Services. Available at: http://www.aoa.gov/aoaroot/aging_statistics/Profile/index.aspx. Accessed April 9, 2014.
72. De Leon SF, Thurston GD, Ito K. (2003) Contribution of respiratory disease to nonrespiratory mortality associations with air pollution. *Am J Respir Crit Care Med* **167**: 1117–1123.
73. Schindler C, Kunzli N, Bongard JP *et al.* (2001) Short-term variation in air pollution and in average lung function among never-smokers: The Swiss study on air pollution and lung diseases in adults (SALPADIA). *Am J Respir Crit Care Med* **163**: 356–361.
74. Celli BR, Halbert RJ, Nordyke RJ *et al.* (2005) Airway obstruction in never smokers: Results from the Third National Health and Nutrition Examination Survey. *Am J Med* **118**: 1364–1372.
75. Hnizdo E, Sullivan PA, Bang KM *et al.* (2002) Association between chronic obstructive pulmonary disease and employment by industry and occupation in the US population: A study of data from the third national health and nutrition examination survey. *Am J Epidemiol* **156**: 738–746.

76. Ely EW, Wheeler AP, Thompson BT *et al.* (2002) Recovery rate and prognosis in older persons who develop acute lung injury and the acute respiratory distress syndrome. *Ann Intern Med* **136**: 25–36.
77. Fry AM, Shay DK, Holman RC *et al.* (2005) Trends in hospitalizations for pneumonia among persons aged 65 years or older in the United States, 1988–2002. *JAMA* **294**: 2712–2719.
78. Miller MR, Hankinson J, Brusasco V *et al.* (2005) Standardisation of spirometry. *Eur Respir J* **26**: 319–338.
79. Pellegrino R, Viegi G, Brusasco V *et al.* (2005) Interpretative strategies for lung function tests. *Eur Respir J* **26**: 948–968.
80. Chan ED, Welsh CH. (1998) Geriatric respiratory medicine. *Chest* **114**: 1704–1733.
81. Hankinson JL, Odencrantz JR, Fedan KB. (1999) Spirometric reference values from a sample of the general U.S. population. *Am J Respir Crit Care Med* **159**: 179–187.
82. Vaz Fragoso CA, Gill TM. (2010) Defining chronic obstructive pulmonary disease in an aging population. *J Am Geriatr Soc* **58**: 2224–2226.
83. Miller MR, Pincock AC. (1988) Predicted values: How should we use them? *Thorax* **43**: 265–267.
84. Official statement of the European Respiratory Society. (1993) Lung volumes and forced ventilatory flows. *Eur Respir J* **6**(S16):5–40.
85. Vaz Fragoso CA, Concato J, McAvay G *et al.* (2010) Chronic obstructive pulmonary disease in older persons: A comparison of two spirometric definitions. *Resp Med* **104**: 1189–1196.
86. Garcia-Rio F, Pino JM, Dorgham A *et al.* (2004) Spirometric reference equations for European females and males aged 65-85 years. *Eur Respir J* **24**: 397–405.
87. Enright PL, Kronmal RA, Higgins M *et al.* (1993) Spirometry reference values for women and men 65–85 years of age: Cardiovascular health study. *Am Rev Respir Dis* **147**: 125–133.
88. Vaz Fragoso CA, Concato J, McAvay G *et al.* (2009) Defining chronic obstructive pulmonary disease in older persons. *Resp Med* **103**: 1468–1476.
89. Cummings SR, Bates D, Black DM. (2002) Clinical use of bone densitometry: Scientific review. *JAMA* **288**: 1889– 1897.
90. Vaz Fragoso CA, Gill TM, McAvay G *et al.* (2011) Evaluating respiratory impairment in middle-aged persons using lambda-mu-sigma derived z-scores. *Respir Care* **56**: 1771–1777.

91. Vaz Fragoso CA, Gill TM, McAvay G *et al.* (2013) Respiratory impairment in older persons: When less means more. *Am J Med* **126**: 49–57.
92. Vaz Fragoso CA, Concato J, McAvay G *et al.* (2012) Respiratory impairment and COPD hospitalization: A competing risk analysis. *Eur Respir J* **40**: 37–44.
93. Mannino DM, Buist AS, Vollmer WM. (2007) Chronic obstructive pulmonary disease in the older adult: What defines abnormal lung function? *Thorax* **62**: 237–241.
94. Mannino DM, Diaz-Guzman E. (2012) Interpreting lung function data using 80% predicted and fixed thresholds identifies patients at increased risk of mortality. *Chest* **141**: 73–80.
95. Singh S, Loke YK, Furberg CD. (2008) Inhaled anticholinergics and risk of major adverse cardiovascular events in patients with chronic obstructive pulmonary disease: A systematic review and meta-analysis. *JAMA* **300**: 1439–1450.
96. Drummond MB, Dasenbrook EC, Pitz MW *et al.* (2008) Inhaled corticosteroids in patients with stable chronic obstructive pulmonary disease: A systematic review and meta-analysis. *JAMA* **300**: 2407–2416.
97. Stephenson A, Seitz D, Bell CM *et al.* (2011) Inhaled anticholinergic drug therapy and the risk of acute urinary retention in chronic obstructive pulmonary disease. *Arch Intern Med* **171**: 914–920.
98. Taylor DR. (2009) The ß-agonist saga and its clinical relevance: On and on it goes. *Am J Respir Crit Care Med* **179**: 976–978.
99. Quanjer PH, Stanojevic S, Cole TJ *et al.* (2012) Multi-ethnic reference values for spirometry for the 3–95 year age range: The global lung function 2012 equations. *Eur Respir J* **40**: 1324–1343.
100. Vaz Fragoso CA, McAvay G, Gill TM *et al.* (2014) Ethnic differences in respiratory impairment. *Thorax* **69**: 55–62.
101. Quanjer PH, Pretto JJ, Brazzale DJ *et al.* (2014) Grading the severity of airways obstruction: New wine in new bottles. *Eur Respir J* **43**: 513–522.
102. Sherman CB, Kern D, Richardson ER *et al.* (1993) Cognitive function and spirometry performance in the elderly. *Am Rev Respir Dis* **148**: 123–126.
103. Allen SC, Yeung P. (2006) Inability to draw intersecting pentagons as a predictor of unsatisfactory spirometry technique in elderly hospital inpatients. *Age and Ageing* **35**: 304–316.

104. Quanjer PH, Lebowitz MD, Gregg I *et al.* (1997) Peak expiratory flow: Conclusions and recommendations of a working party of the European respiratory society. *Eur Respir J* **10**(S24): 2S–8S.
105. Paggiaro PL, Moscato G, Giannini D *et al.* (1997) Relationship between peak expiratory flow and FEV1. *Eur Respir J* **10**(S24): 39S–41S.
106. Cook NR, Albert MS, Berkman LF *et al.* (1995) Interrelationships of peak expiratory flow rate with physical and cognitive function in the elderly: MacArthur foundation studies of aging. *J Gerontol Med Sci* **50**A:M317–M323.
107. Lan T-Y, Melzer D, Tom BDM *et al.* (2002) Performance tests and disability: Developing an objective index of mobility-related limitation in older populations. *J Gerontol Med Sci* **57**: M294–M301.
108. Schaub RT, Munzberg H, Borchelt M *et al.* (2000) Ventilatory capacity and risk for dementia. *J Gerontol Med Sci* **55**A:M677–M683.
109. Cook NR, Evans DA, Scherr PA *et al.* (1989) Peak expiratory flow rate in an elderly population. *Am J Epidemiol* **130**: 66–78.
110. Whitfield KE, Seeman TE, Miles TP *et al.* (1997) Health indices as predictors of cognition among older African Americans: MacArthur studies of successful aging. *Ethnicity Dis* **7**: 127–136.
111. McCallum J, Simons LA, Simons J *et al.* (2005) Patterns and predictors of nursing home placement over 14 years: Dubbo study of elderly Australians. *Australian J Ageing* **24**: 169–173.
112. Cook NR, Evans DA, Scherr PA *et al.* (1991) Peak expiratory flow rate and 5-year mortality in an elderly population. *Am J Epidemiol* **133**: 784–794.
113. Glady CA, Aaron SD, Lunau M *et al.* (2003) Spirometry-based algorithm to direct lung function testing in the pulmonary function laboratory. *Chest* **123**: 1939–1946.
114. Fried TR, Vaz Fragoso CA, Rabow MW. (2012) Caring for the older person with chronic obstructive pulmonary disease. JAMA **308**(12): 1254–1263.

Chapter 3

Aging Lung, Environmental and Genetic Factors — Race, Ethnicity and Gender

Holly Keyt*, Stephanie Levine*, and Claude Jourdan Le Saux*,†,‡

1. Introduction

Not everyone is equal when it comes to aging and the development of age-related pulmonary diseases. Indeed, the lungs of women are affected differently. The susceptibility to the development and progression of age-related pulmonary diseases in women differs from their male counterparts. Race and ethnicity are also factors that influence the gender disparities in aging, although the contribution of these factors is not as straightforward as that for gender.

2. Physiology of the Aging Lung

As part of physiologic aging, the respiratory system sustains changes that affect its ability to respond to challenges from the environment

*University of Texas Health Science Center, Department of Medicine, Division of Pulmonary and Critical Care, 7703 FLoyd Curl Drive, San Antonio Texas 78229, USA.
†University of Texas Health Science Center, Department of Medicine, Division of Cardiology, 7703 FLoyd Curl Drive, San Antonio Texas 78229, USA, E-mail: lesaux@uthscsa.edu
‡Corresponding author.

and exercise. The lungs reach peak function at approximately 20 years of age for women and 25 years of age for men, after which there is a progressive decline in lung function. The age-associated changes that seem to have the most significant impact on functional decline are decreases in elastic recoil, compliance of the chest wall, and respiratory muscle strength,[1] resulting in static air trapping, increased functional residual capacity and increased work of breathing.[2] Forced expiratory flow (FEF) is the flow (or speed) of air coming out of the lung during the middle portion of a forced expiration. Interestingly, FEF depends on age, sex, height, weight and ethnicity. The expiratory flow rates decrease with aging with characteristic changes in flow-volume curves suggestive of increased collapsibility of peripheral airways.[2,3,4] All people experience an annual decline in FEV1 of approximately 20 ml/year in subjects 25–39 years of age.[2] This is increased to 38 ml/year in subjects greater than 65 years of age.[3] The rate of decline is accelerated in women[5] and may make older women more susceptible to expiratory flow limitation and exercise-related dyspnea.[6] The efficiency of alveolar gas exchange decreases progressively with age for a number of reasons. The small increase in anatomic dead space alone cannot account for the uneven pattern of distribution of inspired gas in older subjects that contrasts with the more even distribution in younger subjects. People normally make new alveoli until about age 20. After that, the lungs begin to lose some of their tissue.[7] The number of alveoli decreases and there is a corresponding decrease in lung capillaries.

The majority of elderly persons have some degree of kyphoscoliosis as a result of age-related osteoporosis and vertebral fractures. In one study of 100 chest radiographs from healthy persons aged 75–93 years, 25% had severe kyphoscolisosis and 43% had moderate kyphoscoliosis as a result of partial or complete vertebral fractures.[8] This chest wall deformity contributes to worsened chest wall compliance and affects the force of the diaphragm. Women are particularly susceptible to this age-related change as they have approximately twice the rates of vertebral fractures compared to men of the same age.[9] Symptoms of fatigue or dyspnea can also occur due to weakening of the musculature. Respiratory muscle strength can be measured by transdiaphragmatic pressure (Pdi), maximum voluntary ventilation

(MVV) and maximum inspiratory pressure (MIP).[7] MIP is an index of strength of the diaphragm, which is a measure of inspiratory muscle strength and a determinant of vital capacity. Declines in MIP can lead to inadequate ventilation and impaired clearance of airway secretions, as seen in patients with neuromuscular disease. MVV is also reduced with age and one longitudinal study showed a 12% decline over 6 years in older trained athletes.[10] A likely explanation for reduced diaphragmatic strength with age is related to muscle atrophy and an age-related decrease in fast twitch fibers, responsible for generating higher peak tensions. This age-related decline in diaphragmatic strength may predispose older individuals to diaphragmatic fatigue and ventilatory failure during increased ventilatory load on the respiratory system.

The influence of race/ethnicity in the aging processes is well documented. However it is difficult to tease apart the impact of intrinsic factors (genetic background) from the health and socioeconomic status or the effects of early life events that persist throughout the course of life. However, prolonged exposure to socioeconomic disadvantages over the life course by racial and ethnic minorities lead to the premature onset of chronic disease and more rapid deterioration of general health status including lung-related health.[11] Compared with US-born Whites, US-born Blacks average peak expiratory flow rates that are 37.3 L/m lower and foreign-born Blacks average peak expiratory flow rates that are 63.5 L/m lower. Peak expiratory flow rates of US-born Hispanics are not statistically significantly different from those of the US-born Whites, but foreign-born Hispanics have significantly lower rates.[11] A rigorous evaluation in respiratory impairment, including airflow limitation and restrictive pattern, has established that African Americans had high rates of respiratory impairment associated with mortality but not respiratory symptoms.[12] However this study did not take into consideration the social status of any of the individuals involved in the study.

3. Aging Processes

Different processes have been associated with aging across all organs. The main ones are telomere titration, oxidative stress, increased inflammation and senescence. It is interesting to note that the impact of these factors on aging is gender-dependent. It is well known that telomere titration and oxidative stress are associated with cellular senescence, one of the hallmarks of aging. Both telomere titration and oxidative stress appear to be less pronounced in women.[13]

It is interesting to note that an association between gender and telomere length exists and varies by age.[13,14,15] Although there is contradictory data, telomere length appears to be longer in women.[16–21] A comprehensive systematic review and meta-analyses has demonstrated that telomere length is longer in women.[13] Multiple hypotheses have been postulated to explain this association.[16, 22, 23] One is the action of estrogen.[22] An estrogen-responsive element is present in telomerase reverse transcriptase (hTERT),[16] hence estrogen might stimulate telomerase to add telomere repeats to the ends of chromosomes. Furthermore, telomeres are particularly sensitive to oxidative stress[24] and women produce fewer reactive oxygen species than men.[16] It has been suggested that women might also metabolize reactive oxygen species better because of estrogen,[16] and its antioxidant properties.[25]

Studies of bronchoalveolar lavage (BAL) fluid in elderly adults have demonstrated important age-related changes in both adaptive and innate immunity cellular components.[26, 27] Specifically, increased numbers of neutrophils and total lymphocytes, an increased CD4+/CD8+ T cell ratio, decreased number of B cells, increased IgM and IgA antibodies, as well as decreased vascular endothelial growth factor have been measured.[28] Alveolar macrophages (AM) are a critical aspect of lung-specific immunity and multiple studies have demonstrated important functional changes in AM function with aging.[29] In rat models that have examined macrophage responses, aging has been associated with decreased expression of Toll like receptors,[30,31] decreased generation of nitric oxide,[32] and decreased TNF-alpha release.[33] Although human studies have not been able to replicate all of these results, Zissel and colleagues have demonstrated decreased accessory function in AM of elderly patients, which is necessary for T cell stimulation and activation of the adaptive response.[34] These changes in the immune responses could explain the susceptibility of the elderly to the development of infectious diseases and the lack of response to vaccination.[35] Moreover these alterations of the immune response in the elderly are gender-specific. The profile of cytokines released by T cells stimulated with anti-CD3 plus anti-CD28 antibodies, such as IFN-γ generation, is decreased in older men but increased in older women compared to healthy young subjects, while IL-17 levels were lower for men but showed no difference for women.[36] Most of the studies suggest that in addition to age, in postmenopausal women, changes of the immune system have been attributed to estrogen deprivation.[37] The contribution of age-related alterations in the immune system is one component to take into consideration when comparing men and women.

4. The Environment and the Aging Lung

The respiratory system is an important and dynamic interface between the human body and an increasingly toxic environment. With the passage of time, the lungs sustain frequent and cumulative environmental insults such as exposure to tobacco smoke, air pollution and respiratory infections resulting in a decline in pulmonary function.[2] While this deterioration may be independent of disease pathology,[38] it results in difficulties withstanding environmental injury — a vicious cycle ultimately predisposing the elderly lung to diseases such as cancer, pulmonary fibrosis, asthma and emphysema.

In susceptible individuals, a decline in forced expiratory volume in 1 second (FEV1) is accelerated by environmental exposures.[39] The anatomic and physiologic changes that predispose the aged lung to increased sensitivity to environmental stress are well established. These changes include increased stiffness of the chest wall, structural deformities of the thoracic spine, decreased elastic recoil of the lungs, declining respiratory muscle performance, impaired cough reflex, blunting of the ventilatory response to hypoxia and hypercapnea,[40] and reduced respiratory tract lining antioxidant defense.[41] As a result, the aged respiratory system finds it difficult to clear inhaled particulate matter encountered in the environment such as cigarette smoke, airborne aerosols, coal dust, silica and diesel emissions.[42] As these reactive oxidative species accumulate with time, the cellular defense mechanisms are overwhelmed, ultimately resulting in loss of function, cell death and precipitation of the normal decline in pulmonary function.[42]

In addition to the increased exposure of the pulmonary system to environmental injury and inability to clear particulate matter in the elderly lung, there also seems to be exaggerated inflammatory and pulmonary function responses to environmental insult. Consequently the elderly are at increased risk of morbidity due to environmental stress from air pollution, airborne pathogens, smoking and climate change. The National Morbidity, Mortality and Air Pollution Study (NMMAPS) in the United States (US), covered a wide geographic area with varying levels of air pollution and showed a positive association between the level of particulate matter in the air and the rate of hospital admissions for pneumonia and complications of chronic obstructive pulmonary disease (COPD) in the elderly: For each 10 $\mu g/m^3$ increase in particulate matter, there was a 2% increase in admissions for pneumonia and COPD.[43] The NMMAPS also showed an approximate 0.5% increase in overall mortality for every 10 $\mu g/m^3$ increase in particulate matter in the air measured the day before death.[43] These results are potentially augmented by climate change, through its impact on increasing ground-level ozone production.[42,44]

Another significant source of environmental injury is cigarette smoke, which causes significant morbidity and mortality from direct inhalation as well as through secondhand exposure. Older Americans had a prior smoking rate of 50% in the mid 1960s, which has now decreased to 9%.[12] However, nonsmoking status does not equate to lack of exposure to tobacco smoke. In 2008, among nonsmoking Americans who were greater than 60 years of age, 32% had a documented exposure to secondhand smoke. The US Centers for Disease Control, estimates that 1 of every 5 deaths (more than 480,000 per year) is a result of smoking. Cigarette smoking also has been shown to accelerate age-related declines in forced vital capacity (FVC) and FEV1, an effect even more pronounced amongst women.[42,45] One proposed mechanism for this deterioration is through the induction of senescence in alveolar epithelial cells and impaired re-epithelialization.[42,46] Smoking has also been shown to impair resolution of inflammation.[47] These pathophysiologic changes lead to and/or exacerbate pulmonary diseases such as COPD, lung cancer, interstitial pulmonary fibrosis (IPF) and asthma.

Finally, in many developing countries, people are subjected to the additional environmental stress of biomass fuel combustion. These populations experience a significant burden of disease related to this exposure, including declines in lung function, higher rates of respiratory and cardiovascular morbidity and an increase in overall mortality.[48,49] It is postulated that women are particularly at risk due to increased exposure to indoor solid-fuel-fired cooking and heating stoves. A number of studies were conducted in the 1980s to more specifically describe the health effects of this air pollution. The majority of these studies were done in South Asian homes burning biomass fuels.[50] One study suggests the effects of using biomass fuel are comparable to a 10-year difference in age.[51] Furthermore, decreased lung function is evident in Nepali women who reported more time spent near the stove and chronic obstructive lung disease seems to be associated with daily time spent near the stove for these women.[52]

5. Genetics, Race, and Ethnicity and the Aging Lung

The interactions between genetic ancestry and the aging lung are well known but not well characterized. Despite our reliance on race/ethnic-specific reference standards in quantifying lung function (per the American Thoracic Society/European Respiratory Society guidelines), the definitions of the key variables of race and ethnicity vary worldwide. As illustration, a systematic review of literature regarding lung function and ethnicity, spanning from 1922–2008, showed that only a minority of studies (17.3%) defined race/ethnicity in the methods section even though a majority of the studies (51.2%) reported lower lung capacity in "other race and ethnic groups" compared to "white".[53] Even the COPD Gene study, a large, multicenter observational study designed to identify genetic factors associated with COPD, relies on subjects' self-reported race/ethnicity at enrollment.[54] Our ever-evolving understanding of ethnicity and genetics, combined with the development of ancestry-informative genetic markers, necessitates further research in this area.

The current body of literature is deficient in reports of the aging human lung in the context of race/ethnicity. However, several pulmonary disease processes, which are more prevalent in the geriatric population (COPD, lung cancer, interstitial lung diseases) have been studied with respect to race/ethnicity and will be discussed herewith.

In COPD, a variety of outcomes have traditionally been associated with race/ethnic groups in the US. For example, mortality from COPD is the highest among Caucasians[55]; the rates of hospitalization and emergency department visits due to COPD is highest among African-Americans[55]; and the prevalence of COPD is higher among some Hispanic subgroups compared with African-Americans.[56] However, a large cross-sectional population-based study of adults in the US found that the effect of smoking on markers of COPD (FEV1 to FVC ratio or percent emphysema on imaging) does not vary substantially with respect to genetic ancestry.[57] It is more likely that observed disparities in prior studies may actually be a result of differences in smoking patterns, differential exposure to air pollution or environmental toxins, maternal smoking during pregnancy, low birth weight, and/or exposure to pulmonary irritants during lung development.

Epidemiologic studies of smoking-related lung cancer (the vast majority of lung cancer cases) reveal a striking difference in rates among ethnic/racial groups. Compared to Caucasians, the incidence of lung cancer is substantially higher among Blacks and Native Hawaiians and lower among Japanese Americans and Hispanics.[58] Using the large database of Surveillance, Epidemiology and End Results Program (SEER, http://seer.cancer.gov/statfacts/html/lungb.html), in black men there are 93 new cases of lung cancer per 100,000 persons, compared to 72.4 cases per 100,000 persons in white men and 49.4 cases per 100,000 persons in Asian/Pacific Islander men. This disparity is also observed in death rates due to lung and bronchus cancer (SEER, http://seer.cancer.gov/statfacts/html/lungb.html). The difference in incidence is less striking among women (51.2 cases per 100,000 persons in black women, 53.8 cases per 100,000 persons in white women, 28.1 cases per 100,000 persons in Asian women) (SEER). It has been postulated that part of the significantly increased risk of lung cancer among African Americans is related to metabolism of nicotine and tobacco carcinogens, however, further study of the relationship of genetic ancestry and lung cancer is needed.[59]

In studies of IPF, Caucasians make up the vast majority of subjects, however this is suspected to be largely due to selection bias. A large epidemiologic study published in 2012 identified the ethnic/racial makeup of subjects who died in the US between 1989–2007 and had pulmonary fibrosis as a cause of death, as reported by funeral directors. In this study, 87.2% of decedents were non-Hispanic Caucasian, 5.1% were African-American, 5.4% were Hispanic and 2.2% were from other ethnic/racial groups. Of these subjects, Caucasians died at an older age than African-Americans and Hispanics were the most likely to die from IPF.[60]

In the asthma literature, there are large and persisting disparities in rates of severe asthma exacerbations by race/ethnicity. Traditionally, African-American patients are at the highest risk. In fact, a 2012 study showed that African ancestry was significantly and positively associated with severe exacerbations among male African American subjects.[61] Whether this difference extends to the geriatric population has yet to be studied.

6. Gender and the Aging Lung

Inherent gender-related differences in lung function are apparent throughout the human life span.[62] These differences have been attributed to the action of hormones as well as morphologic/structural differences.[63] Structurally, men have larger airway diameters, larger lung volumes and larger diffusion surfaces. Functionally, women have consistently lower maximal expiratory flow rates and during exercise have increased work of breathing and greater expiratory flow limitation.[63] In the aging population, there is a reduction in lung elastic recoil, vital capacity, diffusion surface area and chest wall compliance. These changes lead to a decrease in maximal expiratory flow rate for both women and men, however, the rate of decrease in maximal expiratory flow rate and lung elastic recoil tends to be greater in men compared to women.[62] Furthermore, women tend to be older at the onset of these decreases in respiratory function.[64]

The role of gender plays in pulmonary diseases is complex, given the multifactorial nature of these diseases and the contributing effects of culture, the environment and behavior. A key factor in many pulmonary diseases is cigarette smoking, which has been shown to be more detrimental to lung function in women than men.[45] When controlled for pack-years smoked, the rate of lung function decline in women is faster than in men; women lose in FEV1, 10.5 ml/pack-year and men lose 8.4 ml/pack-year.[65] It follows, that in smoking-related illnesses, women develop symptoms at a younger age than men and also have a smaller pack-year history.[62] Unfortunately, women are continuing to smoke at significant rates and COPD, which has long been considered a disease of the male smoker, has seen a dramatic rise in the number of women diagnosed each year.[55,66]

The role that sex hormones play with respect to aging and lung function has not been clearly identified. It is has been postulated that pregnancy may have an affect on the variation in aging and lung function that is seen among men and women. Asthma is one pulmonary condition that has been studied with respect to pregnancy.[67] It is well established that asthma control varies for different patients during pregnancy: Approximately one-third of asthmatic women have worse symptoms during pregnancy, one-third have improved symptoms and one-third experience no change.[68] The physiologic mechanisms behind this are unclear. Later in life, women may experience worse asthma severity and worsened asthma quality of life, however, this has not been shown to be associated with menopause and is more likely due to other age-associated comorbidities or age-dependent conditions.[69] More research is needed to clarify the role that sex hormones and pregnancy play in aging. However data are indicating that estrogen may influence the expression of key genes encoding proteins involved in the aging processes such as telomerase TERT. It has been suggested that women might also metabolize reactive oxygen species better because of estrogen,[16] and its antioxidant properties.[25] In that regard, estrogen could have a protective role in the aging process for women.

7. Age-Related Pulmonary Diseases

With the growth of the elderly population, patients affected with pulmonary diseases are increasing. It is unclear how much aging of the respiratory system increases susceptibility of the elderly to the age-related diseases such as cancer, COPD, IPF and respiratory infections. There is little doubt that reduced antioxidant capacity, deteriorating lung mechanics, changes in the composition (cellular and proteins) of lung tissue and declined immunity, all play a role in elevated susceptibility, but how these contributing factors are affected by the ethnicity/race and gender of the patients is still unclear and needs further investigation.

Lung cancer is the leading cause of cancer-related death in both men and women in the US.[70] The incidence of lung cancer in men has declined over the past several years, however, lung cancer in women has continued to rise and kills more women each year than breast, uterine and ovarian cancer combined.[71] Aside from the increased susceptibility to the effects of smoking, a hormonal risk for lung cancer has also been postulated to explain the fact that women who are diagnosed with lung cancer have fewer pack-year smoking histories, present at an earlier age than men and are three times more likely to have lung cancer not associated with smoking.[72,73] Lung cancer also has a relationship with advancing age. Using the large SEER database (http://seer.cancer.gov/statfacts/html/lungb.html), the majority of new cases of lung cancer are diagnosed in persons over the age of 65 years with a median age at diagnosis of 70 years. When examined in terms of gender, more cases occurred in males than females, 72.2 per 100,000 persons versus 51.1 per 100,000 persons, respectively. However, female non-smokers are at increased risk for adenocarcinoma.[74] The percent of lung and bronchus cancer death is highest among people aged 65–84 years, with a median age at death of 72 years. The number of deaths is higher in males compared to females. Patients aged 65 years and older account for 80% of lung cancer deaths and 20% of lung cancer deaths are in patients aged 80 years and older.[75] As discussed earlier, ethnic and racial disparities also exist for both the incidence and death rates associated with lung cancer. Incidence rates per 100,000 persons are 93 in black men, 72.4 in white men, 49.4 in Asian men and 40.4 in Hispanic men and the numbers in women are 51.2, 53.8, 28.1 and 26.1, respectively. For mortality rates, the numbers per 100,000 persons are 78.5 in black men, 63.2 in white men, 35.5 in Asian men and 31.3 in Hispanic men and in women the numbers are 37.2, 40.4, 18.4 and 14.1, respectively (SEERS).

COPD is the third leading cause of death in the US.[55,76] At least 10% of persons aged 65 years and older in the US are diagnosed with COPD, but this may be underestimated due to underutilization of pulmonary function testing.[55] The incidence rates increase with age through 75–79 years of age, with greater incidences in men than women.[77] However due to the increased number of women smoking as well as differences in susceptibility to smoke, the number of elderly women affected with COPD is on the rise. This susceptibility could be dependent on hormonal mechanisms. Indeed it has been shown that female sex hormones influence airway function even during childhood. Tobacco smoke or environmental air pollution exposure can induce a larger reduction in lung function in girls compared to boys.[78]

There does appear to be a race/ethnic difference with respect to COPD. In fact, despite significantly less exposure to tobacco smoke, Mexican Americans with COPD have a similar degree of obstruction compared to European Americans with COPD (15.7 versus. 32.4 pack-years, respectively). More Mexican Americans with COPD report being never-smokers compared to European Americans with COPD. Mexican Americans were also found to have worse functional status and perceived health than European Americans.[79]

IPF is a progressive fibrotic lung disease of unknown etiology that primarily affects older individuals. The prevalence and incidence of IPF increases with advancing age, particularly after the 6th decade.[80] The average survival is 20–30% at 5 years after diagnosis. Older age at presentation is associated with shorter survival time.[81] Co-morbidities also affect the outcomes in older patients with IPF. Pulmonary fibrosis is much more common among men than women, with male: female incidences ranging from 1.4:1 to 2.1:1 and usually occurs between the ages of 50 and 70 years.[82, 83] However, in animal models, fibrosis and mortality seem to be exacerbated by estrogen [84] and *in vitro,* estrogens are known to enhance the release of profibrotic factors in lung fibroblasts.[84] We also know that estrogens promote the expression of TERT and therefore may help with the maintenance of telomere length (see section above). This could be a protective factor and explain the lower rate of disease in women, as mutations and defects in the telomerase complex activity have been heavily correlated with the development and progression of IPF.[85] Very few studies have shown differences in the impact of IPF based on ethnicity/race.[60]

8. Asthma

Aging is an important risk factor for asthma. There is a bimodal distribution with increased diagnosis in patients aged 50–65 years.[86,87] Asthma in the elderly is often underdiagnosed and undertreated. The estimated prevalence of asthma in the elderly is between 4–8%,[81] however, older asthmatic patients die from their asthma more often than younger asthmatic patients and account for up to 50% of deaths due to asthma[55,88]. Comorbidities also contribute to this increase in mortality.[81] Two phenotypes have been described among elderly patients with asthma. Patients with chronic asthma may have more severe airflow limitation and less reversibility than those with late-onset asthma.[89] Pathophysiologic differences may also contribute to the differences between young asthmatics and elderly asthmatics.[89] In a large study conducted in West Texas on 3,021 Hispanic and non-Hispanic Caucasian subjects 65 years and older, the overall prevalence of current asthma and probable asthma were 6.3% and 9.0% respectively. In this study, women had 1.64 times greater odds of current asthma as compared to men. Smoking was also a significant risk factor for asthma with the odds of current asthma 1.78 times greater among past smokers as compared to nonsmokers.[90] The role of menopause in asthma has also been evaluated. However, in a study using propensity score matching and multivariate adjusting, menopause was neither associated with a greater incidence of asthma nor a worse quality of life when compared to non-menopaused women.[69]

9. Conclusions

The respiratory system represents a key interface between the human body and its external environment by responding to challenges such as toxins and infectious agents. As people age, this system experiences a decline in function that is partly explained by differing exposures, genetic factors and male or female sex. It is important to remember that the lungs are not aging in isolation. The stress of aging on the heart and on the kidneys, for example, are most likely influencing the aging of the lungs. To illustrate this concept, abnormal spirometry has been measured in older patients affected with heart failure.[91]

Understanding aging lungs is still under investigation and further research is needed to more clearly elucidate how gender and ethnicity/race contribute to the disparities associated with aging and the development and progression of age-related pulmonary diseases.

References

1. Krumpe PE, Knudson RJ, Parsons G *et al.* (1985) The aging respiratory system. *Clin Geriatr Med* **1**: 143–175.
2. Janssens JP, Pache JC, Nicod LP. (1999) Physiological changes in respiratory function associated with ageing. *Euro Respir J* **13**: 197–205.
3. Ware JH, Dockery DW, Louis TA *et al.* (1990) Longitudinal and cross-sectional estimates of pulmonary function decline in never-smoking adults. *Am J Epidemiol* **132**: 685–700.
4. Brandstetter RD, Kazemi H. (1983) Aging and the respiratory system. *Med Clin North Am* **67**: 419–431.

5. Crapo JD. (1993) The aging lung. In: D Mahler (ed.), pp.1–21. Marcel Dekker, New York.
6. Wilkie SS, Guenette JA, Dominelli PB *et al.* (2012) Effects of an aging pulmonary system on expiratory flow limitation and dyspnoea during exercise in healthy women. *Euro J Appl Physiol* **112**: 2195–2204.
7. Sharma G, Goodwin J. (2006) Effect of aging on respiratory system physiology and immunology. *Clin Interv Aging* **1**: 253–260.
8. Edge JR, Millard FJ, Reid L *et al.* (1964) The radiographic appearances of the chest in persons of advanced age.*Br J Radiol* **37**: 769–774.
9. Gunby MC, Morley JE. (1994) Epidemiology of bone loss with aging. *Clin Geriatr Medicine* **10**: 557–574.
10. McClaran SR, Babcock MA, Pegelow DF *et al.* (1995) Longitudinal effects of aging on lung function at rest and exercise in healthy active fit elderly adults. *J Appl Physiol* **78**: 1957–1968.
11. Haas SA, Krueger PM, Rohlfsen L. (2012) Race/ethnic and nativity disparities in later life physical performance: The role of health and socioeconomic status over the life course. *J Gerontol B, Psychol Sci Soc Sci* **67**: 238–248.
12. Vaz Fragoso CA, McAvay G, Gill TM *et al.*(2014) Ethnic differences in respiratory impairment. *Thorax* **69**: 55–62.
13. Gardner M, Bann D, Wiley L *et al.* (2014) Gender and telomere length: Systematic review and meta-analysis. *Exp Gerontol* **51**: 15–27.
14. Okuda K, Bardeguez A, Gardner JP *et al.* (2002) Telomere length in the newborn. *Pediatr Res* **52**: 377–381.
15. Aubert G, Baerlocher GM, Vulto I *et al.* (2012) Collapse of telomere homeostasis in hematopoietic cells caused by heterozygous mutations in telomerase genes. *PLoS genetics* **8**: e1002696.
16. Nawrot TS, Staessen JA, Gardner JP *et al.* (2004) Telomere length and possible link to X chromosome. *Lancet* **363**: 507–510.
17. Bekaert S, De Meyer T, Rietzschel ER *et al.* (2007) Telomere length and cardiovascular risk factors in a middle-aged population free of overt cardiovascular disease. *Aging cell* **6**: 639–647.
18. Fitzpatrick AL, Kronmal RA, Gardner JP *et al.* (2007) Leukocyte telomere length and cardiovascular disease in the cardiovascular health study. *Am J Epidemiol* **165**: 14–21.
19. Shiels PG, McGlynn LM, MacIntyre A *et al.* (2011) Accelerated telomere attrition is associated with relative household income, diet and inflammation in the pSoBid cohort. *PloS one* **6**: e22521.

20. Adams J, Martin-Ruiz C, Pearce MS *et al.* (2007) No association between socio-economic status and white blood cell telomere length. *Aging cell* **6**: 125–128.
21. Hunt SC, Chen W, Gardner JP *et al.* (2008) Leukocyte telomeres are longer in African Americans than in whites: The National Heart, Lung, and Blood Institute Family Heart Study and the Bogalusa Heart Study. *Aging cell* **7**: 451–458.
22. Mayer S, Bruderlein S, Perner S *et al.* (2006) Sex-specific telomere length profiles and age-dependent erosion dynamics of individual chromosome arms in humans. *Cytogenet Genome Res* **112**: 194–201.
23. Barrett EL, Richardson DS. (2011) Sex differences in telomeres and lifespan. *Aging cell* **10**: 913–921.
24. von Zglinicki T. (2002) Oxidative stress shortens telomeres. *Trends Biochem Sci* **27**: 339–344.
25. Carrero JJ, Stenvinkel P, Fellstrom B *et al.* (2008) Telomere attrition is associated with inflammation, low fetuin-A levels and high mortality in prevalent haemodialysis patients. *J Intern Med* **263**: 302–312.
26. Gomez CR, Boehmer ED, Kovacs EJ. (2005) The aging innate immune system. *Curr Opin Immunol* **17**: 457–462.
27. Weng NP. (2006) Aging of the immune system: How much can the adaptive immune system adapt? *Immun* **24**: 495–499.
28. High K. (2014) Immune Senescence:In M Rojas, S Meiners, C Jourdan Le Saux (eds) *Molecular Aspects of Aging*. Wiley Blackwell, New York.
29. Lloberas J, Celada A. (2002) Effect of aging on macrophage function. *Exp Gerontol* **37**: 1325–1331.
30. Dunston CR, Griffiths HR. (2010) The effect of ageing on macrophage Toll-like receptor-mediated responses in the fight against pathogens. *Clin Exp Immunol* **161**: 407–416.
31. Boehmer ED, Goral J, Faunce DE *et al.* (2004) Age-dependent decrease in Toll-like receptor 4-mediated proinflammatory cytokine production and mitogen-activated protein kinase expression. *J Leukoc Biol* **75**: 342–349.
32. Koike E, Kobayashi T, Mochitate K *et al.* (1999) Effect of aging on nitric oxide production by rat alveolar macrophages. *Exp Gerontol* **34**: 889–894.
33. Corsini E, Battaini F, Lucchi L *et al.* (1999) A defective protein kinase C anchoring system underlying age-associated impairment in TNF-alpha production in rat macrophages. *J Immunol* **163**: 3468–3473.

34. Zissel G, Schlaak M, Muller-Quernheim J. (1999) Age-related decrease in accessory cell function of human alveolar macrophages. *J Invest Medicine* **47**: 51–56.
35. Kovaiou RD, Herndler-Brandstetter D, Grubeck-Loebenstein B. (2007) Age-related changes in immunity: Implications for vaccination in the elderly. *Exp Rev Mol Med* **9**: 1–17.
36. Goetzl EJ, Huang MC, Kon J *et al.* (2010) Gender specificity of altered human immune cytokine profiles in aging. *FASEB J* **24**: 3580–3589.
37. Gameiro C, Romao F. (2010) Changes in the immune system during menopause and aging. *Front Biosci* **2**: 1299–1303.
38. Zeleznik J. (2003) Normative aging of the respiratory system. *Clin Geriatr Med* **19**: 1–18.
39. Fletcher C, PEto R, Tinker C. (1976) *The natural history of chronic bronchitis: An eight year followup of working men in London.* Oxford University Press.
40. Pokorski M, Marczak M. (2003) Ventilatory response to hypoxia in elderly women. *Ann Human Biol* **30**: 53–64.
41. Kelly FJ, Dunster C, Mudway I. (2003) Air pollution and the elderly: oxidant/antioxidant issues worth consideration. *Euro Respir J* **40**: 70s–75s.
42. Wang L, Green FH, Smiley-Jewell SM *et al.* (2010) Susceptibility of the aging lung to environmental injury. *Sem Respir Critic Care Med* **31**: 539–553.
43. Samet JM, Zeger SL, Dominici F *et al.* (2000) The national mMorbidity, mortality, and air pollution study. Part II: Morbidity and mortality from air pollution in the United States. *Res Report* **94**: 5–70.
44. Luber G, McGeehin M. (2008) Climate change and extreme heat events. *Am J Prev Med* **35**: 429–435.
45. Chen Y, Horne SL, Dosman JA. (1991) Increased susceptibility to lung dysfunction in female smokers. *Am Rev Respir Dis* **143**: 1224–1230.
46. Ito K, Barnes PJ. (2009) COPD as a disease of accelerated lung aging. *Chest* **135**: 173–180.
47. Moriyama C, Betsuyaku T, Ito Y *et al.* (2010) Aging enhances susceptibility to cigarette smoke-induced inflammation through bronchiolar chemokines. *Am J Respir Cell Mol Biol* **42**: 304–311.
48. Ezzati M, Kammen DM. (2001) Quantifying the effects of exposure to indoor air pollution from biomass combustion on acute respiratory infections in developing countries. *Environ Health Persp* **109**: 481–488.

49. Smith KR, Mehta S. (2003) The burden of disease from indoor air pollution in developing countries: Comparison of estimates. *Int J Hyg Environ Health* **206**: 279–289.
50. Chen BH, Hong CJ, Pandey MR *et al.* (1990) Indoor air pollution in developing countries. *World Health Stat Q* **43**: 127–138.
51. Sumer H, Turaclar UT, Onarlioglu T *et al.* (2004) The association of biomass fuel combustion on pulmonary function tests in the adult population of Mid-Anatolia. *Soz Praventivmed* **49**: 247–253.
52. Pandey MR. (1984) Domestic smoke pollution and chronic bronchitis in a rural community of the Hill Region of Nepal. *Thorax* **39**: 337–339.
53. Braun L, Wolfgang M, Dickersin K. (2013) Defining race/ethnicity and explaining difference in research studies on lung function. *Euro Respir J* **41**: 1362–1370.
54. Regan EA, Hokanson JE, Murphy JR *et al.* (2010) Genetic epidemiology of COPD (COPDGene) study design. *Copd* **7**: 32–43.
55. Mannino D, Homa D, Akinbami L *et al.* (2002) Chronic Obstructive Pulmonary Disease Surveillance — United States, 1971–2000. *Surveill Summ MMWR* **51**: 1–16.
56. Akinbami L. (2011). Chronic Obstructive Pulmonary Disease among Adults aged 18 and over in the United States, 1998–2009. In: *National Center for Health Statistics,* Brief ND, (ed.). MD, Hyattsville.
57. Powell R, Davidson D, Divers J *et al.* (2013) Genetic ancestry and the relationship of cigarette smoking to lung function and per cent emphysema in four race/ethnic groups: A cross-sectional study. *Thorax* **68**: 634–642.
58. Menck HR, Henderson BE. (1982) Cancer incidence patterns in the Pacific Basin. *Natl Cancer I Monogr* **62**: 101–109.
59. Haiman CA, Stram DO, Wilkens LR *et al.* (2006) Ethnic and racial differences in the smoking-related risk of lung cancer. *New Engl J Med* **354**: 333–342.
60. Swigris JJ, Olson AL, Huie TJ *et al.* (2012) Ethnic and racial differences in the presence of idiopathic pulmonary fibrosis at death. *Respir Med* **106**: 588–593.
61. Rumpel JA, Ahmedani BK, Peterson EL *et al.* (2012) Genetic ancestry and its association with asthma exacerbations among African American subjects with asthma. *J Allergy Clin Immunol* **130**: 1302–1306.
62. Townsend EA, Miller VM, Prakash YS. (2012) Sex differences and sex steroids in lung health and disease. *Endocr Revs* **33**: 1–47.

63. Harms CA. (2006) Does gender affect pulmonary function and exercise capacity? *Respir Physiol Neurobiol* **151**: 124–131.
64. Pelzer AM, Thomson ML. (1966) Effect of age, sex, stature, and smoking habits on human airway conductance. *J Appl Physiol* **21**: 469–476.
65. Prescott E, Osler M, Andersen PK *et al.* (1998) Mortality in women and men in relation to smoking. *Int J Epidemiol* **27**: 27–32.
66. Chapman KR. (2004) Chronic obstructive pulmonary disease: are women more susceptible than men? *Clin Chest Med* **25**: 331–341.
67. Maselli DJ, Adams SG, Peters JI *et al.* (2013) Management of asthma during pregnancy. *Ther Adv Respir Dis* **7**: 87–100.
68. Tamasi L, Horvath I, Bohacs A *et al.* (2011) Asthma in pregnancy-immunological changes and clinical management. *Respir Med* **105**: 159–164.
69. Zein J, Comhair S, Bleecker E *et al.* (2014) The Effect of Aging and Menopause on Asthma Severity in Women. *Chest* **145**: meeting abstract.
70. Shafer D, Albain K. (2009) Lung cancer outcomes in women. *Sem Oncol* **36**: 532–541.
71. Rivera MP, Stover DE. (2004) Gender and lung cancer. *Clin Chest Medicine* **25**: 391–400.
72. Harichand-Herdt S, Ramalingam SS. (2009) Gender-associated differences in lung cancer: Clinical characteristics and treatment outcomes in women. *Sem Oncol* **36**: 572–580.
73. Kabat GC. (1996) Aspects of the epidemiology of lung cancer in smokers and nonsmokers in the United States. *Lung cancer* **15**: 1–20.
74. Wakelee HA, Chang ET, Gomez SL *et al.* (2007) Lung cancer incidence in never smokers. *J Clin Oncol* **25**: 472–478.
75. Jemal A, Siegel R, Xu J *et al.* (2010) Cancer statistics. *Cancer J Clin* **60**: 277–300.
76. 2012. Chronic Obstructive Pulmonary Disease Among Adults — United States, CDS.gov.
77. van Durme YM, Verhamme KM, Stijnen T *et al.* (2009) Prevalence, incidence, and lifetime risk for the development of COPD in the elderly: The Rotterdam study. *Chest* **135**: 368–377.
78. Aryal S, Diaz-Guzman E, Mannino DM. (2013) COPD and gender differences: An update. *Transl Res : Journal Lab Clin Med* **162**: 208–218.
79. Adams SG, Anzueto A, Pugh JA *et al.* (2006) Mexican American elders have similar severities of COPD despite less tobacco exposure than European American elders. *Respir Med* **100**: 1966–1972.

80. Kim DS, Collard HR, King TE. (2006) Classification and natural history of the idiopathic interstitial pneumonias. *Proc Am Thorac Soc* **3**: 285–292.
81. Akgun KM, Crothers K, Pisani M. (2012) Epidemiology and management of common pulmonary diseases in older persons. *J Gerontol A Biol Sci Med Sci* **67**: 276–291.
82. Meltzer EB, Noble PW. (2008) Idiopathic pulmonary fibrosis. *Orphanet J Rare Dis* **3**: 8.
83. Gribbin J, Hubbard RB, Le Jeune I *et al.* (2006) Incidence and mortality of idiopathic pulmonary fibrosis and sarcoidosis in the UK. *Thorax* **61**: 980–985.
84. Gharaee-Kermani M, Hatano K, Nozaki Y *et al.* (2005) Gender-based differences in bleomycin-induced pulmonary fibrosis. *Am J Pathol* **166**: 1593–1606.
85. Diaz de Leon A, Cronkhite JT, Katzenstein AL *et al.* (2010) Telomere lengths, pulmonary fibrosis and telomerase (TERT) mutations. *PloS one* **5**: e10680.
86. Bauer BA, Reed CE, Yunginger JW *et al.* (1997) Incidence and outcomes of asthma in the elderly. A population-based study in Rochester, Minnesota. *Chest* **111**: 303–310.
87. Akinbami LJ, Moorman JE, Liu X. (2011) Asthma prevalence, health care use, and mortality: United States, 2005–2009. *Natl Health Stat Report*: 1–14.
88. Slavin RG, National Institue of H. (2004) The elderly asthmatic patient. *Allergy and Asthma Proc* **25**: 371–373.
89. Hanania NA, King MJ, Braman SS *et al.* (2011) Asthma in the elderly: Current understanding and future research needs — a report of a National Institute on Aging (NIA) workshop. *J Allergy Clin Immunol* **128**: S4–S24.
90. Arif AA, Rohrer JE, Delclos GL. (2005) A population-based study of asthma, quality of life, and occupation among elderly Hispanic and non-Hispanic whites: A cross-sectional investigation. *BMC public health* **5**: 97.
91. Georgiopoulou VV, Kalogeropoulos AP, Psaty BM *et al.* (2011) Lung function and risk for heart failure among older adults: The Health ABC Study. *Am J Med* **124**: 334–341.

Chapter 4
Frailty in Pulmonary and Critical Care Medicine

Cristine E. Berry[*,†] and Enid R. Neptune[‡]

1. Introduction to Frailty

Frailty is a syndrome of decreased physiologic reserve and increased vulnerability to stressors. It is the opposite of vitality or fitness. Decline in physiologic function with aging and consequent effects on homeostasis may increase the risk of frailty, but frailty itself is distinct from chronologic aging. Hence, older adults are more likely to be frail, but not all elders are frail and not all frail are very old.

The concept of frailty is well recognized by clinicians, but objective definitions of frailty have only been developed in recent years. This has supported investigation into the mechanistic underpinnings of frailty and increased knowledge regarding how frailty relates to adverse outcomes. To date, our understanding of its pathophysiology remains very limited. Progress in this field has been challenged by lack of consensus among experts regarding the

*Arizona Respiratory Center, University of Arizona College of Medicine; Tucson, Arizona.
†Section of Pulmonary, Allergy, Critical Care, and Sleep Medicine; Department of Medicine; University of Arizona College of Medicine; Tucson, Arizona.
‡Division of Pulmonary and Critical Care Medicine; Johns Hopkins University School of Medicine; Baltimore, MD.

optimal definition of frailty and appropriate frailty biomarkers.[1] However, there appears to be substantial agreement regarding the basic conceptual framework for the syndrome of frailty, including its multi-dimensional nature and fundamental characteristics of diminished reserve and increase vulnerability to stressors.

Sarcopenia is generally considered to be an essential feature of the frailty syndrome.[2–4] Sarcopenia has been defined by consensus as (1) low muscle mass and (2) low muscle strength and/or physical performance.[5] Tools used in research and clinical practice to diagnose sarcopenia include magnetic resonance imaging (MRI), computed tomography (CT), dual energy X-ray absorptiometry (DXA), bioimpedance analysis (BIA), handgrip strength, knee flexion/extension strength, peak expiratory flow, gait speed, timed get-up-and-go test, and the short physical performance battery (SPPB).[5] It is important to note that while sarcopenia is a key characteristic of frailty, not all individuals with sarcopenia are necessarily frail.

Frailty is thought of as a dynamic continuum, but in general, transitions in frailty status tend toward worsening frailty rather than improvement.[3,6] This may lead to a downward spiral of generalized physiologic decline, ultimately resulting in death. The number of physiologic systems affected, rather than the severity of decline in any one system, appears to be very important in determining frailty risk; however, the observed relationship between the number of abnormal systems and frailty is nonlinear.[7] This suggests the loss of homeostasis and lack of adaptive response to stress that are characteristic of frailty may be due to compromised integration of physiologic systems.

The syndrome of frailty has been recognized as a distinct entity that is independent of both disability and multimorbidity or comorbidity.[8] The landmark study conducted by Fried and colleagues using the Cardiovascular Health Study (CHS) cohort provided strong evidence that frailty is associated with increased risk of disability and is also more common among individuals with multiple comorbid diseases.[9,10] However, they also discovered 26.6% of frail individuals did not have a concomitant significant comorbid condition or activity of

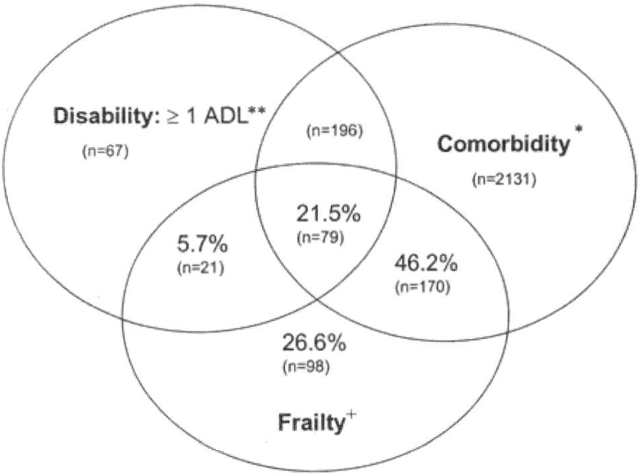

Fig 1. Overlap of Frailty, Disability and Comorbidity among Older Adults in the Cardiovascular Health Study.

This figure is taken from the original publication by Fried and colleagues where the Fried frailty phenotype was first described in Cardiovascular Health Study participants in 2001.[9]

daily living (ADL) disability (Fig 1). There appears to be significant variability in disability status even among individuals where frailty results in death. In a prospective cohort study where frailty was the most common condition leading to death, the trajectories of disability in the year prior to death were very heterogeneous.[11] Therefore, while there may be substantial overlap across frailty, disability and comorbidity in populations, frailty occurs in the absence of comorbidity and disability in some individuals.[9,12] As frailty severity increases, the overlap is likely to be greater.[12] These findings suggest that the factors involved in the development of frailty may be distinct from those involved in its progression.

Frailty appears to be relatively common. Using cross-sectional data from several community-based cohorts, Collard and colleagues found the prevalence of frailty was 10.7% among adults who were age 65 years or older.[13] Frailty prevalence is estimated to be much higher among older adults who are not living independently. Across multiple studies, frailty has been found to be more common in women and as one might expect, its prevalence also increases with age.[9,14] Limited data suggests that frailty may be more common in African Americans and Asians compared with Caucasians and Hispanics.[9,15] Of note, frailty prevalence varies remarkably depending on the operational definition that is used, so differences in frailty prevalence across studies should be examined with this in mind.[16]

Frailty has been associated with a multitude of adverse outcomes across multiple prospective cohort studies (Table 1). Individuals with frailty have demonstrated increased risk of falls, incident disability and hospitalization.[9,14,17–19] There is also a significant relationship between frailty and risk of admission to a long-term care facility.[14,17,18,20,21] Moreover, individuals characterized as intermediate with respect to frailty status demonstrate intermediate levels of risk for these adverse outcomes. Notably, frailty is a strong independent predictor of mortality.[9,14,17–19,21] Frailty as the primary cause of death may be particularly common among the very old.[22]

The biological mechanisms underlying the development and progression of frailty remain poorly understood. Mohler and colleagues recently reviewed the current state of knowledge regarding frailty mechanisms and directions for future research with respect to the development of animal models.[23] In general, there appears to be a strong association between inflammatory comorbid conditions and frailty[24,25] and growing evidence suggests that frailty is related to cytokine dysregulation, manifest in a chronic pro-inflammatory state.[26–31] In particular, elevated serum interleukin-6 levels have been associated with frailty risk and abnormality in frailty-related measurements Figure 2.[27,28,30,31]

Frailty is a multi-dimensional syndrome encompassing physiologic decline in multiple organ systems. This chapter will focus on the impact of frailty syndrome on pulmonary and critical care medicine, but for readers interested in the relationships between frailty and other physiologic systems, please see the recent review by Clegg and colleagues.[3]

Table 1 Adverse outcomes associated with frailty. Frailty has been associated with adverse outcomes across multiple studies. This table describes the landmark studies that examined frailty in community-based cohorts and comes from a recent review of frailty by Clegg and colleagues.[3]

	Year	Country	Participants (n)	Length of follow-up (years)	Falls (HR*/OR† [95% CI])		Worsening disability (HR*/OR† [95% CI])		Hospitalisation (HR*/OR† [95% CI])		Care home admission (HR*/OR† [95% CI])		Mortality (HR*/OR† [95% CI])	
					Intermediate frailty	Severe frailty	Intermediate frailty	Severe frailty	Intermediate frailty	Severe frailty	Intermediate frailty	Severe frailty	Intermediate frailty	Severe frailty
Cardiovascular Health Study (CHS)[3]	2001	USA	5317	7	1.12* (100–1.26)	1.23* (0.99–1.54)	1.55* (1.38–1.75)	1.79* (1.47–2.17)	1.11* (1.03–1.19)	1.27* (1.11–1.46)	NA	NA	1.32* (1.13–1.55)	1.63* (1.27–2.08)
Canadian Study of Health and Aging (C5HA)[92]	2004	Canada	9008	5	NA	NA	NA	NA	NA	NA	2.54† (1-67–3.86)	2.60† (1.36–4.96)	2.54† (1.92–3.37	3.69† (2.26–6.02)
Women's Health and Aging Study (WHAS)[93]	2006	USA	1438	3	0.92* (0-63–1.64)	1.18* (0.63–2.19)	NA	NA	0.99* (0.67–1.47)	0.67* (0.33–1.35)	5.16* (0.81–32.79)	23.98* (4.45–129.2)	3.50* (191–6.39)	6.03* (3.00–12.08)
Study of Osteoporotic Fractures (SOF)[94]	2008	USA	6701	4.5	1.23† (102–1.48)	2.44† (1.95–3.04)	1.89†, (1.66–2.14)	2.79† (2.31–3.37)	NA	NA	NA	NA	1.54† (140–1.69)	2.75* (246–3.07)

HR = hazard ratio. NA = not available. OR = odds ratio. *Hazard ratio. †Odds ratio. The comparator for hazard ratios and odds ratios is people who are not frail.
Table: Covariate-adjusted associations between frailty and adverse outcomes (falls, disability, hospitalisation, care home admission, and mortality) from four large prospective cohort studies

2. Frailty Measurement

Clinicians have long recognized the concept of frailty — *"you know it when you see it"* — but only recently were measurement tools developed and validated that have allowed for the objective assessment of frailty status. In 1999, Rockwood and colleagues described a "fitness to frailty" rules-based scale that predicted institutionalization and mortality among community-dwelling older adults in Canada.[32] Several operational definitions of frailty have emerged since that time[33] and the Fried frailty phenotype and the Rockwood Frailty Index (FI) are among the most highly recognized and validated.

The Fried frailty phenotype was developed from CHS data and was based on five criteria: (1) unintentional weight loss in the prior year (≥10 pounds by self-report or ≥5% measured body weight), (2) physical exhaustion (self-reported 3–4 days per week or most of the time based on US Center for Epidemiological Studies depression scale), (3) low physical activity (lowest quintile of energy expenditure in kcal/week stratified by gender), (4) slow gait speed (lowest quintile of walking time per 15 feet, stratified by gender and height) and (5) low grip strength (lowest quintile stratified by gender and body mass index) (Table 2).[9] The presence of three or more criteria was considered positive for the syndrome of frailty and the presence of 1 or 2 criteria was considered to be an indicator of pre-frailty or intermediate frailty status. This frailty phenotype was a strong predictor of incident disability, falls, fracture, hospitalization and death and it has been validated in other populations.[9,17,19,34–36]

Table 2. Fried frailty phenotype operational definition. The Fried frailty criteria and definition of frailty status come from the original publication by Fried and colleagues examining the Cardiovascular Health Study participants in 2001.[9]

Fried Frailty Criteria	Frailty Status Definition
• Unintentional weight loss	• Frail: ≥3 criteria
• Weak grip strength	• Intermediate/Pre-frail: 1–2 criteria
• Physical exhaustion	• Non-frail: 0 criteria
• Slow gait speed	
• Low physical activity	

In the Study of Osteoporotic Fractures (SOF), Ensrud and colleagues examined a frailty definition that was similar to the Fried phenotype but could be more readily applied in a clinical setting. For the SOF index, frailty is defined by the presence of at least two of the following criteria: (1) unintentional weight loss of 5% or more the past year, (2) inability to rise from a chair five times without using arms and/or (3) a negative response to the question "do you feel full of energy?" The SOF index performs similarly to the Fried phenotype in predicting adverse outcomes.[19,34,36]

The FI was developed by Rockwood and colleagues using data from the Canadian Study of Health and Aging (CSHA). It is based on a cumulative deficit model that incorporates assessment of cognition and psychosocial factors in addition to physical frailty indicators.[21] Each deficit is recorded as present (1) or absent (0) and then the FI is calculated as the proportion of deficits that are present in any given individual. FI varies from study to study with respect to the content and number of deficits involved. Variables included in the FI must be (1) biologically sensible and (2) accumulate with age but (3) not saturate too early.[37] Some studies have derived the FI from a comprehensive geriatric assessment (CGA).[38,39] However, CGA requires significant time and expertise and therefore is not easily transferrable to a research setting. The FI has been shown to predict adverse outcomes in both community-dwelling older adults and hospitalized patients.[18,22,37,38]

In contrast to the Fried phenotype and the Rockwood FI, the Clinical Frailty Scale (CFS) is based on clinical judgment (Tables 3).[40] It has been used predominantly in settings where frailty measurement using the Fried phenotype or FI is impractical, such as clinical encounters where a practitioner's time to assess patients is limited. CFS scores correlate highly with FI and demonstrate similar predictive validity for adverse outcomes.[40]

There has been considerable debate about the optimal instrument for frailty assessment. Some of this debate relates to whether an operational frailty definition should focus on the physical domain alone, which is the basis of the Fried phenotype, or also encompass factors related to cognitive and psychosocial domains.[3,41]

Table 3 The Canadian study of health and aging clinical frailty scale (CFS). CFS was originally described by Rockwood and colleagues in a Canadian community-based cohort of older adults.[40]

CFS score	Description
1	**Very fit** — robust, active, energetic, well motivated and fit; these people commonly exercise regularly and are in the most fit group for their age.
2	**Well** — without active disease, but less fit than people in category 1.
3	**Well, with treated comorbid disease** — disease symptoms are well controlled compared with those in category 4.
4	**Apparently vulnerable** — although not frankly dependent, these people commonly complain of being "slowed up" or have disease symptoms.
5	**Mildly frail** — with limited dependence on others for instrumental activities of daily living.
6	**Moderately frail** — help is needed with both instrumental and non-instrumental activities of daily living.
7	**Severely frail** — completely dependent on others for the activities of daily living, or terminally ill.

Several studies have compared various definitions of frailty in different populations and overall, different frailty indices are highly correlated.[16,18,42–45] However, it has been demonstrated that a cumulative deficit approach such as the FI may have greater ability to discriminate mortality risk compared with the Fried phenotype, which may exhibit a ceiling effect in some populations.[42,44,45] The Fried phenotype has recently been reconstructed from a 5-point scale to a 10-point scale to provide broader distribution and minimize the ceiling effect, but this requires further validation.[10] Because the FI uses historical data rather than physical measurements, it may be more suitable for research involving electronic medical records but less appropriate for intervention studies or research examining biological mechanisms. To date, nearly all of the biological studies in frailty have employed the Fried phenotype.

There is also some limitation to applying the performance-based measures of the Fried phenotype in clinical populations where mobility may be limited, a relevant consideration in persons with chronic respiratory disability.[43] The Survey of Health, Ageing and

Retirement in Europe (SHARE) frailty instrument was developed from the five criteria of the Fried phenotype but is easier to measure in practice because self-reported slowness replaces objective measurement of gait speed. Therefore, it may prove to be a valuable tool for frailty screening in a clinical setting.[46] Frailty defined by the SHARE instrument predicts incident disability and mortality,[47,48] with similar performance to the Fried phenotype in predicting risk of death.[49]

The debate about how to define frailty is likely to be ongoing, as is the case with many other syndromes based on clinical diagnosis. Frailty instruments may differ with respect to content validity, practicability, clinimetric properties and risk prediction[33,42] and these tools may also be based on different conceptual models of frailty and therefore capture distinct groups of older adults.[50] Hence, different frailty instruments may be designated to serve different purposes. Rather than considering the Fried frailty phenotype or the Rockwood FI as alternatives, they are best viewed as complementary.[20]

The field of frailty measurement is continuing to evolve. Increasing availability of sensor-based technologies to assess gait, balance and physical activity may transform assessment of frailty,[23,51] particularly with respect to sensitivity and reliability in the identification of frailty and meaningful changes in frailty status. There are also ongoing efforts towards developing frailty assessment tools that can be administered by telephone or proxy that are valid, reliable and sensitive to change.[52]

3. Frailty and Respiratory Function

Physiologic function of the respiratory system may play an integral role in the syndrome of frailty. Lung function is thought to be so significant to frailty that it was recently suggested that pulmonary function testing could serve as a single objective measure in the assessment of frailty status.[3]

In community-dwelling older adults, lung function impairment and frailty have been associated both cross-sectionally and longitudinally.[53] The CHS enrolled elders (age ≥65 years) in 1989 and followed them for over 10 years with serial assessments that included spirometry. At baseline, CHS participants with frailty demonstrated greater lung function impairment compared to their non-frail counterparts. Among frail participants, risks of airflow limitation (adjusted odds ratio 1.88, 95% CI 1.15–3.09) and restrictive pattern (adjusted OR 3.05; 95% CI 1.19–4.88) on spirometry were significantly higher. For pre-frail CHS participants, there was an intermediate increase in the risk of lung function impairment relative to those who were non-frail, including both airflow limitation (adjusted OR 1.62; 95% CI 1.29–2.04) and restrictive pattern (adjusted OR 1.80; 95% CI 1.37–2.36) (53).

In longitudinal analysis of CHS data, abnormal lung function at baseline predicted incident frailty and the presence of frailty features at baseline predicted the development of lung function impairment.[53] Among CHS participants who had lung function within normal range at baseline, those characterized as frail or pre-frail demonstrated increased risk of developing impairment in lung function during follow-up compared to those who were non-frail (adjusted OR 1.42; 95% CI 1.11–1.82). Likewise, among participants who were non-frail at baseline, those with airflow limitation or restrictive pattern on spirometry demonstrated increased risk of developing frailty features during follow-up (adjusted OR 1.58, 95% CI 1.17–2.13).[53]

It should be noted that these analyses were restricted to white participants who had at least two acceptable spirometry maneuvers according to American Thoracic Society (ATS) standards. This approach is likely to have excluded some participants with frailty or frailty features at baseline or follow-up, as non-acceptable spirometry has been associated with frailty status. In the population-based Rotterdam Study of 2730 participants at least 55 years old, frail subjects were more likely to generate spirometric maneuvers that were not interpretable, independent of age and sex (adjusted OR 1.69; 95% CI 1.08–2.64).[54]

Other studies have also identified a relationship between impaired pulmonary function and features of frailty. For example, in the Lifestyle Interventions and Independence for Elders Study of community-based older adults, low ventilatory capacity was associated with slow gait speed and respiratory muscle weakness was associated with moderate to severe mobility impairment.[55] In the Women's Health and Aging Study II, there was a significant association between baseline FEV_1 and usual gait speed, which was independent of age and other potential confounders.[56]

The reasons for this association between frailty and pulmonary function impairment are likely complex, but shared risk factors and common mechanisms may play a role, including aging and chronic inflammation. Some evidence also suggests that frailty may modify the response to established risk factors that impact lung function and its decline. For example, Eckel and colleagues examined the relationship between ambient air pollution and pulmonary function and they found that CHS participants who were frail or pre-frail had significantly greater decline in forced vital capacity (FVC) for similar air pollution exposure compared to non-frail participants.[57]

Respiratory muscle strength may also influence the relationship between frailty and lung function impairment, given frailty is characterized by sarcopenia. Buchman and colleagues examined the relationships between extremity muscle strength, respiratory muscle strength and lung function in older adults who participated in the Rush Memory and Aging Project. Respiratory muscle strength was assessed by measuring maximal inspiratory pressure (MIP) and maximal expiratory pressure (MEP). They found that extremity muscle strength correlated with both respiratory muscle strength ($r = 0.49$, $p < 0.001$) and lung function ($r = 0.46$, $p < 0.001$). Moreover, respiratory muscle strength was also associated with lung function ($r = 0.50$, $p < 0.001$) and explained 25% of its variability.[58] In this same cohort, it was also demonstrated that both low pulmonary function and reduced respiratory muscle strength at baseline independently predicted incident mobility disability, whether defined by slow gait speed or loss of ability to ambulate.[59] Other studies have also suggested that differences in respiratory muscle strength exist across frailty groups. In a Yale cohort study of 754 community-dwelling older adults, peak expiratory flow rate, a marker of expiratory muscle strength, was inversely associated with frailty. However, this analysis did not account for potential confounding by chronic lung disease or smoking status.[60] In a Brazilian study of 51 community-dwelling older adults, there were no significant differences in FEV_1 or FVC among those characterized as frail, pre-frail, or non-frail. However, compared to non-frail participants, individuals with frailty had significantly lower MIP and MEP, and those characterized as pre-frail demonstrated intermediate reductions in MIP and MEP.[61]

Measurements of physiological function at rest may not be sufficient to adequately demonstrate the impact of frailty on response to stress. Exercise represents a stressor, but there has been limited study of older adults with frailty performing objective exercise testing. A subset of participants in the Women's Health and Aging Study I (WHAS I) performed the seated step test, which is a low-level incremental exercise test with four 3-minute stages that determines exercise capacity by cumulative exercise time ($N = 131$).[62] Cardiac chronotropic index (metabolic reserve/heart rate reserve), FVC and quadriceps strength were also measured. Overall, lower exercise capacity was associated with higher chronotropic index, lower FVC and lower quadriceps strength and frail women had lower exercise capacity compared to non-frail women. When these physiological measurements were incorporated in a linear regression model predicting exercise capacity, only FVC, quadriceps strength and frailty were significantly associated with the outcome. Interestingly, the positive impact of FVC on exercise capacity was only significant in the non-frail participants. This suggests that frailty may affect the coupling of physiologic systems important for exercise, which may also be applicable to the impact of frailty on physiologic response to other stressors.[63]

Frailty and low lung function are both independent predictors of mortality. However, frailty may also modify the relationship between lung function and risk of death. In the CHS, there was a significant interaction between frailty and impairment in pulmonary function (airflow limitation or restrictive pattern) with respect to the outcome of mortality ($p = 0.037$, Fig 3).[53] This effect was independent of age, health status and smoking. However, it may be that

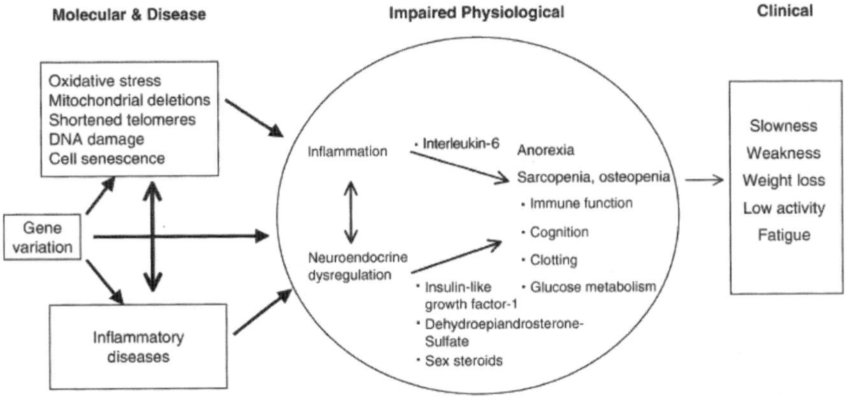

Fig 2. Proposed Frailty Mechanisms and Pathways.

This figure is taken from a publication describing the 2004 proceedings of the American Geriatrics Society/National Institute on Aging Research Conference on Frailty in Older Adults.[2]

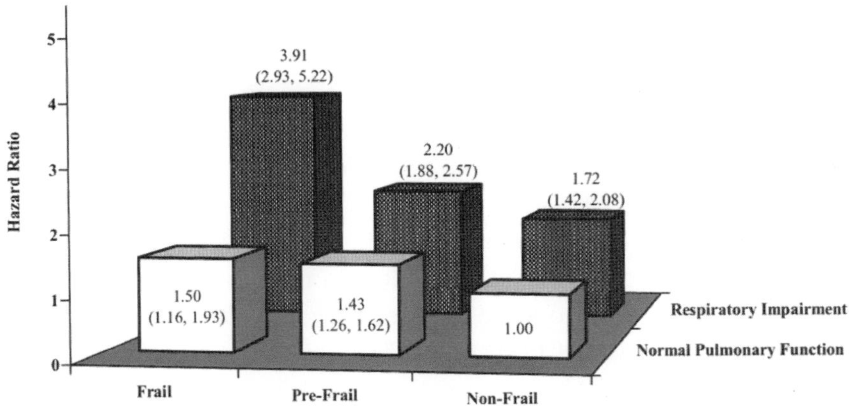

Fig 3. Interaction Between Frailty Status and Respiratory Impairment in Determining Mortality Risk in the Cardiovascular Health Study.

This figure is taken from the publication by Vaz Fragoso and colleagues that first examined the relationship between respiratory impairment and frailty in a community-based cohort.[53] Adjusted HRs and 95% confidence intervals are for all-cause mortality by baseline frailty status and respiratory function. Results were adjusted for age, height, gender, smoking history, body mass index, health status and chronic conditions. The interaction between frailty and respiratory impairment was significant ($p = 0.037$).

this is related to the severity of lung function deficit, assuming there may be a graded effect whereby participants with frailty may have the most severe reduction in FEV_1 compared to the pre-frail and non-frail who may have more mild respiratory impairment. Therefore, further investigation is necessary to better understand the impact of frailty on the relationship between lung function and risk of death.

4. Frailty in Chronic Lung Disease

The vast majority of our knowledge about frailty comes from the study of general populations rather than disease-specific populations, so there is limited evidence regarding the impact of frailty on outcomes in patients with chronic lung diseases. However, it is now clear that chronic medical conditions increase the risk of frailty and chronic lung disease appears to be common in patients with frailty. In CHS participants from whom the Fried frailty phenotype was first described, there was a higher prevalence of chronic lung disease among frail participants compared to pre-frail and non-frail participants. A physician diagnosis of chronic bronchitis, emphysema, or asthma was reported by 14.1% of frail participants and 8.8% of pre-frail participants, compared to 5.8% of their non-frail counterparts ($p < 0.001$).[9]

Park and colleagues examined a highly selected subset of participants from the Third National Health and Nutrition Evaluation Survey (NHANES) who were at least 55 years old and reported a physician diagnosis of COPD and a history of smoking ($n = 211$).[63] They developed FI based on the multi-dimensional Gobbens approach to frailty which they derived from objective physical activity monitoring and from responses to the NHANES questionnaire.[41] The prevalence of frailty based on their definition was 57.8% among the selected participants with COPD. Individuals with respiratory symptoms, especially dyspnea and comorbid diseases, particularly diabetes, were more likely to be frail. Notably, frail participants reported greater healthcare utilization than their non-frail counterparts.

In a study of 1288 older adults in Italy, frailty was measured using the frailty staging system, which combined seven core domains of functioning.[64] Investigators found that the risk of mortality was greater among participants with COPD who also had frailty compared to those participants with COPD who were not frail. Increasing frailty score was an independent predictor of death in the multivariate Cox regression analysis, (adjusted hazard ratio (HR) 1.69 for each unit increase in frailty score, 95% CI 1.42–2.00). When stratified by the presence or absence of COPD, the risk of death increased 36% (adjusted HR 1.36, 95%CI 1.09–1.91) for every unit increase in frailty score among those individuals without COPD, whereas among those with COPD, the risk of death increased 80% for every unit increase in frailty score (adjusted HR 1.80; 95%CI 1.28–2.53). This interaction was not significant after adjusting for multiple potential confounders, including dyspnea, comorbidity and medications.[64]

Although there has been limited investigation of frailty itself in COPD patients, research focusing on distinct frailty features such as sarcopenia and functional limitation has been quite substantial. Muscle dysfunction is common among COPD patients, but the relationships between COPD outcomes and muscle mass, strength and performance measures are variable.[65] In the Health, Aging, and Body Composition (ABC) prospective cohort study, participants with COPD and smokers without COPD demonstrated lower weight, lower fat mass and lower lean mass compared to never-smokers at study enrollment. However, during follow-up, the subsequent trajectories in lean mass loss with aging were similar across all participants, regardless of COPD or smoking status. This suggests the differences in lean mass at baseline must have been due to an earlier life insult, likely from smoking. Interestingly, men with COPD demonstrated a more rapid decline in SPPB scores compared to those without COPD, suggesting that accelerated functional decline over time may occur in COPD in the absence of accelerated decline in lean mass.[66]

Cesari and colleagues examined the relationships between body composition, spirometric lung function and functional capacity in a small clinical cohort of older adults with COPD (n = 71).[67] They found that both lean mass and FEV_1 were positively associated with six minute walk distance, but only FEV_1 remained a significant predictor after adjusting for multiple potential confounders. Similarly, there was no independent relationship between fat-free mass index and six minute walk distance in participants from the Evaluation of COPD Longitudinally to Identify Predictive Surrogate Endpoints (ECLIPSE) study. In spite of the lack of correlation between muscle mass and six minute walk performance, limb muscle strength has a direct relationship with six minute walk distance that is independent of FEV_1 in patients with COPD.[68] Better performance on the SPPB test also predicts greater six minute walk distance in COPD, independent of lung function.[69] In another study of COPD patients, gait speed was a stronger predictor of six minute walk distance than FEV_1.[70] Taken together, such data underscore the challenges of using FEV_1 alone as a marker of COPD severity when considering functional performance.

Limb muscle dysfunction is thought to be important to patient-centered COPD outcomes as it is associated with decreased exercise tolerance, poor quality of life and increased risk of death.[65] Related frailty features including slow gait speed and low physical activity have also been associated with poor outcomes. For example, slow gait speed has been associated with ADL disability in COPD patients.[71] With respect to activity level, a large multicenter study of medical records data demonstrated that self-reported low physical activity at baseline is associated with increased risk of 30-day all-cause rehospitalization in COPD patients.[72] Likewise, a recent single-center study that objectively measured physical activity using actigraphy in a small group of patients after COPD hospitalization showed that low physical activity after discharge is a powerful predictor of 30-day readmission.[73] It may be that low physical activity is a measure of disease severity, but in this study, other typical disease severity parameters like FEV_1 and six minute walk distance were not associated with rehospitalization. Further investigation in a larger number of patients across multiple centers is needed to determine if this phenomenon may be related to frailty.

It remains unclear if the sarcopenia that occurs in some COPD patients is similar to that which occurs in frailty with respect to underlying mechanisms and/or clinical consequences. Given shared mechanisms of chronic inflammation and oxidative stress, it may be that the underlying pathways leading to sarcopenia in frailty and COPD are similar or even interlaced, but further investigation is needed.

Beyond COPD, evidence related the impact of frailty in other chronic lung diseases is limited. A study conducted at Columbia University examined the effects of frailty on six minute walk distance in 95 consecutive patients with end stage lung disease referred for transplant evaluation.[74] Patients included in this analysis had a mean age of 55 years and had a variety of pulmonary diagnoses including interstitial lung disease (49%), COPD (22%), cystic fibrosis (15%) and pulmonary hypertension (9%). Frailty was present in 27% of patients and it was associated with a mean decrease in six minute walk distance of 99 m. This finding was independent of potential confounders including age, gender, height, diagnosis and lung allocation score.

There has been growing interest in the effect of frailty on lung transplant outcomes, as there is evidence that sarcopenia is associated with higher risk of post-transplant mortality in other solid organ transplantation.[75] Hook and colleagues at Columbia University are conducting a prospective single-center cohort study to examine the effect of pre-transplant frailty on post-transplant outcomes.[76] Early findings suggest that the Fried frailty phenotype is common among lung transplant candidates, affecting 29% in their cohort. Among the limited number patients who had undergone lung transplantation at the time the data was reported ($n = 16$), there were only two in-hospital deaths after surgery and both of the participants who died were frail. This is in line with other data indicating preoperative frailty is associated with higher risk of postoperative complications.[77]

Frailty also appears to be related to sleep disturbances and sleep-related breathing disorders. In a large ancillary study associated with the Osteoporotic Fractures in Men cohort, sleep surveys and in-home sleep studies were performed and frailty status was assessed in a similar manner to the Fried phenotype.[78] Investigators found that frailty was associated with poor sleep quality, prolonged sleep latency and reduced sleep efficiency. Moreover, sleep-disordered breathing, defined by a respiratory disturbance index ≥15, was independently associated with frailty status. Interestingly, this finding was confirmed in a different study examining the relationship between sleep-disordered breathing and frailty characteristics in a subset of CHS participants who also participated in the Sleep Heart Health Study, but only among women.[79] Further study of the relationship between sleep-disordered breathing and frailty is warranted, particularly with respect to therapeutic implications and long-term outcomes.

While frailty may be prevalent among older patients with many different diseases, there is evidence to support that frailty may be especially relevant to pulmonary disease. In a cohort of Japanese elders, it was observed that ADL dependency increased the risk of both all-cause and respiratory mortality but not other disease-specific mortality including cancer and cardiovascular.[80] Frailty was not directly assessed in this study, but given strong links between frailty and ADL dependency, this suggests that frailty may confer increased risk of death due to respiratory disease but not necessarily death due to other common causes including cancer and cardiovascular disease. Further investigation of the impact of frailty on respiratory mortality and other important outcomes is necessary to determine the role of frailty in the evaluation and management of respiratory diseases. In particular, greater understanding is needed regarding whether interventions intended to reduce the risk of respiratory morbidity and mortality may be influenced by frailty status in patients with chronic lung disease.

5. Frailty in Critical Illness

Frailty is characterized by decreased physiologic reserve and adaptability and ensuing vulnerability to stressors. This means that frailty may be more readily identifiable in a stressed state such as critical illness. Frailty status may be revealed for the first time in the intensive care unit (ICU), particularly among elderly individuals who lack significant comorbidity.

Frailty appears to be quite common among elders admitted to the ICU. Bagshaw and colleagues conducted a Canadian multicenter study of 421 older adults with critical illness.[81] Frailty was defined by a CFS score >4 immediately before hospital admission and was determined through medical record review and interviews with participants or surrogates. They identified 32.8% of older adults admitted to the ICU as frail. Similarly, Le Maguet *et al* examined frailty in 196 patients from four university-affiliated ICUs in France.[82] They defined frailty using CFS score >4 based on information about patient status one month prior to admission obtained from the participant, surrogates and/or medical record and they also assessed frailty using a derivation of the Fried frailty phenotype adapted for the ICU. Frailty prevalence was 23% using a CFS score >4 and 41% using the adapted Fried phenotype.

Among the ICU patients included in both of these studies, frailty was associated with important short- and long-term outcomes.[81,82] In the Canadian study, frailty status was associated with longer length of stay and higher risk of in-hospital mortality.[81] Frailty was also associated with lower likelihood of being discharged to independent living at home and higher risk of hospital readmission. Over the follow-up period of one year after enrollment, frailty was independently associated with an increased risk of death (adjusted HR 1.81, 95% CI 1.09–3.01).[81] It is worth noting that ICU treatment intensity was not significantly different for participants across frailty categories in this study, even though those with frailty were more likely to have some documentation in the medical record of medical therapy limitation such as a do-not-resuscitate order.

In contrast to the Canadian study, the French study did not find differences in length of stay by frailty status, but this may be related to significant differences in reason for ICU admission between the two studies. In the French study, frailty by adapted Fried criteria predicted ICU mortality, whereas frailty defined by CFS score was associated with an increased risk of mortality at six months.[82] There may have been some effect of end-of-life decision making on the relationship between frailty and mortality in the French study, as the proportion of participants who had care withheld or withdrawn was much higher among those with frailty compared to the non-frail.[82]

The French study investigators acknowledged there was some difficulty in adapting the Fried criteria to the ICU setting, particularly those criteria related to performance and therefore this may have affected their findings.[82] In a small pilot study ($n = 22$), Baldwin and colleagues at Columbia University explored measuring Fried frailty criteria including performance assessment among elderly ICU survivors prior to hospital discharge.[83] There was a very high prevalence of frailty (82%), with the remaining participants meeting pre-frail criteria (18%). Fried frailty score predicted increased risk of ADL disability at one month and mortality at six months in this small study. There was also a trend towards a higher risk of incident disability at one month by frailty score, but it was not statistically significant.[83]

Frailty has also been associated with poor health-related quality of life (HRQL) among elderly ICU survivors. In the same Canadian cohort study, Bagshaw *et al* assessed health status using Short Form-12 (SF-12) and HRQL using EuroQOL at six and twelve months after discharge.[84] Frailty was independently associated with lower HRQL at both time points and lower health status after one year.

Frailty may be an important predictor of outcomes among ICU survivors who require prolonged ventilatory support. In a small single center study of patients transferred from an ICU to a university-based long term care facility for ventilator weaning ($n = 30$), Fried frailty criteria including acute weight loss, handgrip strength and gait speed were assessed.[85] Frailty was defined by having all three criteria and was identified in 57% of participants ($n = 17$). Among frail participants, the majority (76%, $n = 13$) had an unfavorable outcome at 60 days, defined by transfer to a skilled nursing facility, readmission to the ICU, continued stay in the long term care facility, or death.

In conclusion, frailty has been associated with increased risk of adverse outcomes among older adults with critical illness, but the evidence remains limited and is not clearly generalizable to all ICU settings. With increasing recognition that sarcopenia is common among older adults presenting with critical illness and that skeletal muscle wasting is a complication of critical illness,[86,87] further investigation is necessary to understand differences that may exist between prevalent frailty and incident frailty in ICU patients and potential impact on short- and long-term ICU outcomes. Moreover, additional research is needed to guide how frailty assessment may be integrated into prognostic models related to post-ICU disability and mortality.[88] As the evidence grows and our population continues to age, frailty assessment may become a valuable tool incorporated into clinical decision-making strategies for older adults with critical illness.

6. Summary

Frailty is a syndrome of diminished physiologic reserve that is more common among older adults and individuals with comorbid disease. Several studies have demonstrated that frailty is associated with adverse outcomes among community-dwelling older adults, including disability and death. Substantial data suggests there is a relationship between frailty and respiratory function impairment and growing evidence indicates that frailty is an important predictor of adverse outcomes in critical illness. Whether frailty status can inform more rigorous prognostic instruments for lung disease phenotyping is unknown and should be explored. Further research is necessary to establish the mechanism by which frailty contributes to the development and progression of chronic lung disorders and how lung disease predisposes to the onset of frailty.

References

1. Rodriguez-Manas L *et al.* (2013) Searching for an operational definition of frailty: A Delphi method based consensus statement: The frailty operative definition-consensus conference project. *J Gerontol A Biol Sci Med Sci* **68**(1): 62–67.
2. Walston J *et al.* (2006) Research agenda for frailty in older adults: Toward a better understanding of physiology and etiology: Summary

from the American Geriatrics Society/National Institute on Aging Research Conference on Frailty in Older Adults. *J Am Geriatr Soc* **54**(6): 991–1001.

3. Clegg A, Young J, Iliffe S *et al.* (2013) Frailty in elderly people. *Lancet* **381**(9868): 752–762.
4. Cesari M, Landi F, Vellas B *et al.* (2014) Sarcopenia and physical frailty: Two sides of the same coin. *Front Aging Neurosci* **6**: 192.
5. Cruz-Jentoft AJ *et al.* (2010) Sarcopenia: European consensus on definition and diagnosis: Report of the European working group on sarcopenia in older people. *Age Ageing* **39**(4): 412–423.
6. Gill TM, Gahbauer EA, Allore HG *et al.* (2006) Transitions between frailty states among community-living older persons. *Arch Intern Med* **166**(4): 418–423.
7. Fried LP *et al.* (2009) Nonlinear multisystem physiological dysregulation associated with frailty in older women: Implications for etiology and treatment. *J Gerontol A Biol Sci Med Sci* **64**(10): 1049–1057.
8. Fried LP, Ferrucci L, Darer J *et al.* (2004) Untangling the concepts of disability, frailty, and comorbidity: Implications for improved targeting and care. *J Gerontol A Biol Sci Med Sci* **59**(3): 255–263.
9. Fried LP *et al.* (2001) Frailty in older adults: Evidence for a phenotype. *J Gerontol A Biol Sci Med Sci* **56**(3):M146–M156.
10. Sanders JL *et al.* (2011) Measurement of organ structure and function enhances understanding of the physiological basis of frailty: The cardiovascular health study. *J Am Geriatr Soc* **59**(9): 1581–1588.
11. Gill TM, Gahbauer EA, Han L *et al.* (2010) Trajectories of disability in the last year of life. *New Engl J Med* **362**(13): 1173–1180.
12. Theou O, Rockwood MR, Mitnitski A *et al.* (2012) Disability and co-morbidity in relation to frailty: How much do they overlap? *Arch Gerontol Geriatr* **55**(2):e1–e8.
13. Collard RM, Boter H, Schoevers RA *et al.* (2012) Prevalence of frailty in community-dwelling older persons: A systematic review. *J Am Geriatr Soc* **60**(8): 1487–1492.
14. Rockwood K *et al.* (2004) Prevalence, attributes, and outcomes of fitness and frailty in community-dwelling older adults: Report from the Canadian study of health and aging. *J Gerontol A Biol Sci Med Sci* **59**(12): 1310–1317.
15. Cawthon PM *et al.* (2007) Frailty in older men: Prevalence, progression, and relationship with mortality. *J Am Geriatr Soc* **55**(8): 1216–1223.

16. Theou O, Brothers TD, Mitnitski A *et al.* (2013) Operationalization of frailty using eight commonly used scales and comparison of their ability to predict all-cause mortality. *J Am Geriatr Soc* **61**(9):1537–1551.
17. Bandeen-Roche K *et al.* (2006) Phenotype of frailty: Characterization in the women's health and aging studies. *J Gerontol A Biol Sci Med Sci* **61**(3): 262–266.
18. Rockwood K, Andrew M, Mitnitski A. (2007) A comparison of two approaches to measuring frailty in elderly people. *J Gerontol A Biol Sci Med Sci* **62**(7): 738–743.
19. Ensrud KE *et al.* (2008) Comparison of 2 frailty indexes for prediction of falls, disability, fractures, and death in older women. *Arch Intern Med* **168**(4): 382–389.
20. Cesari M, Gambassi G, van Kan GA *et al.* (2014) The frailty phenotype and the frailty index: Different instruments for different purposes. *Age Ageing* **43**(1): 10–12.
21. Rockwood K, Mitnitski A, Song X *et al.* (2006) Long-term risks of death and institutionalization of elderly people in relation to deficit accumulation at age 70. *J Am Geriatr Soc* **54**(6): 975–979.
22. Evans CJ *et al.* (2014) Place and cause of death in centenarians: A population-based observational study in England, 2001 to 2010. *PLoS medicine* **11**(6):e1001653.
23. Mohler MJ, Fain MJ, Wertheimer AM *et al.* (2014) The Frailty syndrome: Clinical measurements and basic underpinnings in humans and animals. *Exp Gerontol* **54**: 6–13.
24. Chang SS, Weiss CO, Xue QL *et al.* (2010) Patterns of comorbid inflammatory diseases in frail older women: The Women's health and aging studies I and II. *J Gerontol A Biol Sci Med Sci* **65**(4): 407–413.
25. Chang SS, Weiss CO, Xue QL *et al.* (2012) Association between inflammatory-related disease burden and frailty: Results from the women's health and aging studies (WHAS) I and II. *Arch Gerontol Geriatr* **54**(1): 9–15.
26. Walston J *et al.* (2002) Frailty and activation of the inflammation and coagulation systems with and without clinical comorbidities: Results from the Cardiovascular Health Study. *Arch Intern Med* **162**(20): 2333–2341.
27. Cohen HJ, Harris T, Pieper CF. (2003) Coagulation and activation of inflammatory pathways in the development of functional decline and mortality in the elderly. *Am J Med* **114**(3): 180–187.

28. Leng SX, Xue QL, Tian J *et al.* (2007) Inflammation and frailty in older women. *J Am Geriatr Soc* **55**(6): 864–871.
29. Bandeen-Roche K, Walston JD, Huang Y *et al.* (2009) Measuring systemic inflammatory regulation in older adults: Evidence and utility. *Rejuv Res* **12**(6): 403–410.
30. Ferrucci L *et al.* (2002) Change in muscle strength explains accelerated decline of physical function in older women with high interleukin-6 serum levels. *J Am Geriatr Soc* **50**(12): 1947–1954.
31. Visser M *et al.* (2002) Relationship of interleukin-6 and tumor necrosis factor-alpha with muscle mass and muscle strength in elderly men and women: The Health ABC Study. *J Gerontol A Biol Sci Med Sci* **57**(5): M326–332.
32. Rockwood K, *et al.* (1999) A brief clinical instrument to classify frailty in elderly people. *Lancet* **353**(9148): 205–206.
33. de Vries NM *et al.* (2011) Outcome instruments to measure frailty: A systematic review. *Ageing Res Rev* **10**(1): 104–114.
34. Ensrud KE *et al.* (2007) Frailty and risk of falls, fracture, and mortality in older women: The study of osteoporotic fractures. J *Gerontol A Biol Sci Med Sci* **62**(7): 744–751.
35. Kiely DK, Cupples LA, Lipsitz LA. (2009) Validation and comparison of two frailty indexes: The MOBILIZE Boston Study. *J Am Geriatr Soc* **57**(9): 1532–1539.
36. Ensrud KE *et al.* (2009) A comparison of frailty indexes for the prediction of falls, disability, fractures, and mortality in older men. *J Am Geriatr Soc* **57**(3): 492–498.
37. Song X, Mitnitski A, Rockwood K. (2010) Prevalence and 10-year outcomes of frailty in older adults in relation to deficit accumulation. *J Am Geriatr Soc* **58**(4): 681–687.
38. Jones DM, Song X, Rockwood K. (2004) Operationalizing a frailty index from a standardized comprehensive geriatric assessment. *J Am Geriatr Soc* **52**(11): 1929–1933.
39. Evans SJ, Sayers M, Mitnitski A *et al.* (2014) The risk of adverse outcomes in hospitalized older patients in relation to a frailty index based on a comprehensive geriatric assessment. *Age Ageing* **43**(1): 127–132.
40. Rockwood K *et al.* (2005) A global clinical measure of fitness and frailty in elderly people. *CMAJ* **173**(5): 489–495.
41. Gobbens RJ, Luijkx KG, Wijnen-Sponselee MT *et al.* (2010) Toward a conceptual definition of frail community dwelling older people. *Nurs Outlook* **58**(2): 76–86.

42. Theou O, Brothers TD, Pena FG *et al.*(2014) Identifying common characteristics of frailty across seven scales. *J Am Geriatr Soc* **62**(5): 901–906.
43. Hubbard RE, O'Mahony MS, Woodhouse KW. (2009) Characterising frailty in the clinical setting. A comparison of different approaches. *Age Ageing* **38**(1): 115–119.
44. Malmstrom TK, Miller DK, Morley JE. (2014) A comparison of four frailty models. *J Am Geriatr Soc* **62**(4): 721–726.
45. Kulminski AM *et al.* (2008) Cumulative deficits better characterize susceptibility to death in elderly people than phenotypic frailty: Lessons from the Cardiovascular Health Study. *J Am Geriatr Soc* **56**(5): 898–903.
46. Romero-Ortuno R, Walsh CD, Lawlor BA *et al.* (2010) A frailty instrument for primary care: Findings from the survey of health, ageing and retirement in Europe (SHARE). *BMC Geriatr* **10**: 57.
47. Romero-Ortuno R. (2011) The Frailty Instrument of the Survey of Health, Ageing and Retirement in Europe (SHARE-FI) predicts mortality beyond age, comorbidities, disability, self-rated health, education and depression. *Euro Geriatr Med* **2**(6): 323–326.
48. Romero-Ortuno R, O'Shea D , Kenny RA. (2011) The SHARE frailty instrument for primary care predicts incident disability in a European population-based sample. *Qual Prim Care* **19**(5): 301–309.
49. Romero-Ortuno R. (2013) The SHARE operationalized frailty phenotype: A comparison of two approaches. *Euro Geriatr Med* 4(4).
50. Cigolle CT, Ofstedal MB, Tian Z *et al.* (2009) Comparing models of frailty: The health and retirement study. *J Am Geriatr Soc* **57**(5): 830–839.
51. Schwenk M, *et al.* (2014) Frailty and technology: A systematic review of gait analysis in those with frailty. *Gerontol* **60**(1): 79–89.
52. Cesari M *et al.* (2014) A self-reported screening tool for detecting community-dwelling older persons with frailty syndrome in the absence of mobility disability: The FiND questionnaire. *PloS one* **9**(7):e101745.
53. Vaz Fragoso CA, Enright PL, McAvay G *et al.* (2012) Frailty and respiratory impairment in older persons. *Am J Med* **125**(1): 79–86.
54. Lahousse L LD, Verlinden VJA, Ziere G *et al.* (2013) Frailty affects quality of spirometry: The Rotterdam study. *Am J Respir Crit Care Med* **187**: A2835.
55. Vaz Fragoso CA *et al.* (2014) Respiratory impairment and dyspnea and their associations with physical inactivity and mobility in sedentary community-dwelling older persons. *J Am Geriatr Soc* **62**(4): 622–628.

56. Berry CE WR, Bandeen-Roche K, Chaves PH *et al.* (2012) Predictors of baseline lung function and lung function decline differ in the Women's Health and Aging Study (WHAS) II. *Am J Respir Crit Care Med* **185**: A6025.
57. Eckel SP, Louis TA, Chaves PH *et al.*(2012) Modification of the association between ambient air pollution and lung function by frailty status among older adults in the Cardiovascular Health Study. *Am J Epidemiol* **176**(3): 214–223.
58. Buchman AS, *et al.* (2008) Respiratory muscle strength predicts decline in mobility in older persons. *Neuroepidemiol* **31**(3): 174–180.
59. Buchman AS, Boyle PA, Leurgans SE *et al.* (2009) Pulmonary function, muscle strength, and incident mobility disability in elders. *Proc Am Thorac Soc* **6**(7): 581 –587.
60. Vaz Fragoso CA, Gahbauer EA, Van Ness PH *et al.* (2007) Reporting peak expiratory flow in older persons. *J Gerontol A Biol Sci Med Sci* **62**(10): 1147–1151.
61. Pegorari MS, Ruas G, Patrizzi LJ. (2013) Relationship between frailty and respiratory function in the community-dwelling elderly. *Braz J Phys Ther* **17**(1): 9–16.
62. Weiss CO, Hoenig HH, Varadhan R *et al.* (2010) Relationships of cardiac, pulmonary, and muscle reserves and frailty to exercise capacity in older women. *J Gerontol A Biol Sci Med Sci* **65**(3): 287–294.
63. Park SK, Richardson CR, Holleman RG *et al.*(2013) Frailty in people with COPD, using the National Health and Nutrition Evaluation Survey dataset (2003–2006). *Heart & lung : J Critic Care* **42**(3): 163–170.
64. Galizia G *et al.* (2011) Role of clinical frailty on long-term mortality of elderly subjects with and without chronic obstructive pulmonary disease. *Aging Clin Exp Res* **23**(2): 118–125.
65. Maltais F *et al.* (2014) An official American Thoracic Society/European Respiratory Society statement: update on limb muscle dysfunction in chronic obstructive pulmonary disease. *Am J Respir Crit Care Med* **189**(9): e15–e62.
66. van den Borst B *et al.* (2011) Is age-related decline in lean mass and physical function accelerated by obstructive lung disease or smoking? *Thorax* **66**(11): 961–969.
67. Cesari M *et al.* (2012) Physical performance, sarcopenia and respiratory function in older patients with chronic obstructive pulmonary disease. *Age Ageing* **41**(2): 237–241.

68. Eisner MD *et al.* (2008) Pulmonary function and the risk of functional limitation in chronic obstructive pulmonary disease. *Am J Epidemiol* **167**(9): 1090–1101.
69. Spruit MA *et al.* (2010) Determinants of poor 6-min walking distance in patients with COPD: The ECLIPSE cohort. *Respir Med* **104**(6): 849–857.
70. Karpman C, DePew ZS, LeBrasseur NK *et al.* (2014) Determinants of gait speed in COPD. *Chest* **146**(1): 104–110.
71. Kluka EM BR, Karpman C. (2014) Gait speed and activities of daily living disability in individuals with COPD. *Am J Respir Crit Care Med* **189**: A5854.
72. Nguyen HQ *et al.* (2014) Associations between physical activity and 30-day readmission risk in chronic obstructive pulmonary disease. *Ann Am Thorac Soc* **11**(5): 695–705.
73. Chawla H, Bulathsinghala C, Tejada JP *et al.* (2014) Physical activity as a predictor of thirty-day hospital re-admission after a discharge for a clinical exacerbation of COPD. *Ann Am Thorac Soc* 11(8):1203–1209.
74. Restivo M PE, Shah L, Robbins H *et al.* (2013) Frailty is independently associated with reduced six-minute walk distance in lung transplant candidates. *Am J Respir Crit Care Med* **187**: A2198.
75. Hook JL, Lederer DJ. (2012) Selecting lung transplant candidates: Where do current guidelines fall short? *Expert Rev Respir Med* **6**(1):51–61.
76. Hook J SJ, Wilt J, Shah L *et al.* (2012) The frailty phenotype in lung transplantation: Preliminary results. *Am J Respir Crit Care Med* **185**: A5328.
77. Makary MA *et al.* (2010) Frailty as a predictor of surgical outcomes in older patients. *JACS* **210**(6): 901–908.
78. Ensrud KE *et al.* (2009) Sleep disturbances and frailty status in older community-dwelling men. *J Am Geriatr Soc* **57**(11): 2085–2093.
79. Endeshaw YW, Unruh ML, Kutner M *et al.* (2009) Sleep-disordered breathing and frailty in the Cardiovascular Health Study Cohort. *Am J Epidemiol* **170**(2): 193–202.
80. Takata Y *et al.* (2013) Activities of daily living dependency and disease-specific mortality during 12-year follow-up in an 80-year-old population. *Aging Clin Exp Res* **25**(2): 193–201.
81. Bagshaw SM *et al.* (2014) Association between frailty and short- and long-term outcomes among critically ill patients: A multicentre prospective cohort study. *CMAJ* **186**(2):E95–E102.

82. Le Maguet P *et al.* (2014) Prevalence and impact of frailty on mortality in elderly ICU patients: A prospective, multicenter, observational study. *Intens Care Med* **40**(5):674–682.
83. Baldwin MR *et al.* (2014) The feasibility of measuring frailty to predict disability and mortality in older medical intensive care unit survivors. *J Crit Care* **29**(3): 401–408.
84. Bagshaw SM SH, McDermid RC, Rolfson D *et al.* (2014) Long-term association between frailty and health-related quality of life among survivors of critical illness: A multi-centre prospective cohort study. *Am J Respir Crit Care Med* **189**: A2182.
85. Bassman GA WC, Beans J, Jenkins T *et al.* (2014) Frailty in intensive care unit survivors receiving prolonged mechanical ventilation at long term care facilities is associated wtih poor outcomes. *Am J Respir Crit Care Med* **189**: A1921.
86. Puthucheary ZA *et al.* (2013) Acute skeletal muscle wasting in critical illness. *JAMA* **310**(15): 1591–1600.
87. Moisey LL *et al.* (2013) Skeletal muscle predicts ventilator-free days, ICU-free days, and mortality in elderly ICU patients. *Crit Care* **17**(5):R206.
88. Baldwin MR *et al.* (2013) A prognostic model for 6-month mortality in elderly survivors of critical illness. *Chest* **143**(4): 910–919.

Chapter 5

Intensive Care Unit Outcomes in Older Adults

Margaret A. Pisani*,†,‡ and Lauren Ferrante*,†

1. Introduction

The global population is expected to increase 38% by the year 2050.[1] This constitutes a change from 6.9 billion persons in 2010 to 9.6 billion in 2050. Projections suggest that worldwide there will be 1.5 billion people aged 65 and older by 2050. Older persons are the fastest growing segment of the United States population. These changes are complex and likely related to both shifts in birth rates and decreases in death rates. According to census data the number of persons aged 60 years and older increased 24.6% from 2000 to 2010.[2] The largest proportion of this increase (29.6%) was in persons aged 85 years and older. Projections from the Department of Health and Human Services Administration on Aging suggest that by 2050 people age 60 and older will constitute 25.5% of the United States population.[2] Along with increases in age, estimates suggest increases in older persons living with disabilities and limitations in

*Department of Internal Medicine, Pulmonary & Critical Care Section, Yale University School of Medicine, 300, Cedar street, New Haven, CT 06510, USA.
†Program on Aging, Yale University School of Medicine, 300 Cedar Street, New Haven, CT 06510, USA.
‡Corresponding author.

activities of daily living (ADL). The current projection is that 21.4% of people age 65 and older will have impairment in ADL.

As the population ages, in turn, the number of older patients being cared for in intensive care units (ICUs) has increased. A study examining the worldwide burden of critical illness found that the mean age of patients admitted to ICUs across 84 countries was 60 years.[3] Patients aged 65 and older make up greater than 45% of the ICU population.[4] Sepsis continues to be a major reason for ICU admission and occurs more frequently in older persons.[3]

While the majority of ICU studies use mortality as their primary outcome, more recently focus has shifted to include functional, cognitive and quality of life outcomes post-discharge. Older patients and their families express willingness to undergo the burden of intensive care if it will prolong life, but are often focused on maintaining function, especially cognitive function.[5,6] With increasing numbers of older persons receiving ICU care; it is important for us to have an understanding of patient-centered outcomes after an episode of critical illness.

This review will discuss (1) risk factors for adverse outcomes after ICU admission, (2) outcomes specifically after sepsis and acute respiratory distress syndrome(ARDS), (3) cognitive outcomes post-ICU, (4) functional outcomes post-ICU and, (5) quality of life outcomes post-ICU.

2. Risk Factors for Adverse ICU Outcomes

There are many potential risk factors that predispose older patients who are admitted to the ICU to poor outcomes including multiple medical comorbidities and frailty.[7] There are also precipitating risk factors including the etiology and severity of their acute illness and aspects of ICU care that put older patients at risk for adverse outcomes after ICU admission.

Many studies have examined survival after ICU admission in older ICU patients reporting short-term hospital survival rates of 60% to 85% depending on the type of ICU (surgical versus medical) and inclusion criteria for the study.[8] Many studies have reported that age greater than 65 years is a risk factor of ICU mortality, but these studies often did not control for admitting diagnosis, important comorbidities and severity of illness.[9–14] When one takes into account severity of illness at ICU admission using the Acute and Chronic Health Evaluation II (APACHE II) scoring system age has less of an impact on survival.[15–18]

The APACHE III Prognostic system is a series of multivariate logistic regression equations designed to predict mortality of patients admitted to ICUs.[19] This severity of illness measure adjusts for acute physiologic abnormalities, comorbidities, age, primary diagnosis and origin of admission. When incorporating APACHE III into mortality models, age accounts for only 3% of the explanatory power in risk for death and acute physiology accounts for between 43% and 86% of the explanatory power in risk for death. A study from Canada demonstrated that patients age 65 and older had higher mortality compared to their younger counterparts, but that age accounted for less than 5% of the variance in absolute risk of death and that APACHE II scores were again most predictive of ICU mortality.[20]

Dementia is the 5th leading cause of death in patients over the age of 65.[21] The physical consequences of dementia predispose patients to infection; especially aspiration pneumonia and urinary tract infections and these are important causes of death in demented patients.[22–25] Research has demonstrated that 49% of older hospitalized persons with dementia received at least one invasive treatment in their last days of life. Dementia or preexisting cognitive impairment is prevalent in older medical ICU patients and has been reported to be between 31% and 42%, depending on the screening instrument that is used.[26]

A study of 395 patients aged 65 years and older examined the impact of preexisting dementia on outcomes from ICU care. Seventeen percent of the study population had evidence of moderate to severe dementia by a well-validated measure based on proxy report. Despite the fact that the patients with dementia were significantly older, had higher APACHE II scores on ICU admission and were more likely to have a Do Not Resuscitate (DNR) and Do Not

Intubate (DNI) order, dementia did not exert significant impact on short-term ICU outcomes.[27] It is difficult to predict who will derive benefit from intensive care. Although multiple studies have attempted to address this issue, lingering questions remain about whether older persons, particularly those with dementia, will benefit from ICU care.

Delirium defined as an acute disorder of attention and global cognitive function characterized by acute onset and fluctuating symptoms is a risk factor for adverse outcomes after critical illness.[28] Multiple studies have demonstrated that dementia and age are two of the strongest risk factors for the development of ICU delirium.[28–31] Other risk factors for delirium include predisposing factors such a functional status, underlying medical comorbidities and cognitive status as well as precipitating factors related to the critical illness including severity of illness, medications, medical procedures, restraints and sleep deprivation.[32]

Delirium is a common disorder among older ICU patients because of their advanced age, critical illness and multiple medical procedures and interventions.[30,31,33–35] Prevalence rates of delirium in older ICU patients range from 30–87% depending on the population studied and the type and frequency of the screening instrument.[29,31,36,37] Delirium leads to poor outcomes, including increased morbidity, mortality, nursing home placement, longer length of ICU and hospital stays, and costlier hospitalizations.[38,39] In addition, there is growing evidence that delirium and delirium duration contribute to long-term cognitive impairment in survivors of critical illness.[40,41]

A multicenter study of patients after acute lung injury identified ICU length of stay and corticosteroid use as risk factors for impairment in physical outcomes.[42] After accounting for patient's baseline status they demonstrated significant impairment in six-minute walk test and SF-36 physical function measures. The caveat to this study was that the mean patient age was 48 years, but one can speculate that older patients would be likely to have similar deficits.

3. Outcomes After Sepsis and Acute Respiratory Distress Syndrome

Age is an important risk factor for sepsis, with respiratory and genitourinary sources as the primary etiologies and more frequently gram-negative infections. A study benchmarking the incidence and mortality of sepsis in the United States utilizing four different methods of database abstraction demonstrated that regardless of the method used there was about a 13% annual increase in the incidence of severe sepsis.[43] In this study mortality rates varied based on the database abstraction method used but all methods demonstrated an increase in total mortality yearly from 2004 to 2008.[43] This likely coincides with increase occurrence in older patients with more comorbidities. In a large study of sepsis in the United States, patient's age 65 and older accounted for 65% of the sepsis cases. Compared to a younger cohort, older patients had a relative risk of 13% for developing sepsis.[44] In addition, older patients died earlier during hospitalization than the younger patients and were more likely to be admitted to a skilled nursing facility upon discharge.

A recent study out of Australia and New Zealand reported a decrease in sepsis mortality even in older subgroups of patients.[45] A study of older patients, mean age of 78.6 years, using Medicare claims data from the Health and Retirement Study describes the outcomes of sepsis cohort.[46] There was significant organ dysfunction among these older patients admitted with sepsis, 42% had renal dysfunction, 23% had cardiovascular dysfunction, 19% had hematologic dysfunction, 10% had respiratory dysfunction and 1% had hepatic dysfunction. Patients with severe sepsis had a 28% 90-day mortality and a 44% 1-year mortality. Among the patients who died in the year after their sepsis hospitalization, 48% died at home, 34% died in a hospital and 18% died in a nursing home. Thirty-four percent enrolled in hospice before their death.

There is some recent evidence that mortality from sepsis and septic shock may be decreasing, even among older patients. Many factors may be at play here including early recognition and treatment of the sepsis and septic shock. Despite suggested mortality decreases sepsis still carries a high burden of morbidity for older patients.

4. Cognitive Outcomes

There is limited data regarding cognitive outcomes in older patients after critical illness. Performing studies to assess cognitive outcomes in this patient population of older ICU survivors is challenging. Older patients may have preexisting cognitive impairment that is not documented at the time of ICU admission. Many large trials conducted in ICU's for sepsis or ARDS did not include older patients. In addition morbidity and mortality are high in older patients after a critical illness and so they are not available for participation in trials post-ICU discharge. A study of cognitive impairment after acute lung injury highlights this point; the mean age of patients was 49 years, range of 40 to 58 years.[47] In this younger group of patients they demonstrated that most patients experienced long-term cognitive and psychiatric morbidity.[47]

A study utilizing the Health and Retirement study, which is a nationally represented survey of US residents from 1998–2006, examined cognitive outcomes in survivors of severe sepsis.[48] The mean age of participants was 77 years and they demonstrated an increase in moderate to severe cognitive impairment of 10.6% points compared to baseline. Severe sepsis was independently associated with tripling of the odds of moderate to severe cognitive impairment. The cognitive impairments in this cohort persisted for the eight years of follow-up.

A larger prospective cohort study of older persons in Seattle, WA demonstrated that community dwelling older patients who experienced a hospital admission relative to participants who were not hospitalized had a hazard ratio for subsequent dementia of 1.4 (95% CI, 1.1 to 1.7; $p=0.001$) and those who required an ICU admission had a hazard ratio of 2.3 (95% CI, 0.9 to 5.7; $p = 0.09$).[49] One limitation to this study is that of the 2929 participants only 41 required ICU admission so they could not reliably examine predictors for developing dementia.

De Rooj *et al.* examined patients aged 80 years and older who survived for at least one year after admission to either a medical or surgical ICU.[50] They found a 17% prevalence of severe cognitive impairment and a 56% prevalence of mild to moderate cognitive impairment. In looking at the data by reason for ICU admission, 25% of medical ICU admissions, 28% of the unplanned surgery admissions and, 11% of the planned surgery admissions had moderate to severe cognitive impairment.[50]

Cognitive impairment and long term brain dysfunction is an important consideration in the growing number of patients who are chronically critically ill. Chronic critical illness is a syndrome of chronic ventilator dependence with associated derangements in other organ systems.[51] For both research and clinical purposes the syndrome of chronic critical illness is defined by the placement of tracheostomy after at least 10 days of failure to wean from a mechanical ventilator.[51] A study examining 385 patients, with a median age of 71 years, who met the definition of chronic critical illness demonstrated high 6-month mortality and long-term brain dysfunction.[40] The 6-month mortality rate in this cohort of chronically ill adults, the majority who were living at home without cognitive impairment prior to hospitalization was 56%. In addition another 28% were living with long-term brain dysfunction.[40]

The numbers of older chronically critically ill patients are growing and in addition to high mortality rates they have significant long-term brain dysfunction. These poor outcomes in older patients who meet the definition of chronic critical illness are important for helping us inform avenues for future research as well as discussions with patients and families about preferences and goals of care.

5. Functional Outcomes

Increasing attention has been paid in recent years to the importance of functional outcomes after critical illness in ICU survivors of all ages. As with cognitive impairment, it is now well established that many ICU survivors experience new or worsening physical impairment after critical illness.[48,52–54] Studies focusing on functional outcomes after critical illness in older adults have been varied in their approach, but largely focus on disability assessments as measured by ADL and instrumental activities of daily living (IADLs). Mobility, which is the third key domain of disability in geriatric assessments,[55,56] has been less of a focus in these studies.

One key feature that many studies of functional outcome in older survivors of critical illness lack is ability to control for pre-ICU functional status. A nationwide study of 516 older adults with sepsis, median age 77 years, demonstrated the presence of many geriatric conditions after hospitalization including low body mass index and decreased ability to walk across a room or lift ten pounds.[57] The prevalence of other geriatric conditions, such as injurious falls, incontinence, chronic pain and vision and hearing impairment were not increased after severe sepsis when a patient's pre-sepsis trajectories were considered.[57]

Several studies have used the Katz ADL index to evaluate disability outcomes after critical illness in older adults.[58–64] The Katz ADL index is a dichotomous instrument that evaluates six activities of ADLs: bathing, dressing, toileting, transferring, continence and feeding.[65] This tool has consistently demonstrated its utility in evaluating functional status in the elderly, though it is less likely to identify small decrements in function. A smaller number of studies evaluated both ADLs and IADLs after critical illness.[66–68] One study only evaluated IADLs.[69] Most of the aforementioned studies that evaluated IADLs utilized the Lawton index; one used the Pfeffer Functional Activities Questionnaire, which can be used in adults with cognitive impairment. The Lawton instrument, which takes 10–15 minutes to administer, assesses eight domains of function: food preparation, shopping, ability to use the telephone, housekeeping, laundry, ability to handle finances, mode of transportation and medication administration.[70]

The aforementioned studies that evaluate disability outcomes with ADL and IADL indices demonstrate that functional decrements are common after critical illness. These studies assessed patients for functional disability at time points ranging from hospital discharge through 4 years after critical illness, with the most common assessments occurring at 6 months and/or 1 year after ICU discharge. Although the prevalence of ADL and IADL decrements varied widely, all studies reported decreased functional disability after critical illness in older adults.

One important fact that has come to light in recent years is the impact of ICU-acquired weakness (ICUAW) on physical dysfunction after critical illness. This condition is caused by many pathophysiologic processes that are not mutually exclusive.[71] Critical illness polyneuropathy (CIN) affects the limbs, especially the lower extremities, in a symmetric distribution, with weakness most notable in the proximal neuromuscular areas. It can affect the muscles of respiration and is an independent predictor of prolonged weaning from mechanical ventilation.[72] Critical illness myopathy (CIM) is a primary myopathy in which electrophysiological studies show reduced amplitude and increased duration of compound muscle action potentials (CMAPs). It occurs more frequently than CIN and exhibits a higher rate of recovery.[73] This condition is also manifested by limb and respiratory muscle weakness, but histopathological examination reveals selective loss of muscle thick filaments, affecting myosin to a greater extent than actin.[74] CIN refers to elements of both CIM and CIP occurring simulataneously.[75] Diagnosis of these conditions can be difficult in the critically ill patient as electromyographic and nerve-conduction testing are not routinely performed in the ICU. However, the diagnosis of ICU-acquired weakness can be made with the use of the Medical Research Council (MRC) scale, which grades the strength of various muscle groups in the upper and lower extremities; a combined score of less than 48 indicates ICU-acquired weakness.[76] Patients who are diagnosed with ICUAW using the MRC scale should be followed with serial examinations and if persistent deficits are noted, axonal and muscle testing can then be pursued. Risk factors for ICUAW include sepsis, persistent systemic inflammation and multisystem organ failure.[76] Glucocorticoids,[74,76,77] neuromuscular blocking agents[78] and hyperglycemia[79] have all been reported as risk factors for ICUAW, though the evidence surrounding these variables is less clear; nevertheless, these agents and conditions should probably be avoided if possible.

Increased attention to the functional deficits noted after critical illness as well as growing interest in the impact of ICUAW has resulted in an increased focus on early mobilization in the ICU and post-ICU rehabilitation programs for all ICU patients. These programs will be especially important for the 1.4 million older adults who survive a critical illness every year and remain at high risk of poor functional outcomes after critical illness.

6. Quality of Life Outcomes

An important patient-centered outcome after critical illness is quality of life. Specifically, health-related quality of life (HRQOL) is defined as the degree to which a patient's health status affects their self-determined evaluation of their satisfaction with their life.[80] Quality of life outcomes after critical illness are particularly relevant for older patients in the ICU and the intensivists who care for them, as both must balance the expected benefit of admitting older patients to the ICU with the burden of disease thereafter.

As an outcome, HRQOLe should describe the sum of the patient's physical and psychological functions, their capacity for meeting their social needs and their own perception of their situation.[81] Multiple instruments have been used over the years to assess HRQOL. One PubMed review of the tools used most frequently between 1995–2004 in ICU studies showed that only three instruments were reported in at least ten articles: The Medical Outcome Study Short Form- 36 (SF-36) in 23, the Nottingham Health Profile (NHP) in 13 and the EuroQoL (EQ) in 10.[82]

The Medical Outcome Study SF-36 is the most commonly used instrument to assess HRQOL. This 36-item questionnaire relies upon patient self-report to assess eight domains: physical functioning, role limitations due to physical problems, bodily pain, general health perceptions, vitality, social functioning, role limitations due to emotional problems and general mental health. The most commonly used scoring system, the SF-36, yields two scores: The Physical Component Summary (PCS) score and the Mental Component Summary

(MSC) score.[83] The total SF-36 score ranges from 0 to 100, with a greater score reflecting a better health-related quality of life. The SF-36 has been validated for assessing HRQOL after critical illness.[83,84] It has also been validated in the primary care setting for the general population.[85,86]

The last systematic review of HRQOL outcomes after critical illness in older adults was performed in 2005.[87] This review identified 16 studies evaluating the outcome of interest over 13 years (1990–2003). Multiple different instruments were used in the various studies; only one HRQOL instrument was used twice in the 16 studies. Ten of the 16 studies demonstrated that HRQOL was relatively good, that patients were satisfied, or that there was no change from premorbid HRQOL. However, this review highlighted the limitations of the HRQOL research in older adults through 2003: Most studies were small, retrospective and lacked a validated HRQOL assessment tool.

Several recent prospective longitudinal studies evaluated HRQOL in older adults admitted to the ICU in order to address the aforementioned gaps in the literature. Khouli[88] enrolled 484 patients aged 65 and older at the time of ICU admission and used an instrument developed by the Centers for Disease Control (CDC)[89] to assess HRQOL during the 30 days prior to ICU admission. When the patient did not have the capacity to answer HRQOL questions reliably, proxies were interviewed. The assessment was repeated at 6 months after hospital discharge. Among the survivors at 6 months, HRQOL had significantly worsened over time in the oldest patients (aged 86.3+, 1 standard deviation above the mean cohort study age) but improved in the youngest (65–69). However, nearly one-third of the patients had died within 6 months of hospital discharge.

In a prospective cohort study, Vest examined contributors to decreased quality of life in ICU survivors' age 60 and older at one-month and one-year after admission.[90] They used SF-12, ADL and depression scales. At one-month both depression and impairment in ADL was associated with decreased QOL. These factors account for 17% of the variability in SF-12 physical component score and 20% of the variability in the SF-12 mental component score.

Hofhuis[91] enrolled patients over age 80 ($n = 129$) and less than age 80 ($n = 620$) at the time of ICU admission. Using SF-36, the investigators assessed each patient's HRQOL with proxy interviews for all patients. The SF-36 was then administered to the patient at ICU discharge, hospital discharge and 3 and 6 months after ICU discharge. Mean SF-36 scores in the octogenarians at 6 months after ICU discharge was comparable to baseline. However, 71 of the 129 octogenarians had died by 6 months after ICU discharge, so the 6-month assessment was only performed in 49 patients. Both studies were performed in a single center and required proxy assessments for a significant part, if not all, of their baseline HRQOL assessments. Both studies also had a significant number of deaths at the time of follow-up — a common limitation of conducting critical care research in older adults. The conflicting results in these two recent studies highlight the need for further research into HRQOL outcomes in older adults after critical illness.

7. Summary

As mortality rates from acute critical illness decrease there is mounting evidence that ICU survivors are experiencing health-related sequelae including functional, cognitive and psychological disturbances. One of the unanswered questions is which group of older

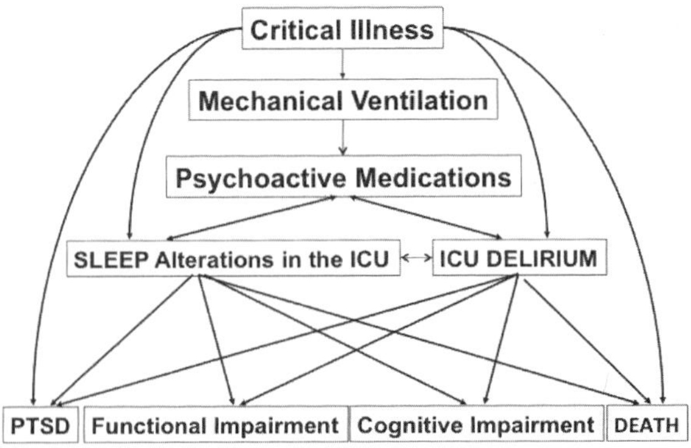

Fig. 1. Schematic of Critical Illness in Older Patients and Outcomes.

patients will benefit from ICU care. In addition patients, their families and physicians need to weigh the burden of treatment against long-term functional and cognitive outcomes even more then against the likelihood of survival.[6] Studies that control baseline function and cognitive status as well as ICU factors are needed to examine long-term functional, cognitive and quality of life outcomes in older ICU patients. This information is important to help inform decision-making and discussions about goals of care and meaningful patient outcomes.

References

1. Kochnar R. (2014) *10 Projections for the global population in 2050.* Available at http://www.pewresearch.org/fact-tank/2014/02/03/10-projections-for-the-global-population-in-2050/.
2. *Aging Statistics: Administration on Aging (AoA).* Available at http://www.aoa.acl.gov/Aging_Statistics/.
3. Vincent JL, Marshall JC, Namendys-Silva SA *et al.* (2014) Assessment of the worldwide burden of critical illness: The Intensive Care Over Nations (ICON) audit. *Lancet. Respir Med* **2**: 380–386.
4. Fuchs L, Chronaki CE, Park S *et al.* (2012) ICU admission characteristics and mortality rates among elderly and very elderly patients. *Intens Care Med* **38**: 1654–1661.
5. Cosgriff JA, Pisani M, Bradley EH *et al.* (2007) The association between treatment preferences and trajectories of care at the end-of-life. *J Gen Intern Med* **22**: 1566–1571.
6. Fried TR, Bradley EH, Towle VR *et al.* (2002) Understanding the treatment preferences of seriously ill patients. *New Engl J Med* **346**: 1061–1066.
7. Pisani MA, Kong SY, Kasl SV *et al.* (2009) Days of delirium are associated with 1-year mortality in an older intensive care unit population. *Am J Respir Crit Care Med* **180**: 1092–1097.
8. Chelluri L, Grenvik A, Silverman M. (1995) Intensive care for critically ill elderly: Mortality, costs, and quality of life. Review of the literature. *Arch Intern Med* **155**: 1013–1022.
9. Kass JE, Castriotta RJ, Malakoff F. (1992) Intensive care unit outcome in the very elderly. *Crit Care Med* **20**: 1666–1671.
10. McLean RF, McIntosh JD, Kung GY *et al.* (1985) Outcome of respiratory intensive care for the elderly. *Crit Care Med* **13**: 625–629.

11. Chelluri L, Pinsky MR, Donahoe MP *et al.* (1993) Long-term outcome of critically ill elderly patients requiring intensive care. *JAMA* **269**: 3119–3123.
12. Chelluri L, Pinsky MR, Grenvik AN. (1992) Outcome of intensive care of the "oldest-old" critically ill patients. *Crit Care Med* **20**: 757–761.
13. Campion EW, Mulley AG, Goldstein RL *et al.* (1981) Medical intensive care for the elderly. A study of current use, costs, and outcomes. *JAMA* **246**: 2052–2056.
14. Tran DD, Groeneveld AB, van der Meulen J *et al.* (1990) Age, chronic disease, sepsis, organ system failure, and mortality in a medical intensive care unit. *Crit Care Medicine* **18**: 474–479.
15. Hanson LC, Danis M. (1991) Use of life-sustaining care for the elderly. *J Am Geriatr Soc* **39**: 772–777.
16. Le Gall JR, Brun-Buisson C, Trunet P *et al.* (1982) Influence of age, previous health status, and severity of acute illness on outcome from intensive care. *Crit Care medicine* **10**: 575–577.
17. Mahul P, Perrot D, Tempelhoff G *et al.* (1991) Short- and long-term prognosis, functional outcome following ICU for elderly. *Intens Care Med* **17**: 7–10.
18. Wu AW, Rubin HR, Rosen MJ. (1990) Are elderly people less responsive to intensive care? *J Am Geriatr Soc* **38**: 621–627.
19. Knaus WA, Wagner DP, Draper EA *et al.* (1991) The APACHE III prognostic system. Risk prediction of hospital mortality for critically ill hospitalized adults. *Chest* **100**: 1619–1636.
20. Rockwood K, Cosway S, Stolee P *et al.* (1994) Increasing the recognition of delirium in elderly patients. *J Am Geriatr Soc* **42**: 252–256.
21. Tejada-Vera B. (2013) Mortality from Alzheimer's disease in the United States: Data for 2000 and 2010. *NCHS data brief*: 1–8.
22. Campbell-Taylor I, Nadon GW, Sclater AL *et al.* (1988) Oro-esophageal tube feeding: An alternative to nasogastric or gastrostomy tubes. *Dysphagia* **2**: 220–221.
23. Lipsky BA, Boyko EJ, Inui TS *et al.* (1986) Risk factors for acquiring pneumococcal infections. *Arch Intern Med* **146**: 2179–2185.
24. Volicer L, Hurley AC. (1995) Risk factors for pneumonia in nursing home residents. *J Am Geriatr Soc* **43**: 1443–1444.
25. Beard CM, Kokmen E, Sigler C *et al.* (1996) Cause of death in Alzheimer's disease. *Ann Epidemiol* **6**: 195–200.

26. Pisani MA, Inouye SK, McNicoll L *et al.* (2003) Screening for preexisting cognitive impairment in older intensive care unit patients: Use of proxy assessment. *J Am Geriatr Soc* **51**: 689–693.
27. Pisani MA, Redlich CA, McNicoll L *et al.* (2005) Short-term outcomes in older intensive care unit patients with dementia. *Crit Care Med* **33**: 1371–1376.
28. Inouye SK. (2006) Delirium in older persons. *New Engl J Med* **354**: 1157–1165.
29. McNicoll L, Pisani MA, Zhang Y *et al.* (2003) Delirium in the intensive care unit: Occurrence and clinical course in older patients. *J Am Geriatr Soc* **51**: 591–598.
30. Pisani MA, Murphy TE, Van Ness PH *et al.* (2007) Characteristics associated with delirium in older patients in a medical intensive care unit. *Arch Intern Med* **167**: 1629–1634.
31. Van Rompaey B, Elseviers MM, Schuurmans MJ *et al.* (2009) Risk factors for delirium in intensive care patients: A prospective cohort study. *Crit Care* **13**: R77.
32. Jones SF, Pisani MA. (2012) ICU delirium: An update. *Curr opin Crit Care* **18**: 146–151.
33. Pandharipande P, Shintani A, Peterson J *et al.* (2006) Lorazepam is an independent risk factor for transitioning to delirium in intensive care unit patients. *Anesthesiol* **104**: 21–26.
34. Ouimet S, Kavanagh BP, Gottfried SB *et al.*(2007) Incidence, risk factors and consequences of ICU delirium. *Intens Care Med* **33**: 66–73.
35. Dubois MJ, Bergeron N, Dumont M *et al.* (2001) Delirium in an intensive care unit: A study of risk factors. *Intens Care Med* **27**: 1297–1304.
36. Thomason JW, Shintani A, Peterson JF *et al.* (2005) Intensive care unit delirium is an independent predictor of longer hospital stay: A prospective analysis of 261 non-ventilated patients. *Crit Care* **9**: R375–R381.
37. Ely EW, Inouye SK, Bernard GR *et al.* (2001) Delirium in mechanically ventilated patients: Validity and reliability of the confusion assessment method for the intensive care unit (CAM-ICU). *JAMA* **286**: 2703–2710.
38. Ely EW, Gautam S, Margolin R *et al.* (2001) The impact of delirium in the intensive care unit on hospital length of stay. *Intens Care Med* **27**: 1892–1900.
39. Milbrandt EB, Deppen S, Harrison PL *et al.* (2004) Costs associated with delirium in mechanically ventilated patients. *Crit Care Med* **32**: 955–962.

40. Hope AA, Morrison RS, Du Q *et al.* (2013) Risk factors for long-term brain dysfunction after chronic critical illness. *Ann Am Thorac Soc* **10**: 315–323.
41. Girard TD, Jackson JC, Pandharipande PP *et al.* (2010) Delirium as a predictor of long-term cognitive impairment in survivors of critical illness. *Critic Care Med* **38**: 1513–1520.
42. Needham DM, Wozniak AW, Hough CL *et al.* (2014) Risk factors for physical impairment after acute lung injury in a national, multicenter study. *Am J RespirCrit Care Med* **189**: 1214–1224.
43. Gaieski DF, Edwards JM, Kallan MJ *et al.* (2013) Benchmarking the incidence and mortality of severe sepsis in the United States. *Crit Care Med* **41**: 1167–1174.
44. Martin GS, Mannino DM, Moss M. (2006) The effect of age on the development and outcome of adult sepsis. *Crit Care Med* **34**: 15–21.
45. Kaukonen KM, Bailey M, Suzuki S *et al.* (2014) Mortality related to severe sepsis and septic shock among critically ill patients in Australia and New Zealand, 2000–2012. *JAMA* **311**: 1308–1316.
46. Prescott HC, Langa KM, Liu V *et al.* (2014) Increased 1-year healthcare use in survivors of severe sepsis. *Am J Respir Crit Care Med* **190**: 62–69.
47. Mikkelsen ME, Christie JD, Lanken PN *et al.* (2012) The adult respiratory distress syndrome cognitive outcomes study: Long-term neuropsychological function in survivors of acute lung injury. *Am J Respir Crit Care Med* **185**: 1307–1315.
48. Iwashyna TJ, Ely EW, Smith DM *et al.* (2010) Long-term cognitive impairment and functional disability among survivors of severe sepsis. *JAMA* **304**: 1787–1794.
49. Ehlenbach WJ, Hough CL, Crane PK *et al.* (2010) Association between acute care and critical illness hospitalization and cognitive function in older adults. *JAMA* **303**: 763–770.
50. de Rooij SE, Govers AC, Korevaar JC *et al.*. (2008) Cognitive, functional, and quality-of-life outcomes of patients aged 80 and older who survived at least 1 year after planned or unplanned surgery or medical intensive care treatment. *J Am Geriatr Soc* **56**: 816–822.
51. Nelson JE, Cox CE, Hope AA *et al.* (2010) Chronic critical illness. *Am J Respir Crit Care Med* **182**: 446–454.
52. Bienvenu OJ, Colantuoni E, Mendez-Tellez PA *et al.* (2012) Depressive symptoms and impaired physical function after acute lung injury: A 2-year longitudinal study. *Am J Respir Crit Care Med* **185**: 517–524.

53. Herridge MS, Tansey CM, Matte A *et al.* (2011) Functional disability 5 years after acute respiratory distress syndrome. *New Engl J Med* **364**: 1293–1304.
54. Unroe M, Kahn JM, Carson SS *et al.* (2010) One-year trajectories of care and resource utilization for recipients of prolonged mechanical ventilation: A cohort study. *Ann Intern Med* **153**: 167–175.
55. Gill TM, Gahbauer EA, Murphy TE *et al.* (2012) Risk factors and precipitants of long-term disability in community mobility: A cohort study of older persons. *Ann Intern Med* **156**: 131–140.
56. Gill TM, Murphy TE, Gahbauer EA *et al.* (2013) The course of disability before and after a serious fall injury. *JAMA Intern Med* **173**: 1780–1786.
57. Iwashyna TJ, Netzer G, Langa KM *et al.* (2012) Spurious inferences about long-term outcomes: The case of severe sepsis and geriatric conditions. *Am J Respir Crit Care Med* **185**: 835–841.
58. Kass JE, Castriotta RJ, Malakoff F. (1992) Intensive-Care unit outcome in the very elderly. *Crit Care Med* **20**: 1666–1671.
59. Chelluri L, Pinsky MR, Donahoe MP *et al.* (1993) Long-term outcome of critically ill elderly patients requiring intensive care. *JAMA* **269**: 3119–3123.
60. Rockwood K, Noseworthy TW, Gibney RTN *et al.* (1993) One-year outcome of elderly and young patients admitted to intensive care units. *Crit Care Med* **21**: 687–691.
61. Montuclard L, Garrouste-Orgeas M, Timsit JF *et al.* (2000) Outcome, functional autonomy and quality of life of elderly patients with a long-term intensive care unit stay. *Crit Care Med.* **28**: 3389–3395.
62. Udekwu P, Gurkin B, Oller D *et al.* (2001) Quality of life and functional level in elderly patients surviving surgical intensive care. *JACS* **193**: 245–249.
63. Balas MC, Happ MB, Yang W *et al.* (2009) Outcomes associated with delirium in older patients in surgical ICUs. *Chest* **135**: 18–25.
64. Barnato AE, Albert SM, Angus DC *et al.* (2011) Disability among elderly survivors of mechanical ventilation. *Am J Respir Crit Care Med* **183**: 1037–1042.
65. Katz S, Ford AB, Moskowitz RW *et al.* (1963) Studies of illness in the aged — The index of Adl — A standardized measure of biological and psychosocial function. *JAMA* **185**: 914–919.
66. Broslawski GE, Elkins M, Algus M. (1995) Functional abilities of elderly survivors of intensive care. *J Am Osteopath Assoc* **95**: 712–717.

67. Daubin C, Chevalier S, Seguin A *et al.* (2011) Predictors of mortality and short-term physical and cognitive dependence in critically ill persons 75 years and older: A prospective cohort study. *Health Qual Life Out* **9**:
68. Jackson JC, Pandharipande PP, Girard TD *et al.* (2014) Depression, post-traumatic stress disorder, and functional disability in survivors of critical illness in the BRAIN-ICU study: A longitudinal cohort study. *Lancet. Respir Med* **2**: 369–379.
69. Boumendil A, Maury E, Reinhard I *et al.* (2004) Prognosis of patients aged 80 years and over admitted in medical intensive care unit. *Intens Care Med* **30**: 647–654.
70. Lawton MP, Brody EM. (1969) Assessment of older people — Self-maintaining and instrumental activities of daily living. *Gerontol* **9**: 179.
71. Kress JP, Hall JB. (2014) ICU-acquired weakness and recovery from critical illness. *New Engl J Med* **370**: 1626–1635.
72. De Jonghe B, Bastuji-Garin S, Sharshar T *et al.* (2004) Does ICU-acquired paresis lengthen weaning from mechanical ventilation? *Intens Care Med* **30**: 1117–1121.
73. Koch S, Spuler S, Deja M *et al.* (2011) Critical illness myopathy is frequent: Accompanying neuropathy protracts ICU discharge. *J Neurol Neurosurg Psychiatry* **82**: 287–293.
74. Derde S, Hermans G, Derese I *et al.* (2012) Muscle atrophy and preferential loss of myosin in prolonged critically ill patients. *Crit Care Med* **40**: 79–89.
75. Stevens RD, Marshall SA, Cornblath DR *et al.* (2009) A framework for diagnosing and classifying intensive care unit-acquired weakness. *Crit Care Med* **37**: S299–S308.
76. De Jonghe B, Sharshar T, Lefaucheur JP *et al.* (2002) Paresis acquired in the intensive care unit — A prospective multicenter study. *JAMA.* **288**: 2859–2867.
77. Herridge MS, Cheung AM, Tansey CM *et al.* (2003) One-year outcomes in survivors of the acute respiratory distress syndrome. *N Engl J Med.* **348**: 683–693.
78. Leatherman JW, Fluegel WL, David WS *et al.* (1996) Muscle weakness in mechanically ventilated patients with severe asthma. *Am J Respir Crit Care Med* **153**: 1686–1690.
79. Van den Berghe G, Wouters P, Weekers F *et al.* (2001) Intensive insulin therapy in critically ill patients. *N Engl J Med* **345**: 1359–1367.

80. Curtis JR. (2003) Measuring health status after critical illness: Where are we and where do we go from here? *Surviv Intens Care* **39**: 181–196.
81. (1994) Quality of life: A tool for decision-making in the ICU. Spanish group for the epidemiological analysis of critical patients (PAEEC). *Intens Care Med.* **20**: 251–252.
82. Capuzzo M, Bertacchini S, Chiani C. (2005) Evaluating quality of life after intensive care. *APICEM.* 843–851.
83. Heyland DK, Hopman W, Coo H *et al.* (2000) Long-term health-related quality of life in survivors of sepsis. Short Form 36: A valid and reliable measure of health-related quality of life. *Crit Care Med* **28**: 3599–3605.
84. Chrispin PS, Scotton H, Rogers J *et al.* (1997) Short Form 36 in the intensive care unit: Assessment of acceptability, reliability and validity of the questionnaire. *Anaesthesia* **52**: 15–23.
85. Brazier JE, Harper R, Jones NMB *et al.* (1992) Validating the sf-36 health survey questionnaire — New outcome measure for primary care. *Br Med J* **305**: 160–164.
86. Jenkinson C, Coulter A, Wright L. (1993) Short form-36 (sf-36) health survey questionnaire — Normative data for adults of working age. *Br Med J* **306**: 1437–1440.
87. Hennessy D, Juzwishin K, Yergens D *et al.* (2005) Outcomes of elderly survivors of intensive care — A review of the literature. *Chest* **127**: 1764–1774.
88. Khouli H, Astua A, Dombrowski W *et al.* (2011) Changes in health-related quality of life and factors predicting long-term outcomes in older adults admitted to intensive care units. *Crit Care Med* **39**:
89. Centers for disease control and prevention, national center for chronic disease prevention and health promotion: Health-Related Quality of Life Methods and Measures. Available at: http://www.cdc.gov/hrqol/methods.htm. Accessed January 24, 2011.
90. Vest MT, Murphy TE, Araujo KL *et al.* (2011) Disability in activities of daily living, depression, and quality of life among older medical ICU survivors: A prospective cohort study. *Health Qual Life Out* **9**: 9.
91. Hofhuis JGM, van Stel HE, Schrijvers AJP *et al.* (2011) Changes of health-related quality of life in critically ill octogenarians a follow-up study. *Chest* **140**: 1473–1483.

Chapter 6

Severe Sepsis, Pneumonia and Aging

Olufunmilayo Falade* and Sachin Yende*,†

1. Introduction

Sepsis is defined as the presence of at least two of the four systemic inflammatory response syndrome (SIRS) criteria (Table 1) developing in response to a documented or suspected infection. However, the terms infection, sepsis and septicemia are often used interchangeably. The clinical presentation of sepsis includes a spectrum of conditions. The least severe manifestation of sepsis includes individuals who have an infection and meet the SIRS criteria and they are often seen in the outpatient setting. At the other end of the spectrum are patients with organ dysfunction or severe sepsis (Table 1) and these patients often require intensive care unit (ICU) admission.

Infectious diseases account for one in three deaths in people who are 65 years and older, with pneumonia, influenza and septicemia listed as the top 10 causes of death according to the Centers for Disease Control (CDC).[1] In this chapter, we will examine the significance and special characteristics of infections and severe sepsis in the older adult. For infections, we focus on pneumonia because

*Department of Critical Care Medicine and CRISMA Laboratory, University of Pittsburgh, PA, USA.

†Veterans Affairs Pittsburgh Healthcare System, Pittsburgh, PA, USA, E-mail: yendes@upmc.edu

Table 1. Criteria for SIRS, sepsis, severe sepsis and septic shock based on the 1991 ACCP/SCCM Consensus conference.

Term	Criteria: 2 out of the 4 following criteria
SIRS	Temperature >38°C or <36°C
	Heart rate >90/min
	Hyperventilation evidenced by respiratory rate >20/min or $PaCO_2$ lower than 32 mmHg
	White blood cell count >12,000 cells/μL or <4,000 cells/μL
Sepsis	SIRS criteria with presumed or proven infection
Severe sepsis	Sepsis with organ dysfunction
Septic shock	Sepsis with hypotension despite adequate fluid resuscitation

it is the most common infectious cause of hospitalization in North America, the most common cause of severe sepsis and a leading cause of death.[2] We will also explore mechanisms and risk factors that increase susceptibility to these infections, including age-related changes of the immune system. Finally, we will discuss the long-term impact of infection in this population and the importance of preventive practices.

2. Public Health Significance

Pneumonia and severe sepsis are major public health problems, particularly in the older adults. Compared to younger individuals, older adults are more likely to be hospitalized for pneumonia and severe sepsis and once hospitalized, they are more likely to die.

Severe sepsis is a leading cause of admission among critically-ill patients in non-coronary ICUs. The incidence of severe sepsis increases disproportionately in older adults with more than half of severe sepsis cases occurring in adults >65 years of age. For instance, hospitalization rates for severe sepsis in those >80 years were approximately 2-fold, 6-fold and 15–19 fold higher as compared to those 65–79 years, 50–64 years and 35–49 years respectively.[3,4] In 2003, the elderly accounted for one of three inpatient stays (13.2 million hospital admissions) totaling almost 329 billion in hospital charges, or 43.6% of the national hospital care costs.[5]

Severe sepsis is regarded as a grave prognostic indicator especially for the elderly. For instance, the 90-day mortality after community-acquired pneumonia (CAP) is 6%. However, the mortality approaches 26% for patients who develop severe sepsis and is 40% for the subset that have septic shock.[6] Old age is considered an independent risk factor for mortality among adults hospitalized for sepsis. Between 1979 and 2002, case fatality increased linearly across age deciles and averaged 27.7% for those 65 years or older as compared to 17.7% for those younger than 65 years.[3] This increase in mortality with age persisted at 90 days and at 1-year after hospital discharge.[7]

3. Key Issues and Risk Factors for Infections

Epidemiologic studies suggest that age is an important risk factor for infection and severe sepsis, but underlying reasons remain unclear. There is likely a complex interplay between age-related clinical and immunologic risk factors, which may contribute to the increased risk. Epidemiologic studies suggest that age-related differences in clinical risk factors, such as higher chronic disease burden and higher rates of institutionalization may explain some of the differences.[8] Both clinical and immunologic risk factors may also contribute to worse outcomes seen in older adults.[9] We will discuss key clinical and immune risk factors below:

3.1. *Burden of chronic disease*

The presence of a chronic disease is a risk factor for infection across all ages, but it plays a unique role in older adults due to the higher prevalence and severity. Adults older than 65 years are twice as likely to have at least one chronic disease compared to younger patients.[3] Diseases, such as chronic kidney disease, heart failure, chronic obstructive pulmonary disease (COPD), cardiovascular disease, diabetes and cancer, are present in as many as 72% of sepsis patients.[3]

A chronic disease can increase the risk of infection in multiple ways depending on the disease type and severity. For instance, patients who have diabetes are prone to infections for several reasons, including an abnormal immune system.[10] Patients with chronic kidney disease have an abnormal immune system and undergo repeated invasive procedures that increase the risk of infections. The chronic diseases also expose patients to repeated contact with the healthcare system, which serves as a risk factor for recurrent infections. Furthermore, a high burden of chronic disease often co-exists with polypharmacy. These individuals are often on multiple immunosuppressive medications, including glucocorticoids and immune modulators, such as methotrexate, which increase their risk for infection. Finally, older adults often engage in high-risk health behaviors. For instance, a history of and the duration of smoking is a well-known risk factor for lower respiratory tract infections.

3.2. *Long-term care facility use and hospitalization*

Nearly a third of people who are 80 years of age and older live in long-term care facilities (LTCF).[11] Older adults living in LTCFs, including nursing homes and assisted living centers, are among the most vulnerable to infectious diseases. These people tend to have a higher burden of chronic disease.

Nursing home residence and hospitalization are each associated with oropharyngeal colonization with gram-negative bacilli. This in combination with depressed cough and impaired mucociliary function leads to increasing rates of pneumonia.[11]

The three most common infections in LTCFs are urinary tract infections, respiratory infections and skin and soft tissue infections. The incidence of infection ranges from 1.8 –13.5 episodes per 1,000 resident care days, resulting in 1.6–3.8 million infections annually.[12] Also, in LTCFs, antibiotic resistance is a growing problem.[13,14] For instance, in a nursing home outbreak of drug resistant gram-negative infections, 46% had antibiotic resistant *Escherichia coli.*[15] The economic cost of treating infections that occur in residents of LTCFs is high and estimated to exceed $1 billion annually.[12] Finally, the risk of mortality with these infections is high (add a percentage or something to give the reader a sense of the magnitude).

3.3. *Immunosenescence*

Changes in the immune system that occurs with age potentially contribute to the increased susceptibility of older persons to infection.[16] Immunosenescence is the age-related progressive alteration of the immune system, which occurs, in both innate and adaptive systems. This includes reduced natural killer(NK) cell toxicity on a per cell basis, reduced number and or function of dendritic cells (DC) in blood, decreased total naive and memory *T* cells, decreased naïve and memory B cells.[17] These immunosenescent changes may accelerate several chronic conditions, they may also contribute to the decreased efficacy of vaccination and independently increase susceptibility to developing an infection in older adults.[18] However, it is important to note that the study of immunosenescence is still evolving and much of the work done is in murine models.

3.4. *Innate immunity*

The innate response comprises of the initial recognition and destruction of pathogens. This response is characterized by its rapid action, lack of immunologic memory and plays a vital role in resistance to infectious disease. This exquisite system is triggered by recognition of a pathogenic antigen and results in activation of a transcription factor NF-kB that is considered the master regulator of the innate immune system. This leads to production of pro-inflammatory cytokines (e.g. TNF and IL[interleukin]-6) that are crucial to activation of downstream cytokines, recruiting immune effector cells, activating coagulation networks and stimulating the adaptive immune response by virtue of their function as Antigen Presenting cells (APCs)[9] The principal cellular components of the innate immune system include neutrophils, monocytes/macrophages, natural killer (NK) cells and DC. These cells are able to recognize pathogens through the use of toll-like receptors (TLRs), which are evolutionarily considered molecules that are expressed on the cell surface of pathogens, such as lipopolysaccharides (LPS) or bacterial flagellin. The activation of the TLRs leads to destruction of the pathogen and the release of inflammatory cytokines, which recruit nearby immune cells and help to activate the adaptive immune system. Although the cells of the innate immune system have traditionally been thought to be spared the effects of immunosenescence, there is increasing evidence that there are several age related changes in the function of the innate immune system. Studies have shown that cytokine and chemokine signaling networks are altered with increasing age and these changes likely contribute to the increased susceptibility to sepsis seen in older adults.[19]

Neutrophils are the predominant phagocytes circulating in blood and these help to clear bacterial and fungal infections. Although the overall number of neutrophils and their chemotactic ability remains intact in old age, studies of aged neutrophils show a decreased response to priming and an increased rate of apoptosis.[20] Also, neutrophils develop decreased phagocytic activity that is important to eradicate *E. coli* and *Staphylococcus aureus* by opsonization.[21]

Monocytes and macrophages function as phagocytes of microbes and are important APCs that initiate the inflammatory response. Although the absolute number of monocytes and macrophages remain stable as we age, the phagocytic function and intracellular killing ability of these cells is reduced in older adults.[21] Furthermore, there are age-related defects in TLR activation, likely related to reduced sensitivity to LPS antigens and the cytokine production by the macrophages is reduced in older adults.[19,21] DCs are important in the cross talk between the innate and adaptive immune system. These cells appear to have decreased cytokine expression in aging mice infected with herpes virus.[22,23] NK cells have also been found to have waning function with age, including decreased cytotoxicity and cytokine expression.[21,23] These changes in the immune system has been a major focus in studies that attempted to understand the role of immunosenescence in increased susceptibility to sepsis and the high morbidity and mortality after sepsis.

3.5. *Adaptive immunity*

The adaptive immune response differs from the innate immunity in the ability to form an immunologic memory. The predominant cells of the adaptive immune system are *T* and *B* cells. *T* cells or thymus-derived lymphocytes, participate in the activation of immune cells and the cell-mediated destruction of infected cells. The *B* cells are derived from the bone marrow and they produce antibodies that attack foreign antigens. Both of these classes of lymphocytes are activated by antigens initially displayed by the APCs of the innate immune system.[7,11] In comparison to the innate immune response, the adaptive immune response is significantly impaired with increasing age.[24] For example, cell-mediated immune responses are diminished as are elements of the humoral immunity.[19,25] The cell-mediated immune responses are profoundly diminished, with CD8+ cells being more affected than CD4+ cells.[19,25] The *B* cell responses and other elements of humoral immunity are also affected by age.[19] The *T* cells in elderly patients generate less IL-2 and they have limited proliferative capacity and impaired signal transduction after engagement with APCs, compared with *T* cells in younger patients.[26] This explains the markedly increased risk of invasive intracellular pathogens, such as West Nile virus and *Listeria monocytogenes* in older adults.[24] The diminished ability of *T* and *B* cells to generate an immune response to new antigens with age is supported epidemiologically as older adults are often the first to be infected with new pathogens, such as West Nile virus.[27] The *T* and *B* cell immunosenescence also has implications on vaccine efficacy in adults at the extremes of age.[28,29] Regardless, older adults are still able to respond appropriately to new antigens and vaccines are an essential preventative measure in older adults, as we would discuss below.

4. Conceptual Model

Several models have been suggested to describe the increased susceptibility and poor outcomes of sepsis in older adults.

4.1. *Cytokine dysregulation and chronic inflammation*

Cytokines are a diverse group of non-antibody proteins released by the immune system to coordinate the migration and activation of immune cells. Studies on age-related cytokine dysregulation have yielded contradictory results. However, there is evidence for alterations in *T* cell and polymorphonuclear cell signaling as an underlying cause of the dysregulation.[30] Circulating levels of various cytokines are higher in older adults, especially IL-6.[31] This phenomenon has been referred to as "inflamm-aging" and has been correlated with chronic disease and functional decline in older adults.[30] The reason for chronic inflammation in older adults is poorly understood. Chronic subclinical infections have been hypothesized to contribute to increased inflammation.

Studies in animal models of pneumonia and in humans suggest that chronic inflammation may increase susceptibility to pneumonia. For instance, increased circulating TNF levels may have a priming effect, it leads to dysfunction of the TLR receptors and increases the translocation of bacteria in the lung.[32]

Despite having similar inflammatory profiles compared to their younger peers at admission for sepsis, older adults had higher circulating IL-6 levels at hospital discharge.[7] Chronic inflammation has been suggested to play a role in dementia and cardiovascular disease.[31] The persistent inflammation after sepsis may accelerate these chronic diseases and worsen long-term outcomes of sepsis patients. Thus, inflamm-aging may play an important role in both susceptibility and long-term outcomes of sepsis in older adults.

4.2. *Immunosuppression*

An alternative model suggests that poor outcomes after sepsis in older adults may be due to immunosuppression or immunoparalysis rather than a hyper inflammatory immune response. Immunsuppression is a complex phenomenon and may be worsening of the adaptive changes observed with aging. It is characterized by increased *T* cell apoptosis, reduced proliferation and increased *T*-cell suppressor activity, reduced HLA-DR expression and antigen presentation by myeloid cells, increased reactive oxygen species and nitric oxide production and reduced *exvivo* cytokine production.[33] These changes may delay the resolution of the primary infection and increase the risk of secondary infections in patients with sepsis; the later may worsen both short and long-term outcomes. Whether immunosuppression is more common in older adults during severe sepsis is unclear. Several molecular pathways, including immune checkpoint proteins, such as CTLA-4 and programmed death (PD)-1 receptor and its ligand, PD-L1, may play a role.[34] Thus, the abnormalities in the adaptive immune system may increase susceptibility to sepsis, increase the risk of organ dysfunction and lead to poor outcomes.

5. Clinical Presentation

The elderly patients routinely present with atypical symptoms that make the prompt and accurate diagnosis of an infection difficult. These patients have a tendency to under report or not report symptoms [35], or have non-specific symptoms, which may lead to delays in treatment.[36] For instance, altered mental status (delirium, somnolence and coma) is common in acutely ill older persons and does not necessarily herald a neurological infection; likewise tachypnea does not always indicate a respiratory infection.[37] Other non-specific signs of sepsis in older adults include anorexia, malaise, falls, urinary incontinence and generalized weakness.[36]

Although fever is a classic sign of infection in most patients, studies examining the clinical manifestations of sepsis in older adults have consistently shown that they are less likely to develop fever. For instance, in a study examining bacteremic patients, 13% of patients >65 years old remained afebrile despite bacteremia, while only 4% of younger patients were found to be afebrile.[37] Furthermore, patients >80 years of age were found to have lower temperatures as compared to those 60–79 years.[38] The elderly experience a noticeable change in temperature from baseline when infected, but the temperature in these patients often does not reach the fever thresholds used in clinical care.[39] This atypical mode of presentation exhibited by older adults often poses a diagnostic challenge and further threatens the ability to diagnose sepsis in a timely manner.

Older patients are more likely than their younger counterparts to have gram-negative infections. For instance, older adults presenting with community-acquired bacteremia are more likely to have *E. coli* as the pathogen as compared to younger adults who are more likely to have *S. aureus*.

The increase in susceptibility, differences in presentation patterns and clinical course, and poor prognostic patterns, including altered immune responses contribute to poorer outcomes seen in older adults. This brings to fore the importance of prevention, early diagnosis and treatment.

6. Pneumonia as a Common Cause of Severe Sepsis

CAP is the fifth leading cause of death in people over the age of 65 years in the United States and an estimated 60,000 die annually.[40] Many of the factors discussed above are important for pneumonia and these factors explain the high incidence and mortality due to pneumonia in older adults.

6.1. *Mechanisms*

The risk factors for the development of pneumonia can be broadly classified into factors that alter host defenses and factors that increase the exposure to bacteria. Age-related effects on pulmonary host defenses include impairments of the mechanical barriers, phagocytic activity and humoral and *T* cell immunity. [41] Older people have less efficient mucocilliary clearance [42], swallowing disorders, aspiration of gastric and oropharyngeal contents [43] and malnutrition.[44] Other independent risk factors for pneumonia include chronic lung, heart and kidney diseases, weight loss, poor functional status, previous history of pneumonia hospitalization, diabetes mellitus, immunosuppression, excess alcohol intake and smoking.[45–48]

Both silent and overt aspiration of oropharyngeal or gastric contents may be an important risk factor for both community-acquired and healthcare associated pneumonia in older people.[49]

The incidence of aspiration increases with impairment of the gag reflex, alteration in level of consciousness, use of nasogastric tubes and endotracheal tubes, and presence of esophageal diseases.[50,51] While some degree of aspiration of gastric and oropharyngeal contents is common in all adults, the impaired immune system in older individuals increases their risk of developing a pneumonia.

Inhalation is another common mechanism of particular importance with legionella and mycobacterium tuberculosis infections. Though less common than aspiration, it is probably an important mechanism in the development of pneumonia. Other mechanisms include hematogenous dissemination, invasion from infections in contiguous structures, such as the pleura or sub diaphragmatic space, direct inoculation after a procedure (e.g. surgery mechanical ventilation) and finally reactivation of pathogens (e.g. *Mycobacterium tuberculosis, Pneumocystis Jiroveci* and cytomegalovirus).

6.2. *Etiology*

Pneumonia is classically describes as being either community or hospital acquired. In 2005, the American Thoracic Society/Infectious Disease Society of America (ATS/IDSA) guidelines suggested a new category of pneumonia called healthcare-associated pneumonia (HCAP).[52] This entity included patients with pneumonia who have recent contact with health care systems, including hospitalization in the last 90 days, residence in NH or LTCFs, recent intravenous antibiotic use, or history of chronic hemodialysis. Thus, hospital-acquired pneumonia (HAP) is a subset of HCAP.

The causative organisms differ in frequency in CAP and HCAP. An infectious etiology was identified in approximately 40% of CAP cases and the frequency did not differ across different age groups.[54] More than 1 etiology was identified in less than 5% of cases. The most common cause of CAP in older adults was viral infection, including human rhinovirus, influenza A/B, human metapneumovirus, respiratory syncytial virus, parainfluenza virus, coronovirus, and adenovirus. *Streptococcus pneumoniae* was the most common bacterial infection (8% of cases in adults over 65 years) and *Staphylococcus aureus* and Enterobacteriaceae accounted for a small proportion of cases (<2%

of cases in adults over 65 years). A typical organisms, such as Mycoplasma and Legionella, were less common compared to younger adults and accounted for 1% of cases.[54,55] The gram-negative enteric bacilli and *P. aeruginosa* appear to be more important etiologic agents in older patients with chronic diseases.[56] Additionally, pneumonia due to gram-negative organisms appears to be more severe, and these patients were more likely to require admission to the ICU.[56]

Unlike CAP, HCAP and HAP have similar etiologic patterns with a higher incidence of multi drug-resistant (MDR) bacteria. The etiologic agents in these cases include *P. aeruginosa,* Enterobactereciae, or methicillin-resistant *S. aureus* (MRSA).[57] The identification of causative agents in the elderly remains a challenge.[58] The commons reasons include difficulty obtaining sputum samples from the patient and limitations of current microbiologic techniques. Additionally, these patients have a high rate of bacterial colonization in the oropharynx, which makes it challenging to distinguish causative pathogens from colonized organisms.

6.3. *Prognostic factors*

Over the years, several scoring systems have been developed either to guide treatment or to predict outcomes in patients with CAP. These scores, such as the Pneumonia severity index (PSI) and the CURB-65,[59,60] emphasize age and higher burden of chronic diseases as poor prognostic factors. Other scores include SMART-COP, IDS/S, SCAP, CORB, REA-ICU and CURXO-80. The clinical role of these scores has been studied extensively.[61,62] Biomarkers, such as Creactive protein level, procalcitonin level, proadrenomedullin and natriuretic peptide have been explored to either independently prognosticate or improve the performance of clinical risk prediction scores in patients with CAP. The value of these biomarkers is unclear in the elderly.

6.4. *Diagnosis and management*

The diagnostic work up includes assessment of disease severity and identification of causative organism using sputum microscopy, imaging and radiography. The cornerstone of management is early diagnosis and therapy targeting potential organisms as judged by patient risk factors. Early antibiotics and resuscitation is key.

7. Long Term Outcomes

Traditional measurements of success in the care of patients with sepsis has been to reduce short-term morbidity and mortality, but it has become clear that severe sepsis survivorship is complex with morbidity and mortality continuing beyond the traditional 90 days used in studies. Patients with severe sepsis have ongoing mortality for several months after the initial hospitalization. For instance, the one-year mortality for severe sepsis patients who survive the first three months is 40%.[63,64] These studies largely focused on patients over 65 years of age. While it seems intuitive that older patients have a higher chronic disease burden and are therefore more likely to incur higher morbidity and mortality, several studies have shown that the increased long-term mortality is independent of the pre-infection health status.[64,65] The reasons for this high long-term mortality are poorly understood. Furthermore, there is increasing evidence that the adverse long-term outcomes are not limited to increased mortality. Severe sepsis may worsen chronic disease burden by both unmasking pre-existing subclinical disease and may increase the risk of emergence of new health conditions. This relationship is thought to be bidirectional and has been shown in common chronic diseases, such as dementia and cardiovascular disease. [66,67] For instance, individuals with heart disease are at higher risk of hospitalization for pneumonia and once hospitalized, they are at increased risk of a cardiovascular event.[68] Similarly, a severe sepsis hospitalization is associated with increased risk of long-term cognitive impairment and functional disability, but patients with pre-existing cognitive impairment are also at risk for severe sepsis.[65] These findings have important implications to understand mechanisms underlying the complex interplay between chronic diseases and infection and for the management of these patients.

8. Preventive and Therapeutic Strategies

Infection control programs play a vital role in the early identification of outbreaks in LTCFs and preventing antimicrobial resistance. Because older patients are frequently exposed to infections, implementation of infection control strategies is fundamental to the prevention of sepsis in this population. The infection control programs include strategies to minimize use of indwelling catheters, disinfection of premises, appropriate use of personal protective equipment and early recognition of ongoing infections.

Widespread vaccination is another effective strategy against infectious diseases. Across all age groups vaccines are the most effective means of preventing morbidity and mortality due to infectious diseases.[18] The increased vulnerability to infection in the elderly makes them an important target population for vaccination. In older adults the CDC recommends vaccination against influenza, pneumococcal disease, herpes zoster, diphtheria, pertussis and tetanus (table X). Influenza and pneumococcal vaccines will go a long way towards reducing the incidence of severe pneumonia in the elderly. Vaccines may not elicit an adequate immunologic response in older adults due to immunosenescence and a higher vaccine dose may be beneficial.[69]

There is increasing evidence that severe sepsis survivors have increased burden of chronic disease.[65,66] The complexity of survivorship leads to increased health care utilization possibly as a result of recurrent infectious processes, cardiovascular events and related health conditions.[70] In light of this, it seems prudent to suggest aggressive post discharge monitoring with provision of required supportive care, including physical and occupational therapy, follow-up primary care visits, tight control of cardiovascular risk factors and palliative and supportive care. The effect of these interventions on outcomes is unclear.

9. Conclusion

Pneumonia and severe sepsis are major public health problems in the elderly. Innate and adaptive immune abnormalities may explain increased susceptibility to infections and severe sepsis. There have been significant improvements in the care of severe sepsis patients over the last decade leading to increased survivorship. Ways to improve long-term outcomes for severe sepsis survivors must be explored and adopted.

References

1. Centers for Disease Control and Prevention (2011). 10 leading causes of death by age group, United States . Office of statistics and programming, National Center for Injury Prevention and Control, CDC WISQARS.
2. Mayr FB, Yende S, Angus DC. (2014) Epidemiology of severe sepsis. *Virulence* **5**: 4–11.
3. Martin GS, Mannino DM, Moss M. (2006) The effect of age on the development and outcome of adult sepsis. *Crit Care Med* **34**: 15–21.
4. Dombrovskiy VY, Martin AA, Sunderram J *et al.* (2007) Rapid increase in hospitalization and mortality rates for severe sepsis in the United States: A trend analysis from 1993 to 2003. *Crit Care Med* **35**: 1244–1250.
5. Russo CA, Elixhauser A. (2006). Hospitalizations in the elderly population, 2003: Statistical brief #6. In *Healthcare Cost and Utilization Project (HCUP) Statistical Briefs.* Rockville MD.
6. Kellum JA, Kong L, Fink MP *et al.* (2007) Understanding the inflammatory cytokine response in pneumonia and sepsis: Results of the genetic and inflammatory markers of sepsis (GenIMS) Study. *Arch Intern Med* **167**: 1655–1663.
7. Kale S, Yende S, Kong L *et al.* (2010) The effects of age on inflammatory and coagulation-fibrinolysis response in patients hospitalized for pneumonia. *PloS one* **5**: e13852.
8. Sogaard M, Schonheyder HC, Riis A *et al.* (2008) Short-term mortality in relation to age and comorbidity in older adults with community-acquired bacteremia: A population-based cohort study. *J Am Geriatr Soc* **56**: 1593–1600.
9. Kale SS, Yende S. (2011) Effects of Aging on Inflammation and Hemostasis through the continuum of critical illness. *Aging Dis* **2**: 501–511.
10. Rajagopalan S. (2005) Serious infections in elderly patients with diabetes mellitus. *Clin Infect Dis* **40**: 990–996.

11. Girard TD, Ely EW. (2007) Bacteremia and sepsis in older adults. *Clin Geriatr Med* **23**: 633–647.
12. Strausbaugh LJ, Joseph CL. (2000) The burden of infection in long-term care. *Infect Control Hosp Epidemiol* **21**: 674–679.
13. Rajagopalan S, Yoshikawa TT. (2001) Antimicrobial therapy in the elderly. *Med Clin North Am* **85**: 133–147.
14. Nicolle LE. (2012) Antimicrobial resistance in long-term care facilities. *Future Microbiol* **7**: 171–174.
15. Wiener J, Quinn JP, Bradford PA *et al.* (1999) Multiple antibiotic-resistant Klebsiella and Escherichia coli in nursing homes. *JAMA* **281**: 517–523.
16. Opal SM, Girard TD, Ely EW. (2005) The immunopathogenesis of sepsis in elderly patients. *Clin Infect Dis* **41**: S504–S512.
17. Frasca D, Blomberg BB. (2011) Aging affects human B cell responses. *J Clin Immunol* **31**: 430–435.
18. Weinberger B, Grubeck-Loebenstein B. (2012) Vaccines for the elderly. *Clin Microbiol Infect* **18** : 100–108.
19. Weksler ME, Goodhardt M, Szabo P. (2002) The effect of age on B cell development and humoral immunity. *Springer Semin Immunopathol* **24**: 35–52.
20. Gomez CR, Nomellini V, Faunce DE *et al.* (2008) Innate immunity and aging. *Exp Gerontol* **43**: 718–728.
21. Weiskopf D, Weinberger B, Grubeck-Loebenstein B. (2009) The aging of the immune system. *Transplant Int* **22**: 1041–1050.
22. Stout-Delgado HW, Yang X, Walker WE *et al.* (2008) Aging impairs IFN regulatory factor 7 up-regulation in plasmacytoid dendritic cells during TLR9 activation. *J Immunol* **181**: 6747–6756.
23. Panda A, Arjona A, Sapey E *et al.* (2009) Human innate immunosenescence: Causes and consequences for immunity in old age. *Trends Immunol* **30**: 325–333.
24. Grubeck-Loebenstein B, Wick G. (2002) The aging of the immune system. *Adv Immunol* **80**: 243–284.
25. Fry AM, Shay DK, Holman RC *et al.* (2005) Trends in hospitalizations for pneumonia among persons aged 65 years or older in the United States, 1988–2002. *JAMA* **294**: 2712–2719.
26. Douek DC, Koup RA. (2000) Evidence for thymic function in the elderly. *Vaccine* **18**: 1638–1641.
27. Nash D, Mostashari F, Fine A *et al.* (2001) The outbreak of West Nile virus infection in the New York City area in 1999. *New Engl J Med* **344**: 1807–1814.

28. Aspinall R, Del Giudice G, Effros RB *et al.* (2007) Challenges for vaccination in the elderly. *Immunity Ageing* **4**: 9.
29. Grubeck-Loebenstein B, Della Bella S, Iorio AM *et al.* (2009) Immunosenescence and vaccine failure in the elderly. *Aging Clin Exp Res* **21**: 201–209.
30. Fulop T, Le Page A, Fortin C *et al.* (2014) Cellular signaling in the aging immune system. *Curr Opin Immunol* **29**: 105–111.
31. Krabbe KS, Pedersen M, Bruunsgaard H. (2004) Inflammatory mediators in the elderly. *Exp Gerontol* **39**: 687–699.
32. Hinojosa E, Boyd AR, Orihuela CJ. (2009) Age-associated inflammation and toll-like receptor dysfunction prime the lungs for pneumococcal pneumonia. *J Infect Dis* **200**: 546–554.
33. Hotchkiss RS, Monneret G, Payen D. (2013) Sepsis-induced immunosuppression: From cellular dysfunctions to immunotherapy. *Nat Revs. Immunol* **13**: 862–874.
34. Hotchkiss RS, Moldawer LL. (2014) Parallels between cancer and infectious disease. *New Engl J Med* **371**: 380–383.
35. Beloosesky Y, Weiss A, Hershkovitz A *et al.* (2000) Atypical illness presentation in the elderly. *IMAJ* **2**: 540–543.
36. Chassagne P, Perol MB, Doucet J *et al.* (1996) Is presentation of bacteremia in the elderly the same as in younger patients? *Am J Med* **100**: 65–70.
37. Gleckman R, Hibert D. (1982) Afebrile bacteremia. A phenomenon in geriatric patients. *JAMA* **248**: 1478–1481.
38. Leibovici L, Pitlik SD, Konisberger H *et al.* (1993) Bloodstream infections in patients older than eighty years. *Age Ageing* **22**: 431–442.
39. Castle SC, Norman DC, Yeh M *et al.* (1991) Fever response in elderly nursing home residents: Are the older truly colder? *J Am Geriatr Soc* **39**: 853–857.
40. Loeb M. (2004) Pneumonia in the elderly. *Curr Opin Infect Dis* **17**: 127–130.
41. Meyer KC. (2001) The role of immunity in susceptibility to respiratory infection in the aging lung. *Respir Physiol* **128**: 23–31.
42. Ho JC, Chan KN, Hu W *et al.* (2001) The effect of aging on nasal mucociliary clearance, beat frequency, and ultrastructure of respiratory cilia. *Am J Respir Crit Care Med* **163**: 983–988.
43. Marik PE, Kaplan D. (2003) Aspiration pneumonia and dysphagia in the elderly. *Chest* **124**: 328–336.
44. Riquelme R, Torres A, El-Ebiary M *et al.* (1996) Community-acquired pneumonia in the elderly: A multivariate analysis of risk and prognostic factors. *Am J Respir Crit Care Med* **154**: 1450–1455.

45. Jackson ML, Nelson JC, Jackson LA. (2009) Risk factors for community-acquired pneumonia in immunocompetent seniors. *J Am Geriatr Soc* **57**: 882–888.
46. Vila-Corcoles A, Ochoa-Gondar O, Rodriguez-Blanco T *et al.* (2009) Epidemiology of community-acquired pneumonia in older adults: A population-based study. *Respir Med* **103**: 309–316.
47. Skull SA, Andrews RM, Byrnes GB *et al.* (2009) Hospitalized community-acquired pneumonia in the elderly: An Australian case-cohort study. *Epidemiol Infect* **137**: 194–202.
48. Farr BM, Woodhead MA, Macfarlane JT *et al.* (2000) Risk factors for community-acquired pneumonia diagnosed by general practitioners in the community. *Respir Medicine* **94**: 422–427.
49. Yamaya M, Yanai M, Ohrui T *et al.* (2001) Interventions to prevent pneumonia among older adults. *J Am Geriatr Soc* **49**: 85–90.
50. Huxley EJ, Viroslav J, Gray WR *et al.* (1978) Pharyngeal aspiration in normal adults and patients with depressed consciousness. *Am J Med* **64**: 564–568.
51. Craven DE, Steger KA, Barber TW. (1991) Preventing nosocomial pneumonia: State-of-the-art and perspectives for the 1990s. *Am J Med* **91**: 44S–53S.
52. American Thoracic Society; Infectious Diseases Society of America. Guidelines for the management of adults with hospital-acquired, ventilator-associated, and healthcare-associated pneumonia. *Am J Respir Crit Care Med* **2005 Feb 15; 171**(4): 388–416.
53. Jokinen C, Heiskanen L, Juvonen H *et al.* (2001) Microbial etiology of community-acquired pneumonia in the adult population of 4 municipalities in eastern Finland. *Clin Infect Dis* **32**: 1141–1154.
54. Jain S, Self WH, Wunderink RG *et al.* (2015) Community-Acquired pneumonia requiring hospitalization among U.S. adults. *N Engl J Med.* 373(5): 415–427; doi: 10.1056/NEJMoa1500245.
55. Mandell LA. (2009) Severe community-acquired pneumonia (CAP) and the infectious diseases society of America/American Thoracic Society CAP guidelines prediction rule: Validated or not. *Clin Infect Dis* **48**: 386–388.
56. Ruiz M, Ewig S, Marcos MA *et al.* (1999) Etiology of community-acquired pneumonia: Impact of age, comorbidity, and severity. *Am J Respir Crit Care Med* **160**: 397–405.

57. Falcone M, Blasi F, Menichetti F *et al.* (2012) Pneumonia in frail older patients: An up to date. *Intern Emerg Med* **7**: 415–424.
58. Venkatesan P, Gladman J, Macfarlane JT *et al.* (1990) A hospital study of community acquired pneumonia in the elderly. *Thorax* **45**: 254–258.
59. Fine MJ, Auble TE, Yealy DM *et al.* (1997) A prediction rule to identify low-risk patients with community-acquired pneumonia. *New Engl J Med* **336**: 243–250.
60. Lim WS, van der Eerden MM, Laing R *et al.* (2003) Defining community acquired pneumonia severity on presentation to hospital: An international derivation and validation study. *Thorax* **58**: 377–382.
61. Naito T, Suda T, Yasuda K *et al.* (2006) A validation and potential modification of the pneumonia severity index in elderly patients with community-acquired pneumonia. *J Am Geriatr Soc* **54**: 1212–1219.
62. Lim WS, Macfarlane JT. (2001) Defining prognostic factors in the elderly with community acquired pneumonia: A case controlled study of patients aged > or = 75 yrs. *Euro Respir J* **17**: 200–205.
63. Winters BD, Eberlein M, Leung J *et al.* (2010) Long-term mortality and quality of life in sepsis: A systematic review. *Crit Care Med* **38**: 1276–1283.
64. Yende S, Angus DC, Ali IS *et al.* (2007) Influence of Comorbid Conditions on Long-Term Mortality After Pneumonia in Older People. *J Am Geriatr Soc* **55**: 518–525.
65. Iwashyna TJ, Ely EW, Smith DM *et al.* (2010) Long-term cognitive impairment and functional disability among survivors of severe sepsis. *JAMA* **304**: 1787–1794.
66. Yende S, Iwashyna TJ, Angus DC. (2014) Interplay between sepsis and chronic health. *Trends Mol Med* **20**: 234–238.
67. Shah FA, Pike F, Alvarez K *et al.* (2013) Bidirectional relationship between cognitive function and pneumonia. *Am J Respir Crit Care Med* **188**: 586–592.
68. Corrales-Medina VF, Musher DM, Shachkina S *et al.* (2013) Acute pneumonia and the cardiovascular system. *Lancet* **381**: 496–505.
69. Fuoco MA. (2014). *High-dose flu vaccine found more effective for the elderly.* Available at http://www.post-gazette.com/news/health/2014/12/18/High-dose-flu-vaccine-found-more-effective-for-elderly/stories/201412170206.
70. Prescott HC, Langa KM, Liu V *et al.* (2014) Increased one-year health care utilization in survivors of severe sepsis. *Am J Respir Crit Care Med.*

Chapter 7
Sepsis and Acute Lung Injury in Aging

Anup Srivastava*, Yao Wong*, Shruti Erramilli*,
and Praveen Mannam*,†

1. Introduction

The world's population is growing and aging. Declining birth rates in the developing countries, combined with low birth rates in developed countries, are projected to increase the population of people over 65, so that by 2050 they will outnumber the population aged 0–4 by 2.5 times. The aging of the world population has immense implications for the health care system with increased burden of disease and health care costs. Aging is associated with increased susceptibility to sepsis and acute lung injury (ALI), and respiratory infections are the most common cause of sepsis in the elderly.[1] Lung is the major portal of entry for infectious pathogens in elderly. Lungs are the most common organs to fail in sepsis, and ALI likely contributes to other organ failure and leads to death. Hence understanding the age related changes in sepsis and ALI will lead us to a better understanding of these lethal diseases.

* Pulmonary, Critical Care and Sleep Medicine, Department of Internal Medicine, Yale University School of Medicine. 333 Cedar Street, P.O. Box 208057, New Haven, Connecticut 06520-8057, USA.
† Corresponding author: praveen.mannam@yale.edu

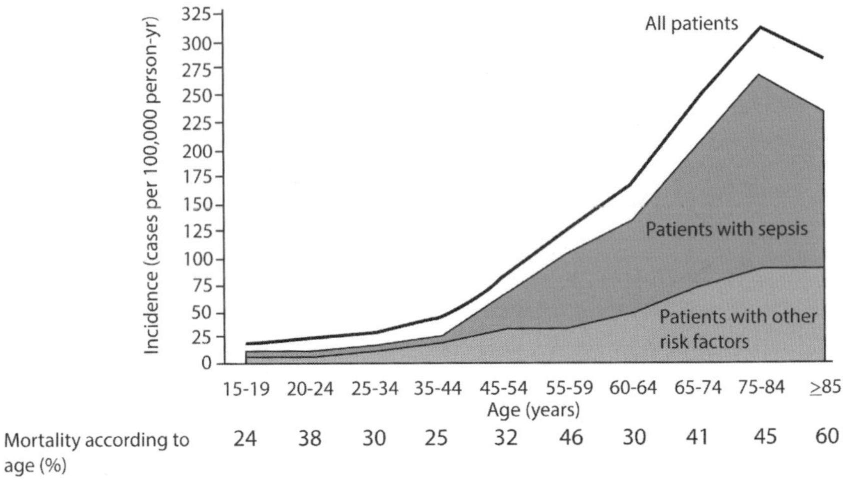

Fig 1. Sepsis is the Major Cause of Acute Lung Injury in Elderly.
Age- and Risk-Specific Incidence of and Age-Specific Mortality from ALI. (Adapted from Ref. 2.)

As people age the incidence and mortality of lung injury rapidly increases. It appears that sepsis is the leading driver of age related incidence of ALI. The incidence of sepsis increases in elderly and this raise parallels the increase in incidence of sepsis to a remarkable degree[2] (Fig. 1). Since there is such as strong association between sepsis and development of ALI in the elderly we will discuss them together in this chapter. We will first analyze the causes of increased susceptibility to sepsis and lung injury in the elderly and then discuss the underlying pathophysiologic abnormalities that predispose the elderly to increased sepsis, ALI and finally consider the long-term sequelae of sepsis and ALI in the elderly population.

2. Epidemiology of Sepsis and ALI in the Elderly

Sepsis can be considered a disease of the aged, with 65% of sepsis cases occurring in patients older than 65 years and 80% of deaths due to sepsis are in this age group.[1,3] Older patients are twice as likely to die of ALI compared with younger patients and have greater difficulty achieving liberation from the ventilator and being discharged from the intensive care unit.[4]

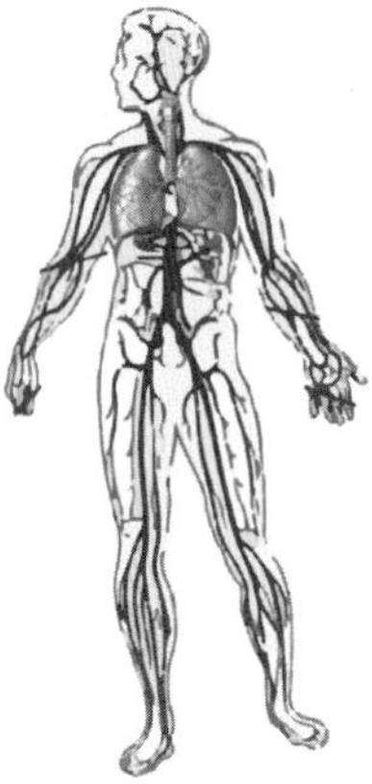

Fig 2. Risk Factor for Sepsis and Acute Lung Injury in Elderly.
The elderly are predisposed to developing infections and dying from sepsis and ALI because of various factors.

The elderly are more susceptible to developing infections and succumbing to sepsis and ALI because of a variety of factors including comorbid illnesses, exposure to instrumentation and procedures, immunosenescence, malnutrition, poor performance status, decline in cardiopulmonary reserve, and higher rates of withdrawal of support[2,5–7] (Fig. 2). Infections to which the aged are particularly vulnerable are lung related such as pneumonia, influenza and tuberculosis.[8] Paradoxically the patients at the extremes of age appear to have the lower incidence of ALI compared to patients in 60–80 years of age. Patients who live to be >80 years of age could have been selected for genetically protective mechanisms against ALI development.[9]

3. Physiologic Changes that Predispose to Sepsis and ALI in Elderly

The aging lung is associated with changes in the mechanics and normal physiologic mechanisms that predispose the elderly to increased susceptibility to infection and lung injury.[10] There is a diminished ability to respond adaptively to stress, which may be related to structural and physiologic changes that accompany aging.

These changes include (1) decreases in the ventilatory capacity secondary to alterations in the structure of the thoracic cage and muscle efficiency and (2) diminished capacity to clear mucus due to reduced cough strength and mucociliary function.[11]

The structure of the thoracic cavity is altered with age by narrowing of the intervertebral disk space causing kyphosis or curvature of the spine. Kyphosis decreases the space between the ribs and creates a smaller chest cavity.[12,13] In addition aging is associated with a decrease in muscle mass and function, a condition known as sarcopenia.[14] This can affect the diaphragm and reduces both ventilation and the expulsive, non-ventilatory force that is essential for airway clearance.[15,16] Aging is also associated with reduced inspiratory and expiratory respiratory muscle strength. It is estimated that overall muscle function in the body decreases by 2% annually with aging[17,18] and the decrease in muscle fiber strength can be as much as 20% by age 70.[19–21] Sarcopenia may occur due to multiple causes such as apoptosis, hormone changes associated with aging and mitochondrial dysfunction.[22,23] There is also evidence that the muscles of elderly individuals have a decline in oxidative phosphorylation and less mitochondrial adenosine triphosphate (ATP) reserves.[24] When an older person develops a lung infection he will not be able to meet the metabolic demands for oxygen due to decreased respiratory muscle strength and decreased cellular energy reserve, leading to an increased risk of respiratory failure.[25]

With aging there is a decreased ability to clear mucus from the lungs due to reduced cough strength and alterations in the body's ability to clear particles in the airways. The decrease in the strength of the inspiratory and expiratory respiratory muscles with aging reduces an individual's ability to generate the force required for an effective cough.[15,26] The mucociliary clearance refers to the action of ciliated cells along the upper and lower airway in clearing mucus and foreign particles out of the lungs.[27] In the elderly, ciliary dysfunction is associated with a decrease in clearance of particles from the lung.[28,29] Thus a combination of decreased ventilatory capacity and an inability to clear airway secretions make the elderly more prone for respiratory infections and lung failure.

4. Pathologic Processes Relevant to Elderly in Sepsis and ALI

Sepsis and ALI in the elderly are caused by interrelated mechanisms such as inflammation, apoptosis, mitochondrial dysfunction, oxidative stress, autophagy and proteostasis, coagulation abnormalities and endothelial dysfunction. These pathologic processes feed into each other and contribute to the high mortality and morbidity of sepsis and ALI in the older population (Fig. 3).

4.1. *Inflammatory and apoptotic responses*

Sepsis is a complex response to infection, which consists of an exaggerated systemic inflammatory response syndrome (SIRS). Increasingly it is recognized that there also exists an anti inflammatory response known as a "compensated anti-inflammatory response" (CARS).[30,31] It was thought that SIRS, the initial reaction to sepsis, is responsible for clearance of the offending infection. SIRS is followed by CARS, which brings the immune response to baseline

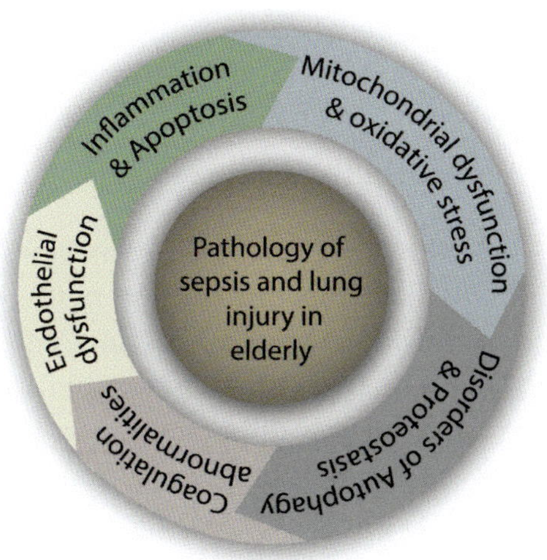

Fig 3. Pathologic Process Involved in Sepsis and Lung Injury in Elderly.
Sepsis and Acute Lung Injury in the Elderly are Caused by Interrelated Pathologic Processes.

without damage to the organism. However the temporal sequence of these two events is not well known. They are not mutually exclusive events and they may coexist at the same time during the septic response.[32] Aging is associated with a lethal combination of inappropriate inflammatory SIRS as well as an immunosuppressive CARS, resulting in an exaggerated susceptibility to sepsis.[33] Inoue S *et al.* used Klotho knockout mice, which are deficient in the *KL* gene. These mice are widely used as a model of accelerated aging. Klotho deficient mice subject to cecal ligation and puncture (CLP) showed worse survival with increased inflammatory cytokine release, release impaired bacterial clearance. They also showed increased apoptosis of lymphocytes, which is indicative of CARS.[34,35] Recent studies demonstrate a synergism between aging and sepsis in promoting apoptosis. There was higher splenic apoptosis and inflammatory response in older septic mice compared to WT mice.[49,50] Combination of infection and aging has been shown to induce a disproportionate increase in the apoptosis of rapidly dividing cells.[51] FasL is a type-II transmembrane protein that belongs to the tumor necrosis factor (TNF) family. The Fas/Fas-L pathway plays an role in lipopolysaccharide (LPS) induced accelerated splenic apoptosis and hyper inflammation in aged rats.[36] In contrast other investigators have found that aged mouse myeloid cells exhibited decreased phagocytosis, reactive oxygen species production, and chemotaxis.[37] Aged mice also had an attenuated cytokine response to the gram-negative respiratory pathogen, *Francisella novicida* when compared to young mice.[38]

Adipocytes in the white adipose tissue contribute to the inflammatory cytokine interleukin-6 (IL-6) production in the aged mice during systemic inflammation induced by LPS.[39] Sphingosine kinase-1 (Sphk-1) a proinflammatory enzyme present in neutrophils and macrophages contributes to age-related hyper inflammation in LPS model of sepsis by generation of TNFα.[40] The stress-mediated induction of interleukin-1β, interleukin-6, and interleukin-10 (IL-1β, IL-6, and IL-10) in the circulating blood tended to be higher with aging in both CLP and LPS models.[41] Aged animals had decreased survival from CLP and had increased plasma cytokines as compared with younger counterparts. In the face of similar CLP insult, aged mice could not be rescued with antibiotics, whereas young mice saw significant benefit.[42] The inflammatory cytokines and chemokines- TNFα, IL-1β, macrophage inflammatory protein-1α, macrophage inflammatory protein-2, and keratinocyte-derived chemokine were significantly higher in 65-week-old mice along with sustained neutrophilia when compared to 11-week-old mice at 72 hrs after LPS exposure.[43]

The p38 MAP kinase pathway (MAPK) appears to be particularly important in determining age related susceptibility to sepsis and lung injury. Activation of p38 and its upstream activator, MAP kinase kinase (MKK), peaked at 24 hrs after LPS and was sustained longer in aged mice[44] and it is known that MKK is a critical mediator of sepsis and lung injury.[45–47] The p38 MAPK was activated in epithelial cells and alveolar macrophages during lung aging with a corresponding increase in pro-inflammatory cytokines and decrease in antioxidant capacity.[48] Inhibition of the MKK-p38 pathway may offer therapeutic targets to reduce the incidence and mortality of sepsis and ALI in the elderly.

The lung appears to be particularly susceptible to the age related increases in inflammatory responses and the pulmonary environment becomes more inflammatory with increasing age. The hyper reactive systemic inflammatory response seen in aged individuals after LPS administration is accompanied by an exacerbated pulmonary inflammatory response, which may contribute to the higher mortality seen in the aged.[52] The lungs of old mice have elevated levels of proinflammatory cytokines and a resident population of highly activated pulmonary macrophages.[53] Aging is also associated with defects in various defense mechanisms and alterations in responses that lead to increased susceptibility to infection and development of lung injury. The enzyme heme oxygenase-1 (HO-1) is induced in the lung after stress and has a cytoprotective role against oxidant damage.[54] There are age-related defects in HO-1 induction in the whole lungs and in alveolar macrophages in response to LPS[55] indicating a mechanism by which aged lungs are more susceptible to injury.

Aging is also associated with worse outcomes after viral infections. Aged mice had a slower recovery, a prolonged period of morbidity and more persistent viral load in lung after influenza infection. Corresponding to the poor clearance of the virus from the lungs of aged mice, there was delayed activation of innate immune cells and detection of cytokines and chemokines in the supernatants of lung homogenates. This resulted in slower activation of the adaptive immune response and prolonged illness in aged animals.[56] In another study aged mice infected with influenza showed higher morbidity and higher necrosis of bronchiolar and alveolar epithelia.[57]

Stem cells are involved in resolution of lung injury. The best studied to date are bone marrow derived mesenchymal stem cells (MSCs) that appear to have immunomodulatory and reparative properties through paracrine secretion of factor or even transfer of mitochondria to injured cells. Engraftment and differentiation into lung cells does not appear to be a major factor in the action of MSCs in reducing ALI.[58,59] Strong pre-clinical data has led to initiation of Phase1 clinical studies using MSCs for treatment of ALI. Aging MSCs fail to protect against LPS induced lung injury because of impaired migration and anti-inflammatory response indicating the reason why the elderly are more susceptible to sepsis induced lung injury.[60]

4.2. *Mitochondrial dysfunction and oxidative stress*

Sepsis and lung injury may be viewed as mitochondrial disorders. Mitochondria are essential hubs of innate immune signaling and are thought to be mediators of inflammatory responses,[61–64] and the mitochondria are dysfunctional in patients with sepsis and lung injury.[65,66] The paradigm that organ failure in sepsis is due to failure of mitochondrial bioenergetics and ATP production is supported by recent studies.[67–69] Restoration of alveolar epithelial ATP through transfer of mitochondria from bone-marrow-derived stromal cells protected against LPS induced lung injury.[58] A study of the metabolome and proteome in septic patients found that mitochondrial functions such as the β oxidation and the citric acid cycle are major determinants of sepsis outcomes.[70] The plasma metabolome and lung transcriptome of monkeys infected with *E.Coli* infection showed that defects in β oxidation and mitochondrial metabolism lead to lung injury and death.[71] In addition dysfunctional mitochondria are sources of damage-associated molecular patterns (DAMPs) such as reactive oxygen species, mitochondrial transcription factor A (TFAM), ATP and mitochondrial DNA that initiate an inflammatory response further exacerbating organ injury.[64,72–74] Aged mice exhibit a higher degree of CLP sepsis-associated multiple organ dysfunction, tissue inflammation and oxidative stress. In addition bioenergetic analysis in isolated liver mitochondria from mice subjected to sham or CLP operation showed a significant worsening of sepsis-induced mitochondrial function in aged mice.[75] Reduced extracellular superoxide dismutase in combination with increased oxidative/nitrosative damage and altered cytoskeletal protein function due to tyrosine nitration may contribute to augmented lung injury in the aged with SIRS.[76]

The inflammasome is a multiprotein complex that regulates the release of pro-inflammatory cytokines such as IL-1β in response to pathogens and endogenous danger signals. The inflammasome is associated with ALI in humans and ventilator associated lung injury in mice.[77,78] We recently identified a protective role for PTEN-induced putative kinase 1 (Pink1, a mitochondria assoicated protein involved in mitophagy) and NLR Family, Pyrin Domain Containing 3 (NLRP3, a component of the inflammasome complex) against hyperoxic lung injury.[79] Since mitochondrial function regulates inflammasome activation, this pathway may be a target of therapies to reduce lung injury in aged.[61,80]

4.3. *Disorders of autophagy and proteostasis*

There is emerging evidence to suggest that impaired proteostasis in the lung is crucial for development of lung injury and may have implications for development of ALI in the elderly.[81–83] In a recent study of mice subjected to CLP and LPS induced lung injury the authors noted age related decrease in the proteasome expression, increase in ubiquitinated proteins and activation of the endoplasmic reticulum unfolded protein response (UPR). This indicates proteostasis imbalance, leading to augmented NF-κB mediated inflammation in sepsis and ALI.[81] In addition to the well-known endoplasmic reticulum UPR, it is now recognized that the mitochondria has a distinct UPR response (UPRmt) mediated by the transcription factor ATFS-1 and chaperones such as mitochondrial Hsp70 (mtHsp70) and Hsp60 among others.[84] This mechanism is responsible for maintaining mitochondrial integrity in face of stress and immune responses. Its role in the context of ALI is not well understood and would be an interesting avenue of research for therapies.

Autophagy is a process by which the cells remove misfolded or aggregated proteins and clear damaged organelles. The role of autophagy has also received considerable attention recently with a study showing that induction of autophagy in the lung prevents lung injury and multi organ failure. This study suggests that lung protection via autophagy is critical and likely important for sepsis treatment because it prevents failure of additional organs. These findings are relevant as the lung is the organ that often shows the first signs of dysfunction in septic patients and drives the failure of other target organs, particularly the kidney and the liver.[85] However in certain situations such as H5N1 infection, inhibition of autophagy may lead to amelioration of lung injury by reducing cell death.[86] The protective versus deleterious effect of autophagy modulation in the lung may be specific to the etiology of injury and there is a need for more studies to elucidate this role.

4.4. *Disorders of coagulation*

Older mice are more susceptible to CLP sepsis and LPS exposure[87] and showed higher physiologic derangements such as hypothermia, hypoglycemia, coagulation abnormalities and severe tissue damage compared to younger mice.[88,89] Protein C is a factor that regulates coagulation by arresting thrombin generation and subsequent fibrin formation. In aged mice the protein C activation is suppressed and contributes to enhanced coagulation and mortality in sepsis.[90,91] In humans use of recombinant activated protein C, Drotrecogin Alfa Activated (DrotAA), in the PROWESS trial showed higher 28 day survival in older >75 year patients (15.5% absolute reduction compared to 6.1% absolute risk reduction in the whole study). The authors also found reductions in mortality at 2-years and reduced morbidity, as assessed by vasopressor-, ventilator-, ICU-, and hospital-free days.

In addition, there is no evidence of increased bleeding risk in this elderly population.[92,93] A follow-up study (ADDRESS trial) showed that DrotAA is not effective in patients at low risk for sepsis-induced mortality, while it may still be effective in patients with high risk for sepsis induced mortality and the elderly.[94,95] DrotAA is off-market now but these results suggest that targeting coagulation pathways using other methods may be useful in elderly.

4.5. *Endothelial dysfunction*

Aging is associated with endothelial dysfunction even in the absence of extra stresses.[96,97] Given the importance of the endothelium in sepsis, it is not surprising that it may play an important role in the age related susceptibility to sepsis. In a recent study aged mice subject to CLP exhibited a higher degree of sepsis-associated multiple organ dysfunction syndrome (MODS), inflammation, oxidative stress and endothelial dysfunction.[75] Aging increases sensitivity of microvascular endothelial cells to oxidative stress and cellular damage induced by inflammatory factors present in the circulation during sepsis.[98]

5. Long Term Outcomes in Elderly Survivors of Sepsis and Lung Injury

A striking feature of the high incidence of sepsis and lung injury in elderly is the effect on long-term outcomes. Severe sepsis in older population is associated with profound and enduring new cognitive impairment and functional disability among survivors.[99,100] Given the high incidence of sepsis in patients 65 years and older, it is estimated that nearly 20,000 new cases/year of moderate to severe cognitive impairment in elderly may be attributed to sepsis.[99] In patients who survived ALI, cognitive changes have been reported in 25–55% of patients 1 year after discharge.[101–104] These defects appear to persist for long term and may be permanent. In a long term follow up study, 47% of ALI survivors showed neurocognitive defects 2 years after discharge[105] and 23.9% of survivors up to 6 years after discharge.[106]

The etiology of cognitive dysfunction induced by sepsis and ALI may be attributable to neuro-inflammation, perfusion abnormalities, and mitochondrial dysfunction.[107,108] In a mouse-based study, CLP sepsis induced severe hippocampal mitochondrial damage and injury associated with cognitive decline. A mitochondrial targeted antioxidant peptide reduced the intensity of mitochondrial dysfunction and cognitive dysfunction after sepsis, indicating a possible therapeutic mechanism.[109]

In addition to cognitive decline, sepsis and lung injury is associated with long-term sequelae of functional disability. This decline in function appears more prominent in the elderly. In a 5 year follow up of survivors of ALI even relatively young patients (median age of 44) had persistent exercise limitations and a reduced physical quality of life. However the elder patients in this study had slower rate of recovery than younger patients and neither group returned to normal predicted levels of physical function at 5 years.[110] Mechanical ventilation in elderly patients is associated with a greater increase in disability compared to non-ventilated patients.[111] The presence of pre existing disability in elderly predicts their post ICU status. Among older persons with critical illness, more than half died within 1 month or experienced significant functional decline over the following year, with particularly poor outcomes in those who had high levels of premorbid disability.[112] In this study, mechanical ventilation and shock are most significantly associated with 30 day and 1 year mortality among the elderly.

6. Summary

The aging of the world population has immense implications for the future of our health and heath resource utilization. Sepsis and ALI are major causes of mortality and morbidity in this group of patients. The causes of increased susceptibility to sepsis and ALI in the elderly are varied and multifactorial. They range from age related physiologic changes in lung function and immunity to pathologic processes that affect the elderly. Indeed the pathologic processes that are implicated in age related susceptibility to sepsis and ALI such as mitochondrial dysfunction, immune dysregulation, disorders of autophagy and proteostasis are known to underpin the aging process itself and many of the diseases of aging. Study of the mechanisms of sepsis and ALI in aging is still in its infancy, but a better understanding of these processes will not only help in development of effective therapies for these devastating illnesses, but also shed light on means to achieve healthy aging for all.

References

1. Martin GS, Mannino DM, Moss M. (2006) The effect of age on the development and outcome of adult sepsis. *Crit Care Med* **34**(1): 15–21.
2. Rubenfeld GD, Caldwell E, Peabody E *et al.* (2005) Incidence and outcomes of acute lung injury. *New Engl J Med* **353**(16): 1685–1693.
3. Angus DC, Linde-Zwirble WT, Lidicker J *et al.* (2001) Epidemiology of severe sepsis in the United States: Analysis of incidence, outcome, and associated costs of care. *Crit Care Med* **29**(7): 1303–1310.
4. Ely EW, Wheeler AP, Thompson BT *et al.* (2002) Recovery rate and prognosis in older persons who develop acute lung injury and the acute respiratory distress syndrome. *Ann Intern Med* **136**(1): 25–36.
5. Girard TD, Opal SM, Ely EW. (2005) Insights into severe sepsis in older patients: From epidemiology to evidence-based management. *Clin Infect Dis* **40**(5): 719–727.
6. Gee MH,Gottlieb JE, Albertine KH, *et al.* (1990) Physiology of aging related to outcome in the adult respiratory distress syndrome. *J Appl Physiol* **69**(3): 822–829.
7. Suchyta MR, Clemmer TP, Elliott CG *et al.* (1997) Increased mortality of older patients with acute respiratory distress syndrome. *Chest* **111**(5): 1334–1339.
8. Yoshikawa TT. (1981) Important infections in elderly persons. *West J Med* **135**(6): 441–445.
9. Johnston CJ, Rubenfeld GD, Hudson LD. (2003) Effect of age on the development of ARDS in trauma patients. *Chest* **124**(2): 653–659.
10. Krumpe PE, Knudson RJ, Parsons G *et al.*(1985) The aging respiratory system. *Clin Geriatr Med* **1**(1): 143–175.
11. Lowery EM, Brubaker AL, Kuhlmann EK *et al.* (2013) The aging lung. *Clin Interv Aging*, 8: 1489–1496.

12. Bartynski WS, Heller MT, Grahovac SZ. (2005) Severe thoracic kyphosis in the older patient in the absence of vertebral fracture: Association of extreme curve with age. *AJNR* 26(8): 2077–2085.
13. Sharma G, Goodwin J. (2006) Effect of aging on respiratory system physiology and immunology. *Clin Interv Aging* **1**(3): 253–260.
14. Mobasheri A, Mendes AF. (2013) Physiology and pathophysiology of musculoskeletal aging: Current research trends and future priorities. *Front Physiol* **4**: 73.
15. Tolep K, Higgins N, Muza S *et al.* (1995) Comparison of diaphragm strength between healthy adult elderly and young men. *Am J Respir Crit Care Med* **152**(2): 677–682.
16. Greising SM, Mantilla CB, Gorman BA *et al.* (2013) Diaphragm muscle sarcopenia in aging mice. *Exp Gerontol* **48**(9): 881–887.
17. Brown M, Hasser EM. (1996) Complexity of age-related change in skeletal muscle. *J Gerontol A Biol Sci Med Sci* **51**(2):B117–B123.
18. Arora NS, Rochester DF. (1982) Effect of body weight and muscularity on human diaphragm muscle mass, thickness, and area. *J Appl Physiol: Respir Environ Exercise Physiol* **52**(1): 64–70.
19. Chen HI, Kuo CS. (1989) Relationship between respiratory muscle function and age, sex, and other factors. *J Appl Physiol* **66**(2): 943–948.
20. Berry JK, Vitalo CA, Larson JL *et al.* (1996) Respiratory muscle strength in older adults. *Nursing Res* **45**(3): 154–159.
21. Faulkner JA, Brooks SV, Zerba E. (1990) Skeletal muscle weakness and fatigue in old age: Underlying mechanisms. *Annu Rev Gerontol Geriatr* **10**: 147–166.
22. Marcell TJ (2003) Sarcopenia: Causes, consequences, and preventions. *J Gerontol A Biol Sci Med Sci* **58**(10):M911–M916.
23. Calvani R, Joseph, A-M, Adhihetty PJ *et al.* (2013) Mitochondrial pathways in sarcopenia of aging and disuse muscle atrophy. *Biol Chem* **394**(3): 393–414.
24. Desler C, Hansen TL, Frederiksen JB *et al.* (2012) Is there a link between Mitochondrial Reserve Respiratory Capacity and Aging? *J Aging Res* **2012**: 192503.
25. Sevransky JE, Haponik, EF (2003) Respiratory failure in elderly patients. *Clin Geriatr Med* **19**(1): 205–224.
26. Kim J, Davenport P, Sapienza C. (2009) Effect of expiratory muscle strength training on elderly cough function. *Arch Gerontol Geriatr* **48**(3): 361–366.

27. Tilley AE, Walters MS, Shaykhiev R *et al.* (2015) Cilia dysfunction in lung disease. *Annu Rev Physiol* **77**: 379–406.
28. Svartengren M. (2005) Long-term clearance from small airways decreases with age. *Euro Respir J* **26**(4): 609–615.
29. Proença de O-M, Janaína BC, Heráclito G *et al.* (2013) Aging, Diabetes, and hypertension are associated with decreased nasal mucociliary clearance. *CHEST* **143**(4): 1091.
30. Bone RC. (1996) Sir Isaac Newton, sepsis, SIRS, and CARS. *Crit Care Med* **24**(7): 1125–1128.
31. Ward NS, Casserly B, Ayala A.(2008) The compensatory anti-inflammatory response syndrome (CARS) in critically ill patients. *Clin Chest Med* **29**(4): 617–625.
32. Buras JA, Holzmann B, Sitkovsky M. (2005) Animal models of sepsis: Setting the stage. *Nat Rev. Drug discovery* **4**(10): 854–865.
33. Nomellini V, Gomez CR, Gamelli, RL. (2009) Aging and animal models of systemic insult: trauma, burn, and sepsis. *Shock* **31**(1): 11–20.
34. Inoue S, Sato T, Suzuki-Utsunomiya, K *et al.* (2013) Sepsis-induced hypercytokinemia and lymphocyte apoptosis in aging-accelerated Klotho knockout mice. *Shock* **39**(3): 311–316.
35. Inoue S, Suzuki K, Komori Y *et al.* (2014) Persistent inflammation and T cell exhaustion in severe sepsis in the elderly. *Crit Care* **18**(3): R130.
36. Zhou M, Wu R, Dong W *et al.* (2010) Accelerated apoptosis contributes to aging-related hyperinflammation in endotoxemia. *Int J Mol Med* **25**(6): 929–935.
37. Nacionales DC, Gentile LF, Vanzant E *et al.* (2014) Aged mice are unable to mount an effective myeloid response to sepsis. *J Immunol* **19**(2): 612–622.
38. Mares CA, Sharma J, Ojeda SS *et al.* (2010) Attenuated response of aged mice to respiratory Francisella novicida is characterized by reduced cell death and absence of subsequent hypercytokinemia. *PloS one* **5**(11): e14088.
39. Starr ME, Evers BM, Saito H. (2009) Age-associated increase in cytokine production during systemic inflammation: Adipose tissue as a major source of IL-6. *J Gerontol A Biol Sci Med Sci* **64**(7): 723–730.
40. Lufrano M, Jacob A, Zhou M *et al.* (2013) Sphingosine kinase-1 mediates endotoxemia-induced hyperinflammation in aged animals. *Mol Med Rep* **8**(2): 645–649.

41. Saito H, Sherwood ER, Varma TK *et al.* (2003) Effects of aging on mortality, hypothermia, and cytokine induction in mice with endotoxemia or sepsis. *Mech Ageing Dev* **124**(10–12): 1047–1058.
42. Turnbull IR, Wlzorek JJ, Osborne D *et al.* (2003) Effects of age on mortality and antibiotic efficacy in cecal ligation and puncture. *Shock* **19**(4): 310–313.
43. Ito Y, Betsuyaku T, Nasuhara Y *et al.* (2007) Lipopolysaccharide-induced neutrophilic inflammation in the lungs differs with age. *Exp Lung Res* **33**(7): 375–384.
44. Ren X, Du H, Li Y *et al.* (2014) Age-related activation of MKK/p38/NF-κB signaling pathway in lung: From mouse to human. *Exp Gerontol* **57**: 29–40.
45. Mannam P, Zhang X, Shan P *et al.* (2013) Endothelial MKK3 is a critical mediator of lethal murine endotoxemia and acute lung injury. *J Immunology* **190**(3): 1264–1275.
46. Mannam P, Shinn AS, Srivastava A *et al.* (2014) MKK3 regulates mitochondrial biogenesis and mitophagy in sepsis-induced lung injury. *Am J Physiol. Lung cell Mol Physiol* **306**(7): L604–L619.
47. Srivastava A, Shinn, AS, Lee PJ *et al.* (2015) MKK3 mediates inflammatory response through modulation of mitochondrial function. *Free Radic Biol Med* 83: 139–148.
48. Li Z, Li J, Bu X *et al.* (2011) Age-induced augmentation of p38 MAPK phosphorylation in mouse lung. *Exp Gerontol* **46**(8): 694–702.
49. Turnbull IR, Buchman TG, Javadi P *et al.* (2004) Age disproportionately increases sepsis-induced apoptosis in the spleen and gut epithelium. *Shock* **22**(4): 364–368.
50. Turnbull IR, Clark AT, Stromberg PE *et al.* (2009) Effects of aging on the immunopathologic response to sepsis. *Crit Care Med* **37**(3): 1018–1023.
51. De Gaudio A, Rinaldi S, Chelazzi C *et al.* (2009) Pathophysiology of sepsis in the elderly: Clinical impact and therapeutic considerations. *Curr Drug Targets* **10**(1): 60–70.
52. Gomez CR, Hirano S, Cutro BT *et al.* (2007) Advanced age exacerbates the pulmonary inflammatory response after lipopolysaccharide exposure. *Crit Care Med* **35**(1): 246–251.
53. Canan CH, Gokhale NS, Carruthers B *et al.* (2014) Characterization of lung inflammation and its impact on macrophage function in aging. *J Leukoc Biol* **96**(3): 473–480.

54. Mannam P, Srivastava A, Sugunaraj JP *et al.* (2014) Oxidants in acute and chronic lung disease. *J Blood Lymph* **4**. pii: 1000128.
55. Ito Y, Betsuyaku T, Moriyama C *et al.* (2009) Aging affects lipopolysaccharide-induced upregulation of heme oxygenase-1 in the lungs and alveolar macrophages.' *Biogerontol* **10**(2): 173–180.
56. Toapanta FR, Ross TM. (2009) Impaired immune responses in the lungs of aged mice following influenza infection. *Respir Res* **10**(1): 112.
57. Yin Lu, Zheng D, Limmon GV *et al.* (2014) Aging exacerbates damage and delays repair of alveolar epithelia following influenza viral pneumonia. *Respir Res* **15**(1): 116.
58. Islam MN, Das SR, Emin MT *et al.* (2012) Mitochondrial transfer from bone-marrow-derived stromal cells to pulmonary alveoli protects against acute lung injury. *Nat Med* **18**(5): 759–765.
59. Lee JW, Fang X, Krasnodembskaya A *et al.* (2011) Concise review: Mesenchymal stem cells for acute lung injury: Role of paracrine soluble factors. *Stem cells* **29**(6): 913–919.
60. Bustos ML, Huleihel L, Kapetanaki MG *et al.* (2014) Aging mesenchymal stem cells fail to protect because of impaired migration and antiinflammatory response. *Am J Respir Crit Care Med* **189**(7): 787–798.
61. Kepp O, Galluzzi L, Kroemer G. (2011) Mitochondrial control of the NLRP3 inflammasome. *Nat Immunol* **12**(3): 199–200.
62. West AP, Shadel GS, Ghosh S. (2011) Mitochondria in innate immune responses. *Nat Rev. Immunol* **11**(6): 389–402.
63. West AP, Brodsky IE, Rahner C *et al.* (2011) TLR signalling augments macrophage bactericidal activity through mitochondrial ROS. *Nat* **472**(7344): 476–480.
64. Zhang Q, Raoof M, Chen Y *et al.* (2010) Circulating mitochondrial DAMPs cause inflammatory responses to injury. *Nat* **464**(7285): 104–107.
65. Brealey D, Brand M, Hargreaves I *et al.* (2002) Association between mitochondrial dysfunction and severity and outcome of septic shock. *Lancet* **360**(9328) : 219–223.
66. Carré JE, Orban J-C, Re L *et al.* (2010) Survival in critical illness is associated with early activation of mitochondrial biogenesis. *Am J Respir Crit Care Med* **182**(6): 745–751.
67. Belikova L, Lukaszewicz AC, Faivre V *et al.* (2007) Oxygen consumption of human peripheral blood mononuclear cells in severe human sepsis. *Crit Care Med* **35**(12): 2702–2708.

68. Japiassú AM, Santiago ASA, d'Avila JCP *et al.* (2011) Bioenergetic failure of human peripheral blood monocytes in patients with septic shock is mediated by reduced F1Fo adenosine-5'-triphosphate synthase activity. *Crit Care Med* **39**(5): 1056–1063.
69. Deutschman CS, Tracey KJ. (2014) Sepsis: Current dogma and new perspectives. *Immunity* **40**(4): 463–475.
70. Langley RJ, Tsalik EL, van Velkinburgh JC *et al.* (2013) An integrated clinico-metabolomic model improves prediction of death in sepsis. *Sci Transl Med* **5**(195): 195ra95.
71. Langley RJ, Tipper JL, Bruse S *et al.* (2014) Integrative 'omic analysis of experimental bacteremia identifies a metabolic signature that distinguishes human sepsis from SIRS. *Am J Respir Crit Care Med* **190**(4): 445–455.
72. Cauwels A, Rogge E, Vandendriessche B *et al.* (2014) Extracellular ATP drives systemic inflammation, tissue damage and mortality. *Cell Death Dis* **5**: e1102.
73. Chaung WW, Wu R, Ji Y *et al.* (2012) Mitochondrial transcription factor A is a proinflammatory mediator in hemorrhagic shock. *Int J Mol Med* **30**(1): 199–203.
74. Krysko DV, Agostinis P, Krysko O *et al.* (2011) Emerging role of damage-associated molecular patterns derived from mitochondria in inflammation. *Trends Immunol* **32**(4): 157–164.
75. Coletta C, Módis K, Oláh G *et al.* (2014) Endothelial dysfunction is a potential contributor to multiple organ failure and mortality in aged mice subjected to septic shock: Preclinical studies in a murine model of cecal ligation and puncture. *Crit* **18**(5): 511.
76. Starr ME, Ueda J, Yamamoto S *et al.* (2011) The effects of aging on pulmonary oxidative damage, protein nitration, and extracellular superoxide dismutase down-regulation during systemic inflammation. *Free Radical Biol Med* **50**(2): 371–380.
77. Dolinay T, Kim YS, Howrylak J *et al.* (2012) Inflammasome-regulated cytokines are critical mediators of acute lung injury. *Am J Respir Crit Care Med* **185**(11): 1225–1234.
78. Kuipers MT, Aslami H, Janczy JR *et al.* (2012) Ventilator-induced lung injury is mediated by the NLRP3 inflammasome. *Anesthesiol* **116**(5): 1104–1115.
79. Zhang Y, Sauler M, Shinn AS *et al.* (2014) Endothelial PINK1 mediates the protective effects of NLRP3 deficiency during lethal oxidant injury. *J Immunol* **192**(11): 5296–5304.

80. Nakahira K, Haspel JA, Rathinam VA *et al.* (2011) Autophagy proteins regulate innate immune responses by inhibiting the release of mitochondrial DNA mediated by the NALP3 inflammasome. *Nat Immunol* **12**(3): 222–230.
81. Bodas M, Min T, Vij N. (2010) Early-age-related changes in proteostasis augment immunopathogenesis of sepsis and acute lung injury. *PloS one* **5**(11): e15480.
82. Lozon TI, Altemeier WA. (2014) *CHOP Deficient Mice Have Augmented Lung Injury with Hyperoxia.', in C28. Extracellular Stress Regulatory Mechanisms And Disease.* American Thoracic Society International Conference Abstracts, American Thoracic Society, p. A4168.
83. Osorio F, Lambrecht B, Janssens S. (2013) The UPR and lung disease. *Semin Immunopathol* **35**(3): 293–306.
84. Pellegrino MW, Nargund AM, Haynes, CM (2013) Signaling the mitochondrial unfolded protein response. *Biochimica et biophysica acta* **1833**(2): 410–416.
85. Figueiredo N, Chora A, Raquel H *et al.* (2013) Anthracyclines induce DNA damage response-mediated protection against severe sepsis. *Immunity* **39**(5): 874–884.
86. Sun Y, Li C, Shu Y *et al.* (2012) Inhibition of autophagy ameliorates acute lung injury caused by avian influenza A H5N1 infection. *Sci Signal* **5**(212): 16.
87. Hyde SR, Stith RD McCallum RE. (1990) Mortality and bacteriology of sepsis following cecal ligation and puncture in aged mice. *Infect Immun* **58**(3): 619–624.
88. Knook DL, Brouwer A. (1989) Kupffer cells and the acute phase response: The effect of aging. *Immunol Invest* **18**(1–4): 339–350.
89. Hyde SR, McCallum RE. (1992) Lipopolysaccharide-tumor necrosis factor-glucocorticoid interactions during cecal ligation and puncture-induced sepsis in mature versus senescent mice. *Infect Immun* **60**(3): 976–982.
90. Starr ME, Ueda J, Takahashi H *et al.* (2010) Age-dependent vulnerability to endotoxemia is associated with reduction of anticoagulant factors activated protein C and thrombomodulin. *Blood* **115**(23): 4886–4893.
91. Starr ME, Takahashi H, Okamura D *et al.* (2015) Increased coagulation and suppressed generation of activated protein C in aged mice during intra-abdominal sepsis. *Am J Physiol* **308**(2): H83–H91.

92. Ely EW, Angus DC, Williams MD *et al.* (2003) Drotrecogin alfa (activated) treatment of older patients with severe sepsis. *Clin Infect Dis* **37**(2): 187–195.
93. Bernard GR, Vincent JL, Laterre PF *et al.* (2001) Efficacy and safety of recombinant human activated protein C for severe sepsis. *New Engl J Med* **44**(10): 699–709.
94. Abraham E, Laterre P-F, Garg R *et al.* (2005) Drotrecogin alfa (activated) for adults with severe sepsis and a low risk of death. *New Engl J Med* **353**(13): 1332–1341.
95. Alexander SL, Ernst FR (2006) Use of drotrecogin alfa (activated) in older patients with severe sepsis. *Pharmacotherapy* **26**(4): 533–538.
96. Herrera MD, Mingorance C, Rodríguez-Rodríguez R *et al.* (2010) Endothelial dysfunction and aging: An update. *Ageing Res Rev* **9**(2): 142–152.
97. Ungvari Z, Buffenstein R, Austad SN *et al.* (2008) Oxidative stress in vascular senescence: Lessons from successfully aging species. *Front Biosci* **13**: 5056–5070.
98. Tucsek Z, Gautam T, Sonntag WE *et al.* (2013) Aging exacerbates microvascular endothelial damage induced by circulating factors present in the serum of septic patients. *J Gerontol A Biol Sci Med Sci* **68**(6): 652–660.
99. Iwashyna TJ, Ely EW, Smith DM *et al.*(2010) Long-term cognitive impairment and functional disability among survivors of severe sepsis. *JAMA* **304**(16): 1787–1794.
100. Pandharipande PP, Girard TD, Jackson JC *et al.* (2013) Long-term cognitive impairment after critical illness. *New Engl J Med* **369**(14): 1306–1316.
101. Needham DM, Dinglas VD, Morris PE *et al.* (2013) Physical and cognitive performance of patients with acute lung injury 1 year after initial trophic versus full enteral feeding EDEN Trial follow-up. *Am J Respir Crit Care Med* **188**: 567–576.
102. Hopkins RO, Weaver LK, Pope D *et al.* (1999) Neuropsychological sequelae and impaired health status in survivors of severe acute respiratory distress syndrome. *Am J Respir Critical Care Med* **160**(1): 50–56.
103. Hopkins RO, Weaver LK, Chan KJ *et al.*(2004) Quality of life, emotional, and cognitive function following acute respiratory distress syndrome. *JINS* **10**(7): 1005–1017.

104. Mikkelsen ME, Christie JD, Lanken PN *et al.* (2012) The adult respiratory distress syndrome cognitive outcomes study: Long-term neuropsychological function in survivors of acute lung injury. *Am J Respir Critl Care Med* **185**(12): 1307–1315.
105. Hopkins RO, Weaver LK, Collingridge D *et al.* (2005) Two-year cognitive, emotional, and quality-of-life outcomes in acute respiratory distress syndrome. *Am J Respir Crit Care Med* **171**: 340–347.
106. Rothenhäusler HB, Ehrentraut S, Stoll C *et al.* (2001) The relationship between cognitive performance and employment and health status in long-term survivors of the acute respiratory distress syndrome: Results of an exploratory study. *Gen Hosp Psychiat* **23**(2): 90–96.
107. Bozza, FA, D'Avila JC, Ritter C *et al.* (2013) Bioenergetics, mitochondrial dysfunction, and oxidative stress in the pathophysiology of septic encephalopathy. *Shock* **39**: 10–16.
108. Annane D, Sharshar T (2015) Cognitive decline after sepsis. *Lancet. Respir Med* **3**(1): 61–69.
109. Wu J, Zhang M, Hao S *et al.* (2014) Mitochondria-targeted peptide reverses mitochondrial dysfunction and cognitive deficits in sepsis-associated encephalopathy. *Mol Neurobiol* 52(1): 783–791.
110. Herridge MS, Tansey CM, Matté A *et al.* (2011) Functional disability 5 years after acute respiratory distress syndrome. *New Engl J Med* **364**(14): 1293–1304.
111. Barnato AE, Albert SM, Angus DC *et al.* (2011) Disability among elderly survivors of mechanical ventilation. *Am J Respir Crit Care Med* **183**(8): 1037–1042.
112. Ferrante LE, Pisani MA, Murphy, TE *et al.* (2015) Functional trajectories among older persons before and after critical illness. *JAMA Intern Med* 175(4): 523–529.

Chapter 8

Acute Respiratory Distress Syndrome: The Role of Mesenchymal Stem Cells and Arising Complications Due to an Aging Lung

John Sembrat*, Maria G. Kapetanaki*,†, and Mauricio Rojas*,†,‡,§,¶

1. Introduction

Aging, a normal and unavoidable biological process, is believed to be the result of accumulated cellular damage associated with the loss of the cell's ability to repair DNA damage and ensure somatic stability during proliferation. Among other grieves, aging cells are

*Vascular Medical Institute University of Pittsburgh, 200 Lothrop Street, Pittsburgh,15261 PA, USA.

†Division of Pulmonary Medicine, Allergy and Critical Care Medicine University of Pittsburgh, 200 Lothrop Street, Pittsburgh,15261 PA, USA.

‡Simmons Center for Interstitial Lung Disease University of Pittsburgh, 200 Lothrop Street, Pittsburgh, 15261 PA, USA.

§McGowan Institute for Regenerative Medicine University of Pittsburgh, 200 Lothrop Street, Pittsburgh, 15261 PA, USA.

¶Corresponding author.

challenged by increased oxidative stress, mitochondrial dysfunction, telomere shortening and weakened cell repair mechanisms, all leading to the organism's inability to cope with exogenous insults such as chemical or smoke inhalations or endogenous insults such as immune activation. In relation to human health, aging not only increases ones susceptibility to injury but also adversely affects the healing process. As the lung acts as one of the body's main interfaces with the environment it is especially prone to injury[1] a trait that makes it particularly interesting for studying the effects of aging on the onset and progression of multiple lung diseases.

The Acute Respiratory Distress Syndrome (ARDS) is the most frequent cause of respiratory failure in critical care medicine representing 78.9 cases per 100,000 person-years with a mortality rate of 38.5%. [2,3] The term acute refers to the rapid onset of the injury which can happen within minutes or hours. The disease usually develops in response to either direct or indirect lung injury.[4] Due to lung endothelial and epithelial cell damage and increased microvascular permeability, ARDS results in strenuous breathing, necessitating the intubation and respiratory support.[5] Similar to other diseases, advanced age has been implicated as a major risk factor for morbidity and mortality of ARDS patients.[6]

Despite the imperative need, there are only a few existing clinical interventions that can benefit ARDS patients mainly by offering supportive care and mechanical ventilation. In recent years, multipotent mesenchymal stromal cells or mesenchymal stem cells (MSCs) have been employed experimentally in treating a growing number of diseases including organ injury and ARDS is no exception. Numerous animal studies have shown that the infusion of exogenous MSCs can be beneficial in the treatment of ARDS.[7–12] It is generally accepted that MSCs' healing properties result from their paracrine function such as the secretion of growth factors and cytokines which can modulate the inflammatory and immune response to lung injury. The present chapter will focus on the MSCs' protective and curative properties in response to ARDS as well as on the impact of aging in both the disease severity and MSCs' healing capacity.

2. Acute Respiratory Distress Syndrome

The disease: First described in a 1967 seminal publication by Ashbaugh *et al.* [13] the definition of ARDS has evolved over the following decades and was most recently updated in 2012. The Berlin Definition of ARDS is now based on 4 individual criteria for diagnosing the disease pertinent to the timing of symptoms, the radiographic evidence, the origin of lung edema and the oxygenation impairment.[4,14]

The etiology: The causes of ARDS are often divided into two categories: (1) *direct lung injury* which includes assaults such as bacterial or viral pneumonia, aspiration of gastric contents, pulmonary contusion, inhalation injury and near drowning, or (2) *indirect lung injury* which includes sepsis, severe trauma with multiple shock and multiple transfusions, drug overdose and cardiopulmonary bypass.[15]

The pathophysiology: Regardless of the etiology, the pathophysiological response in ARDS involves altered permeability of both the endothelial and epithelial barriers in alveoli, uncontrolled activation of the coagulation pathways, marked changes in inflammation and inappropriate activation and accumulation of leukocytes and platelets.[4] The most important cause of ARDS is lung endothelium injury and increased vascular permeability in the microcirculation of the lungs that lead to protein-rich pulmonary edema in the alveolar spaces (reviewed in[5,6]). While there are many proposed mechanisms of lung endothelium injury, perhaps the most explored and best understood is neutrophil-dependent lung injury. Neutrophil migration and activation, as a natural innate immune response to both infectious and noninfectious lung injuries, is a result of chemotactic factors released by activated macrophages, endothelial and epithelial cells.[16] Once situated at the lung microvasculature, neutrophils release pro-inflammatory cytokines, reactive oxygen species (ROS), pro-coagulant molecules and proteases, all causing damage to the capillary-alveolar membrane leading to edema.[5,17] The increase of neutrophil concentration in the bronchoalveolar lavage (BAL) fluid of ARDS patients correlates with the severity of the disease while neutrophil depletion protects against capillary-alveolar permeability in induced ARDS.[17,18]

The age factor: Similar to many diseases, age plays a major role in the body's ability to recover from ARDS. Incidence rates of morbidity and mortality increase dramatically with age with studies reporting 306 per 100,000 person-years for people from 75 to 84 years, compared to 16 per 100,000 person-years in teenagers between 15 and 19 years.[19] The term "normal", in reference to the lung, is often used to describe lungs that are free of disease and/or injury. However, when one refers to an aging normal lung, it is necessary to acknowledge that there are distinct biological differences from a young normal lung such as loss of lung volume, terminal airway closure resulting in decreased arterial P_{O2}, reduced adrenergic control of cardiovascular function, perturbed autonomic processes and decreased lung compliance. In addition to age, genetic and environmental factors as well as cigarette smoking and alcohol abuse have been reported to increase the severity and susceptibility to ARDS[4,20–22] but their analysis as risk factors is beyond the scope of this chapter.

3. Mesenchymal Stem Cells

The cells: Stem cells are unspecialized cells capable of self-renewal for extended periods of time and with the ability to divide and differentiate into organ and tissue specific cells under proper physiological conditions. In addition to these characteristics, stem cells play an important role in the repair of aged and injured tissue. Three types of stem cells are currently used in research: (1) embryonic stems cells derived from the pre-implantation human embryo human; (2) induced-pluripotent stem cells (iPSCs) which are specialized adult cells that have been reprogrammed to assume a more stem cell-like state; and (3) adult or somatic stem cells derived from different tissue sources with the ability to differentiate into specialized cells.

The cells were first described as Colony-Forming Unit-Fibroblastic (CFU-F) by Friedenstein *et al.* in a landmark publication in 1966 and they were later named MSCs by Caplan *et al.* They are a group of bone marrow-derived stem cells that are multipotent, self-renewing and able to support hematopoiesis while they can still differentiate into muscle, bone, fat, fibroblasts and cartilage.[23,24] Due to the lack of an MSC specific cell marker, the characterization of MSCs has been slow. However, it is generally accepted that to be labeled an MSC, cells must: (1) adhere to plastic; (2) express CD44, CD73, CD90 and CD105; (3) lack expression of hematopoietic markers CD45, CD34 and CD31; and finally (4) have the ability to differentiate into osteoblasts, adipocytes and chondroblasts *in vitro.*[25] Although they were originally isolated from bone marrow, it is now known that MSCs can be isolated from a number of tissue sources including fat, placental tissue, tendons, umbilical cord blood and skeletal muscle.[26]

The function: Mainly because of their immunomodulatory and anti-inflammatory capacities and less due to their differentiation ability, the interest in MSCs and consequently the research regarding their biological and therapeutic properties has increased greatly in recent years. It appears that one of their most appealing characteristics is that they can mobilize to the injury site where they can perform their beneficial role. It has been repeatedly shown that exogenous MSCs can home to sites of damage in the lung[27], myocardium[28–30], brain[31], skeletal muscle[32] and kidney.[33] The mechanisms of MSC activation, migration and homing as well as their reparatory effects are just beginning to unravel.

Once at the site of injury, MSCs are able to produce and secrete a multitude of molecules that are essential for wound healing such as chemokines and angiogenic factors.[34] It is shown that in vitro cultured MSCs secrete vascular endothelial growth factor (VEGF), hepatocyte growth factor (HGF), monocyte chemotactic protein-1 (MCP-1), interleukin-6 (IL-6) and transforming growth factor-beta1 (TGF-1).[35] Arno *et al.* demonstrated that MSCs derived from Wharton's Jelly aid in wound repair by paracrine signaling and increased expression of TGF-β2, hypoxia-inducible factor-1a and plaminogen activator inhibitor-1. All these genes are implicated in re-epithelialization, neovascularization and remodeling.[36]

Although their ability to mediate repair by assuming tissue specific phenotypes is controversial, there is *in vitro* evidence that MSCs derived from GFP (+) mice, when co-cultured with heat shock-injured small airway epithelial cells from a wild-type mice, can differentiate into cells that are morphologically and phenotypically similar to the epithelial cells seen in the bronchial epithelium.[37]

In ARDS: In recent years, MSCs have become an attractive therapy in the treatment of numerous diseases including ARDS due to their interaction with immune cells and modulation of pro and anti-inflammatory cytokines. Owing to their origins in the bone marrow and their low expression of major-histocompatibility complexes, MSCs have become known as immuno-privileged cells and often shift the immune response to a more tolerant and anti-inflammatory type. Multiple studies have demonstrated that the administration of MSCs following injury helps with several aspects of ARDS (for a review see[6]). Notably, MSC exposure to an ARDS microenvironment either *in vitro* (serum from LPS-treated animals or ARDS patients) or *in vivo* (infusion of exogenous MSCs in ARDS animal models) results in enhanced production of anti-inflammatory with a parallel reduction of pro-inflammatory cytokines.[7,38–40] In addition to their anti-inflammatory capacity, there is accumulating evidence from *in vivo* and *ex vivo* models that MSCs are able to restore vascular and epithelial permeability with significant improvement of pulmonary edema.[12,38,41] Alleviation of pulmonary edema is a major target for therapies aimed at treating ARDS and it has recently been shown that microvesicles/exosomes secreted by human MSCs ameliorate several ARDS-related phenomena in mice via keratinocyte growth factor (KFG).[42] Administration of exogenous MSCs has also promoted bacterial clearance both in a mouse model of Gram-negative pneumonia, through the secretion of antimicrobial peptides and in mouse model of sepsis which is a common component of ARDS.[41,43]

On top of their immunomodulatory and antimicrobial properties, a study conducted in 2010 by Spees *et al.* showed that MSCs could transfer functional mitochondria to epithelial cells containing dysfunctional mitochondria. Additional confirmation of this phenomenon was provided by Islam *et al.* in 2012 when in a mouse model of lung injury mitochondria from human MSCs were transferred to the epithelium conferring lung protection against acute lung injury.[44,45] To complete the list of their beneficial effects, MSCs are able to modulate the host's antioxidant response to protect against lung injury due to ARDS-related oxidative stress. More specifically, injected MSCs enhance the production of anti-oxidant enzymes which results in a significant decrease in the host's BAL glutathione levels.[46]

The age factor: Similar to somatic cells, stem cells experience both physiological aging due to natural causes such as telomere shortening and premature aging in response to various factors such as biological toxins and chemical agents.[47] MSCs from elderly donors exhibit characteristics seen in MSCs cultured *in vitro* for extended periods of time, suggesting that aging and replicative senescence share some common regulatory mechanisms.[48] MSCs from elderly donors not only come in lower numbers but they also lack the characteristic spindle-like morphology of young MSCs, they proliferate at slower rates and a large percentage stain positive for senescence-associated beta-galactosidase.[49] [50,51] At a closer look, they suffer more oxidative damage because of elevated ROS, they have different methylation patterns which affect cell differentiation and they have shorter telomeres because they lack the telomerase enzyme.[52–54] A 2008 study by Wagner *et al.* showed that long term culture of MSCs was associated with changes in the global gene expression profile involved a marked down regulation of genes involved in cell cycle, DNA replication mitosis and repair. Interestingly, these gene expression changes are also seen in MSCs isolated from young and old donors.[55] Several groups have explored the changes in the transcriptional profiles of MSCs derived from old animals or humans and their findings are summarized in Table1.

MSCs from old mice are characterized by a quiescent state with low metabolic activity and are primarily in the G0 phase of the cell cycle. This quiescent state is maintained by both extrinsic and intrinsic mechanisms and has been postulated to be a way of preserving their long-term proliferative potential and genomic integrity. Once stem cells become quiescent, they no longer go through DNA damage checkpoints and as a result they accumulate DNA damage and become genomically unstable, both conditions leading to faster stem cell depletion or exhaustion.[56,57] In addition to intrinsic

Table 1

Publication	Molecule	Organism
40	Global mRNA profiles	mouse
64	interleukin-1, iNOS, mitogen-activated protein kinase/p38, ERK1/2, c-fos, c-jun NF-κB, myc, interleukin-4 receptor 45 miRNAs	human
65	WNT3A, SFRF4, FZD8, CTNNB1, LEF1. FZD6, LRP6, FOSL1	human
66	HSP70, HSF1 mir-766, mir-558 mir-125b, mir-let-7f, mir-222, mir-221, mir-199-3p, mir-23a	Rhesus macaque
67	TGFbeta1 BMP2/4	mouse
54	p53, p21	
68	Trp53, Cdkn1, Rb1, Ccdne1, Ccdnd1, Mdm2, Chek2, Fas, Bax, Bad, Casp8, Apaf1, IGF-1, VEGF, HGF, Angpt1 E2F1, Brca1, Myc, Flt1	mouse
69	CCNE1, ERCC2, TGM2, RPL29, EPB41L3, TCEAL7, IL13RA2, MFAP5, ROBO1, S100A4, STEAP3, UBE2E2, CCND2, CDKN2B, DCN, PODN, TP53INP1, DRAM1, TGFBR3, RPS6KA2, PTGER4, FBXO32, SULF1, DBC1, HEXA, HEXB, ADAMTS5, COL8A2, GPNMB, TNFAIP6, CTSK, SPP1	human
70	IL-6	human
51	RUNX2, Osterix, ALKP, BSP, OC	human

MSC aging, it is becoming more and more evident that extrinsic MSC aging originating at the cells' microenvironment is equally important in shaping the function of MSCs. Friedenstein *et al.* showed that the number of colony forming units (CFU) from old transplants was increased by three fold when the transplants were previously implanted in young mice versus old mice.[58] More recently, the parabiotic pairing of old and young mice resulted in the restoration of Delta-1 and Notch signaling in the skeletal muscle stem cells of the old animals with significant improvement in their regenerative capacity which was compromised as animals aged.[59] Parabiosis studies have demonstrated that a broad improvement in tissue maintenance and repair could be promoted in an old mammal by factors from the young parabiont by boosting the regenerative capacity of tissue stem cells.[60]

Aged MSCs in disease: Because of the important role of MSCs in injury repair, an age-dependent functional decline would have a significant impact on an organism's ability to repair itself. Recent studies by our group and others have documented that stem cells play a crucial role in injury repair and restoration of organ function and that there are appreciable differences in the functionality of young versus old stem cells.[40] While it is clear that age defines the stem cells' ability to respond to injury, the exact mechanisms underlying this link are just starting to emerge. Although it may seem as a reasonable assumption, it is still unclear whether and how much aging of MSCs contributes to the increased disease susceptibility and more severe symptoms of older organisms. Are "aged" MSCs somehow compromised in their ability to respond to injury and mediate tissue repair? A study using a mouse progeria model has provided the first direct evidence that the muscle-derived stem/progenitor cells (MDSPCs) from old and progeroid (Ercc1/- and Ercc1/D) have lost their regenerative potential presumably due to accumulated DNA damage.[61] Our group has used the same progeria model to investigate susceptibility to lung injury (unpublished data) and we were able to establish that Ercc1/D 12-week-old mice have an increased susceptibility to injury and lung fibrosis after bleomycin treatment. As expected, the infusion of young WT B-MSCs, but not natural old B-MSCs or murine embryonic fibroblasts, resulted in the increase of the lifespan of the more severe Ercc1 mutants (Ercc1-/-). Similarly, the administration of human or murine MSC from aged donors showed a significant decrease of cardiac regenerative capacity in a rat model for cardiomyopathy and in senescent mice after myocardial infarction respectively.[62,63]

A recent study by our group has revealed that MSCs from old mice have significant changes in their transcriptional expression profiles, which may account for the old animals' more severe inflammation in response to lung injury. MSCs from old animals have decreased expression of several genes that are implicated in their activation, their migration and their anti-inflammatory properties. *In vitro* activation experiments suggest that MSCs from old animals are hardly stimulated by cytokines and show a lesser migratory ability upon chemokine signaling, both of which coincide with a downregulation of the respective cellular receptors. Adding to the *in vitro* data, *in vivo* experiments both with parabionts as well as intravenous administration confirmed that MSC from old individuals had compromised mobility and immunomodulatory properties resulting in the loss of their beneficial protective effects.[40]

4. Conclusions

Since the original publications in 2007, multiple groups have demonstrated in multiple pre-clinical models the advantage of the use of MSCs as a therapy to reduce the severity of ARDS (Table 1). More importantly the use of MSCs in ADRS has already translated into clinic. The supporting data clearly support the clinical application of MSCs, different to what occurs on other lung diseases, like pulmonary fibrosis. At this moment the most important aspect is the safety of the patients. Only a serious and rigorous process of isolation, characterization and expansion of MSCs can achieve this and reduce to the minimum any possible secondary effect by the systemic or local infusion of MSCs, Futhermore, it has become evident in this chapter that age should be consider a critical factor that is going to determine the biological activity of the MSCs.

References

1. Wang L, Green, FH, Smiley-Jewell SM *et al.* (2010) Susceptibility of the aging lung to environmental injury. *Semin Respir Crit Care Med* **31**: 539–553.
2. Rojas M, Cardenes N, Kocyildirim E *et al.* (2014) Human adult bone marrow-derived stem cells decrease severity of lipopolysaccharide-

induced acute respiratory distress syndrome in sheep. *Stem Cell Research Ther* **5**: 42.

3. Bice T, Cox CE, Carson SS. (2013) Cost and health care utilization in ARDS–different from other critical illness? *Semin Respir Critical Care Med* **34**: 529–536.
4. Matthay MA, Ware LB, Zimmerman GA. (2012) The acute respiratory distress syndrome, *J Clin Invest* **122**: 2731–2740.
5. Matthay MA, Zemans RL. (2011) The acute respiratory distress syndrome: Pathogenesis and treatment. *Annu Rev Pathol* **6**: 147–163.
6. Cardenes N, Caceres E, Romagnoli M *et al.* (2013) Mesenchymal stem cells: A promising therapy for the acute respiratory distress syndrome. *Respir* **85**: 267–278.
7. Gupta N, Su X, Popov B *et al.* (2007) Intrapulmonary delivery of bone marrow-derived mesenchymal stem cells improves survival and attenuates endotoxin-induced acute lung injury in mice. *J Immunol* **179**: 1855–1863.
8. Nemeth K, Leelahavanichkul A, Yuen PS *et al.* (2009) Bone marrow stromal cells attenuate sepsis via prostaglandin E(2)-dependent reprogramming of host macrophages to increase their interleukin-10 production. *Nat Med* **15**: 42–49.
9. Van Haaften T, Byrne R, Bonnet S *et al.* (2009) Airway delivery of mesenchymal stem cells prevents arrested alveolar growth in neonatal lung injury in rats. *Am J Respir Crit Care Med* **180**: 1131–1142.
10. Aslam M, Baveja R, Liang OD *et al.* (2009) Bone marrow stromal cells attenuate lung injury in a murine model of neonatal chronic lung disease. *Am J Respir Crit Care Med* **180**: 1122–1130.
11. Abman SH, Matthay MA. (2009) Mesenchymal stem cells for the prevention of bronchopulmonary dysplasia: Delivering the secretome. *Am J Respir Crit Care Med* **180**: 1039–1041.
12. Lee JW, Fang X, Gupta N *et al.* (2009) Allogeneic human mesenchymal stem cells for treatment of E. coli endotoxin-induced acute lung injury in the *ex vivo* perfused human lung. *Proc Natl Acad Sci USA* **106**: 16357–16362.
13. Ashbaugh DG, Bigelow DB, Petty TL *et al.* (1967) Acute respiratory distress in adults, *Lancet* **2**: 319–323.
14. Force ADT, Ranieri VM, Rubenfeld GD *et al.* (2012) Acute respiratory distress syndrome: The Berlin definition. *JAMA* **307**: 2526–2533.
15. Ware LB, Matthay MA. (2000) The acute respiratory distress syndrome. *N Engl J Med* **342**: 1334–1349.

16. Soehnlein O, Oehmcke S, Ma X *et al.* (2008) Neutrophil degranulation mediates severe lung damage triggered by streptococcal M1 protein. *Eur Respir J* **32**: 405–412.
17. Matthay MA, Zimmerman GA. (2005) Acute lung injury and the acute respiratory distress syndrome: Four decades of inquiry into pathogenesis and rational management. *Am J Respir Cell Mol Biol* **33**: 319–327.
18. Williams AE, Chambers RC. (2014) The mercurial nature of neutrophils: Still an enigma in ARDS? *Am J Physiol Lung Cell Mol Physiol* **306**: L217–L230.
19. Rubenfeld GD, Caldwell E, Peabody E *et al.* (2005) Incidence and outcomes of acute lung injury. *New Engl J Med* **353**: 1685–1693.
20. Moss M, Bucher B, Moore FA *et al.* (1996) The role of chronic alcohol abuse in the development of acute respiratory distress syndrome in adults. *JAMA* **275**: 50–54.
21. Calfee CS, Matthay MA, Eisner MD *et al.* (2011) Active and passive cigarette smoking and acute lung injury after severe blunt trauma. *Am J Respir Crit Care Med* **183**: 1660–1665.
22. Mizgerd JP. (2008) Acute lower respiratory tract infection. *N Engl J Med* **358**: 716–727.
23. Friedenstein AJ, Piatetzky, S, II, Petrakova KV. (1966) Osteogenesis in transplants of bone marrow cells. *J Embryol ExpMorphol* **16**: 381–390.
24. Caplan AI. (1991) Mesenchymal stem cells. *J Orthop Res* **9**: 641–650.
25. Dominici M, Le Blanc K, Muelle I *et al.* (2006) Minimal criteria for defining multipotent mesenchymal stromal cells. The International Society for Cellular Therapy position statement. *Cytotherapy* **8**: 315–317.
26. Gotts JE, Matthay MA. (2011) Mesenchymal stem cells and acute lung injury. *Crit Care Clin* **27**: 719–733.
27. Mei SH, McCarter SD, Deng Y *et al.* (2007) Prevention of LPS-induced acute lung injury in mice by mesenchymal stem cells overexpressing angiopoietin 1. *PLoS Med* **4**: e269.
28. Wu Y, Zhao RC. (2012) The role of chemokines in mesenchymal stem cell homing to myocardium. *Stem Cell Rev* **8**: 243–250.
29. Shim W, Mehta A, Lim SY *et al.* (2011) G-CSF for stem cell therapy in acute myocardial infarction: Friend or foe? *Cardiovasc Res* **89**: 20–30.
30. Bartsch K, Al-Ali H, Reinhardt A *et al.* (2009) Mesenchymal stem cells remain host-derived independent of the source of the stem-cell graft and conditioning regimen used. *Transplantation* **87**: 217–221.
31. Ji JF, He BP, Dheen ST *et al.* (2004) Interactions of chemokines and chemokine receptors mediate the migration of mesenchymal stem

cells to the impaired site in the brain after hypoglossal nerve injury. *Stem Cells* **22**: 415–427.
32. De Bari C, Dell'Accio F, Vandenabeele F *et al.* (2003) Skeletal muscle repair by adult human mesenchymal stem cells from synovial membrane. *J Cell Biol* **160**: 909–918.
33. Morigi M, Imberti B, Zoja C *et al.* (2004) Mesenchymal stem cells are renotropic, helping to repair the kidney and improve function in acute renal failure. *J Am Soc Nephrol* **15**: 1794–1804.
34. Schinkothe T, Bloch W, Schmidt A. (2008) In vitro secreting profile of human mesenchymal stem cells. *Stem cells Dev* **17**: 199–206.
35. Kwon HM, Hur SM, Park KY *et al.* (2014) Multiple paracrine factors secreted by mesenchymal stem cells contribute to angiogenesis. *Vascular Pharmacol.*
36. Arno AI, Amini-Nik S, Blit PH *et al.* (2014) Human Wharton's jelly-mesenchymal stem cells promote skin wound healing through paracrine signaling. *Stem Cell Res Ther* **5**: 28.
37. Spees JL, Olson SD, Ylostalo *et al.* (2003) Differentiation, cell fusion and nuclear fusion during ex vivo repair of epithelium by human adult stem cells from bone marrow stroma. *Proc Natl Acad Sci USA* **100**: 2397–2402.
38. Xu J, Mora A, Shim H *et al.* (2007) Role of the SDF-1/CXCR4 axis in the pathogenesis of lung injury and fibrosis. *Am J Respir Cell Mol Biol* **37**: 291–299.
39. Rojas M, Xu J, Woods CR *et al.* (2005) Bone marrow-derived mesenchymal stem cells in repair of the injured lung. *Am J Respir Cell Mol Biol* **33**: 145–152.
40. Bustos ML, Huleihel L, Kapetanaki MG *et al.* (2014) Aging mesenchymal stem cells fail to protect because of impaired migration and antiinflammatory response. *Am J Respir Crit Care Med* **189**: 787–798.
41. Gupta N, Krasnodembskaya A, Kapetanaki M *et al.* (2012) Mesenchymal stem cells enhance survival and bacterial clearance in murine Escherichia coli pneumonia. *Thorax* **67**: 533–539.
42. Zhu YG, Feng XM, Abbott J *et al.* (2014) Human mesenchymal stem cell microvesicles for treatment of Escherichia coli endotoxin-induced acute lung injury in mice. *Stem Cells* **32**: 116–125.
43. Mei SH, Haitsma, JJ, Dos Santos CC *et al.* (2010) Mesenchymal stem cells reduce inflammation while enhancing bacterial clearance and improving survival in sepsis. *Am J Respir Crit Care Med* **182**: 1047–1057.

44. Spees JL, Olson SD, Whitney MJ *et al.* (2006) Mitochondrial transfer between cells can rescue aerobic respiration. *Proc Natl Acad Sci USA* **103**: 1283–1288.
45. Islam MN, Das SR, Emin MT *et al.* (2012) Mitochondrial transfer from bone-marrow-derived stromal cells to pulmonary alveoli protects against acute lung injury. *Nat Med* **18**: 759–765.
46. Shalaby SM, El-Shal AS, Abd-Allah SH *et al.* (2014) Mesenchymal stromal cell injection protects against oxidative stress in Escherichia coli-induced acute lung injury in mice. *Cytotherapy* **16**: 764–775.
47. Stochaj U, Kodiha M, Shum-Tim D *et al.* (2013) Implications of multipotent mesenchymal stromal cell aging. *Regen Med* **8**: 211–222.
48. Fossett E, Khan WS, Pastides P *et al.* (2012) The effects of ageing on proliferation potential, differentiation potential and cell surface characterisation of human mesenchymal stem cells. *Curr Stem Cell Res Ther* **7**: 282–286.
49. Baxter MA, Wynn RF, Jowitt SN *et al.* (2004) Study of telomere length reveals rapid aging of human marrow stromal cells following in vitro expansion. *Stem Cells* **22**: 675–682.
50. Roobrouck VD, Ulloa-Montoya F, Verfaillie CM. (2008) Self-renewal and differentiation capacity of young and aged stem cells. *Exp Cell Res* **314:** 1937–1944.
51. Zhou S, Greenberger JS, Epperly MW *et al.* (2008) Age-related intrinsic changes in human bone-marrow-derived mesenchymal stem cells and their differentiation to osteoblasts. *Aging Cell* **7**: 335–343.
52. Bork S, Pfister S, Witt H *et al.* (2010) DNA methylation pattern changes upon long-term culture and aging of human mesenchymal stromal cells. *Aging Cell* **9**: 54–63.
53. Choumerianou DM, Martimianaki G, Stiakaki E *et al.* (2010) Comparative study of stemness characteristics of mesenchymal cells from bone marrow of children and adults. *Cytotherapy* **12**: 881–887.
54. Stolzing A, Jones E, McGonagle D *et al.* (2008) Age-related changes in human bone marrow-derived mesenchymal stem cells: Consequences for cell therapies. *Mech Ageing Dev* **129**: 163–173.
55. Wagner W, Horn P, Castoldi M *et al.* (2008) Replicative senescence of mesenchymal stem cells: A continuous and organized process. *PLoS One* **3**: e2213.
56. Sethe S, Scutt A, Stolzing A. (2006) Aging of mesenchymal stem cells. *Ageing Res Rev* **5**: 91–116.

57. Rossi DJ, SeitaJ, Czechowicz A *et al.* (2007) Hematopoietic stem cell quiescence attenuates DNA damage response and permits DNA damage accumulation during aging. *Cell Cycle* **6**: 2371–2376.
58. Friedenstein AJ, Latzinik NV, Gorskaya YF *et al.* (1992) Bone marrow stromal colony formation requires stimulation by haemopoietic cells. *Bone Miner* **18**: 199–213.
59. Conboy IM, Conboy MJ, Wagers AJ *et al.* (2005) Rejuvenation of aged progenitor cells by exposure to a young systemic environment. *Nature* **433**: 760–764.
60. Conboy IM, Rando TA. (2012) Heterochronic parabiosis for the study of the effects of aging on stem cells and their niches. *Cell Cycle* **11**: 2260–2267.
61. Lavasani M, Robinson AR, Lu A *et al.* (2012) Muscle-derived stem/progenitor cell dysfunction limits healthspan and lifespan in a murine progeria model. *Nat Commun* **3**: 608.
62. Fan M, Chen W, Liu W *et al.* The effect of age on the efficacy of human mesenchymal stem cell transplantation after a myocardial infarction. *Rejuvenation Res* **13**: 429–438.
63. Khan M, Mohsin S, Khan S N *et al.* Repair of senescent myocardium by mesenchymal stem cells is dependent on the age of donor mice. *J Cell Mol Med* **15**: 1515–1527.
64. Pandey AC, Semon JA, Kaushal D *et al.* (2011) MicroRNA profiling reveals age-dependent differential expression of nuclear factor kappaB and mitogen-activated protein kinase in adipose and bone marrow-derived human mesenchymal stem cells. *Stem Cell Res Ther* **2**: 49.
65. Brunt KR, Zhang Y, Mihic A *et al.* (2012) Role of WNT/beta-catenin signaling in rejuvenating myogenic differentiation of aged mesenchymal stem cells from cardiac patients. *Am J Pathol* **181**: 2067–2078.
66. Yu JM, Wu X, Gimble JM *et al.* (2011) Age-related changes in mesenchymal stem cells derived from rhesus macaque bone marrow. *Aging Cell* **10**: 66–79.
67. Moerman EJ, Teng K, Lipschitz, DA *et al.* (2004) Aging activates adipogenic and suppresses osteogenic programs in mesenchymal marrow stroma/stem cells: The role of PPAR-gamma2 transcription factor and TGF-beta/BMP signaling pathways. *Aging Cell* **3**: 379–389.
68. Wilson A, Shehadeh LA, Yu H *et al.* (2010) Age-related molecular genetic changes of murine bone marrow mesenchymal stem cells. *BMC genomics* **11**: 229.

69. Jiang SS, Chen CH, Tseng KY *et al.* (2011) Gene expression profiling suggests a pathological role of human bone marrow-derived mesenchymal stem cells in aging-related skeletal diseases. *Aging* **3**: 672–684.
70. Cheleuitte D, Mizuno S, Glowacki J. (1998) *In vitro* secretion of cytokines by human bone marrow: Effects of age and estrogen status. *J Clin Endocrinol Metabol* **83**: 2043–2051.

Chapter 9

The Aging Immune System, Vaccine Efficacy, and the Lung

Jenna M. Bartley* and Laura Haynes*,†

1. Introduction

It is well known that aging can lead to drastic changes in immune function. The progressive decline in immune response with aging, coined immunosenescence, affects both innate and adaptive immunity. This is associated with increased susceptibility to infections, poor response to vaccination, and increased prevalence of cancers, autoimmune and chronic diseases.[1] While previously less studied than the adaptive immune system, aging decrements to the innate immune system include alteration in the functional capacity of neutrophils, natural killer (NK) cells, macrophages, and dendritic cells (DCs).[2] The adaptive immune response from *B* and *T* lymphocytes is also altered with aging leading to diminished response to infections, as well as vaccines, at both the humoral and cell-mediated level.[1] Morbidity and mortality from infectious diseases is significantly increased in the elderly[1] with influenza and

* Center on Aging and Department of Immunology, UConn Health, 263 Farmington Ave, Farmington, CT 06030, United States.
† Corresponding author: E-mail: lhaynes@uchu.edu

pneumonia being the seventh leading cause of death among persons over 65 years old in the United States,[3] yet decreased vaccine efficacy in the elderly mitigates the protective potential. Along with immunosenescence, increased basal levels of inflammation due to a more pro-inflammatory cytokine milieu with aging, or "inflamm-aging", leads to further immune dysregulation and susceptibility to infection and disease.[4]

The lung utilizes both innate and adaptive immunity for protection against pathogens, thus immunosenescence of both arms of the immune system have vast effects on pulmonary immunity in the aging population. Additionally, structural changes to the lung with age, such as reduced inspiratory and expiratory muscle strength, reduced cough strength and mucociliary dysfunction, lead to poor airway clearance likely allowing increased pathogen entry into the lung, further stressing the already compromised aged immune system. Since the elderly are at greater risk for morbidity and mortality due to these pulmonary infections, prophylactic treatment *via* vaccination becomes particularly valuable for protection; however the diminished vaccine response in the elderly due to immunosenescence presents a great challenge. Recent research on improving vaccine efficacy with aging has focused on better understanding aspects and mechanisms of immunosenescence in order to better engineer vaccines to protect aging populations.

2. The Aging Innate Immune System

While the adaptive immune system is commonly the focus of immunosenescence and vaccine research, the innate immune system is also very important for vaccine response and similarly is partly responsible for decreased vaccine efficacy with aging. Immunosenescence affects innate immunity in multiple ways. Innate immune cell migratory ability, function, and signaling patterns are altered in elderly.[2,5] At the expense of lymphopoiesis, hematopoietic stem cells are biased towards myeloid differentiation in both mice[6,7] and humans.[8] Thus unlike lymphoid cells, most studies do not show considerable decreases in myeloid cell number with age.[9] Regardless of stability in frequency, functional alterations severely diminish the efficiency of the aged innate immune system.

2.1. *Neutrophils*

Most studies agree that neutrophil numbers remain stable[10] (or decrease slightly)[11] in aging, however their functional capacity is decreased. Neutrophil chemokinesis and chemotaxis is impaired with age[12–14] leading to altered migration, as well as delayed egress from tissue. Indeed, compared to their young counterparts, aged mice have increased pulmonary endothelial intercellular adhesionmolecule-1 (ICAM-1),[15] keratinocyte chemoattractant (KC) levels,[16] neutrophil infiltration[15,16] and prolonged pulmonary inflammation[16] after burn injuries. Similarly, aged mice have increased pulmonary production of macrophage inflammatory protein 2 (MIP-2)and KC accompanied by increased neutrophil infiltration and interleukin (IL)-1B production after intraperitoneal lipopolysaccharide (LPS, derived from *Pseudomonas aeruginosa*) administration.[17] However, an initial delayed and reduced neutrophil infiltration and cytokine-induced neutrophil chemoattractant (CINC) gene expression was observed in the lung tissue of aged rats following *P. aeruginosa* inoculation.[18] When further time points were analyzed following a sub-lethal influenza infection in aged mice, neutrophil peak infiltration was delayed, but elevations were prolonged compared to young mice well into the resolution phase of the infection[19] These differences in results exemplify the variation in response due to different types and magnitude of infection and injury among different animal models and could also be partially explained by different timing of sampling as neutrophils have a relatively short life-span so slight timing differences could have more drastic impacts on results. Nonetheless, studies indicate that neutrophil migration is altered with aging. As neutrophils are strong mediators of inflammation and the predominant peripheral blood phagocyte, their regulation is essential for optimal pathogen clearance and infection resolution where deregulated responses can lead to further tissue damage from both delayed and/or prolonged inflammation. Along with migratory dysfunction, most studies report decrements in neutrophil phagocytic ability[12–14,20] and neutrophil oxidative burst capacity[12,13,20] in the elderly. Neutrophils also produce and secrete cytokines and chemokines, as well as have the ability to present antigens to aid in the immune response, however the influence of aging on these functions have yet to be determined.[12] Neutrophils represent the beginning steps of recruitment and activation of both the innate and adaptive immunity, thus decreases in their functional capacity not only have impacts in eliminating pathogens, but also on signaling the adaptive immune response.[20]

2.2. *Monocytes/Macrophages*

Discrepancies exist in the literature regarding the alteration in the number of circulating monocytes in the elderly; some show stability,[21] while others show decreases[11] or increases[22] with age. This likely is attributed to the heterogeneity of monocyte subsets and specific classification methods, as well as difference in health status and age delineations. Though literature varies based on the specific subsets classification, increased circulating CD16+ monocytes are generally observed with aging,[21,23] more specifically the expansion of intermediate (CD14++CD16+) and nonclassical (CD14+CD16++) monocytes.[21,23,24] These phenotypic changes are accompanied by altered functional capacity due to changes in surface receptor expression and function. There is a reduction in HLA-DR, CX_3CR1, CD62L, and CD11b expression in monocytes from older adults potentially leading to decreased survival and migration.[11,21,24]

Similarly, both murine and human studies confirm functional defects in macrophages with aging, though specifics vary with tissue type and activation states.[25–27] Similar to neutrophils, in general, aged macrophages have reduced chemotactic activity,[28] as well as phagocytic capacity.[2,25] Toll-like receptor (TLR) signaling and cytokine production is dysregulated in aged macrophages. TLR gene expression is decreased in aged murine splenic and peritoneal macrophages[29] and TLR-induced cytokine production of tumor necrosis factor (TNF), IL-6, and IL-1β is reduced, though species and tissue specific differences exist.[5,29] A robust inflammatory response is necessary to limit replication and clear the pathogen, as well as aid in the recruitment and activation of other immune cells. Interestingly and seemingly contradictory, despite a diminished pro-inflammatory response upon stimulation, basal levels of pro-inflammatory cytokine production seem to be elevated.[4,30] In fact, the constitutive inflammation due to chronic macrophage activation was originally described as the central instigator of inflamm-aging,[4] though further research revealing great heterogeneity in phenotype and function of macrophages proved the situation more complex and multiple other cell types and tissues have been implicated.

Though it was previously thought that tissue macrophages only rose from circulating monocytes, it is now well-established that resident tissue macrophages are embryonically derived and distinct between tissues.[31] Further, resident tissue macrophages have tissue specific function and are transcriptionally distinct.[31,32] The lung contains both alveolar and interstitial macrophages (among others) that have distinct phenotypic and functional differences, though age-associated dysregulated macrophage function seems to be evident in both populations, likely contributing to the increased cases of morbidity and mortality due to respiratory infections in the elderly. Delayed and diminished monocyte chemotactic protein-1 (MCP-1) expression in the lung is accompanied by a decrease in lung macrophage numbers within 24 hrs after *P. aeruginosa* infection.[18] However, following sublethal influenza infection, macrophage numbers seem to be similar initially, but are prolonged through the resolution phase of the infection in aged mice.[19] In totality, research points to an initial delayed and diminished, but then prolonged macrophage infiltration in the lung following infection. This pattern is also seen in most inflammatory cytokines in lung homogenate as well.[19] Congruently, alveolar macrophages exhibit aged-associated delayed and diminished TLR2 induced TNFα and IL-6 production following infection with live *Streptococcus pneumonia*, leading to increased bacterial growth in the lung and increased mortality in mice.[33] While responsiveness of aged macrophages seems to be diminished, the elevated basal levels of inflammation, specifically TNFα, IL-1β, IL-6 and others, are present in aged lung tissue compared to young.[34–36]

Along with their phagocytic and pro-inflammatory functions, macrophages function as antigen presenting cells (APC) and this ability is also less efficient with aging.[2,37] Aged murine macrophages have decreased major histocompatibility complex (MHC) Class II expression[38] and inteferon (IFN)-γ induced MHC Class II expression is impaired.[38] Additionally, there is an increased production of prostaglandin E_2 (PGE_2),[39,40] which inhibits MHC Class II expression on both macrophages and *B* cells.[40] PGE_2 also decreases IL-12 production from macrophages and impairs *T* cell proliferation, cytotoxicity and IL-2 production.[40] Further, necessary co-stimulatory signals on macrophages seem to follow the same delayed and diminished pattern seen in infiltration and cytokine production.[19,41] In monocytes from aged humans, dysregulated cytokine production[42] is accompanied by reduced up regulation of CD80 with TLR stimulation.[41] Importantly, decreased CD80 upregulation upon stimulation predicted future seroconversion and seroprotection to influenza immunization,[41] directly linking defective aged innate immune response and vaccine efficacy. Additionally, CD40 upregulation is delayed in lung interstitial macrophages of aged mice during influenza infection.[19] This was associated with a delayed and decreased levels of $IL\text{-}12_{p70}$ and chemokines in the lungs of aged mice implying a delay in full activation.[19] The diminished ability for antigen presentation and reduced up regulation of costimulatory signals, along with dysregulated infiltration and inflammatory cytokine production from macrophages leaves the elderly with delayed inflammatory responses, resulting in decreased help from other immune cells and the inability to quickly and efficiently invoke the adaptive immune response and prime *T* cells for a more robust response to both infections and vaccines.

2.3. *Dendritic cells*

While macrophages are able to present antigens, DCs are considered the most potent APC to prime *T* cells and are considered a critical component for initiation of adaptive immunity. DCs are very heterogeneous; myeloid (mDCs) and plasmacytoid DCs (pDCs) are the two major subpopulations. They vary in lineage precursors, phenotypic presentation, TLR expression, cytokine production, though plasticity exists even after differentiation.[43–45] While pDCs are important for host defense against pathogens and type I IFN production, mDCs are crucial for facilitating *T* cell responses, though these functions are not exclusive to either subtype.[2] It is currently unclear if the number of DCs change with aging. Some research reports decreased pDCs in elderly,[22,46] while others report maintenance.[47] Similarly, mDCs were shown to be maintained,[46,47] or decreased[22] in the elderly. These conflicting results may be due to differences in subject population parameters and health status or phenotypic classification.

Functional changes in DCs with aging are multi-factorial; gene arrays revealed altered molecular patterns in multiple aspects of DC function from elderly individuals.[48] More specifically, murine and human studies detected alterations in DC phagocytic capacity, migration, cytokine secretion and antigen presentation with aging. DCs sense pathogens *via* Pattern Recognition Receptors (PRR) leading to their uptake and capture, as well as subsequent DC maturation, activation and migration. Additionally, phagocytosis of self, particularly apoptotic cells, by DCs is essential to maintain self-tolerance. Monocyte-derived DCs from elderly subjects have less efficient antigen uptake through micropinocytosis and endocytosis.[47] Further, uptake of apoptotic cells is also impaired in aged individuals.[47] Phagocytosis of apoptotic cells is generally considered anti-inflammatory; age-associated accumulation of apoptotic cells and debris due to inefficient clearance can lead to pro-inflammatory responses, systemic inflammation and even autoimmunity.[49]

DCs must migrate to nonlymphoid tissue, as well as local lymph nodes in order to activate *B* and *T* cells. Inflammatory signals first cause the chemotaxis of immature DCs into sites of inflammation and/or infections, then following maturation and activation, chemokine receptors change and DCs migrate to secondary lymphoid organs. Both DC migration and homing ability is impaired with aging.[19,47,50] In fact, defective pulmonary migration is reported both with delayed mDC infiltration in the lung following influenza,[19] as well as diminished migration of respiratory DCs to the draining lymph node in response to several respiratory viral pathogens.[51] Corresponding to the inflamm-aging hypothesis, prostaglandin D_2 (PGD_2) expression is elevated in aged murine lung and is associated with reduced migration to the draining lymph node, decreased C-C chemokine receptor type 7 (CCR7) upregulation and decreased *T* cell proliferation.[51] Treatment with a PGD_2 antagonist diminished this effect and restored DC migration close to the level of young mice,[51] though it is important to note that cell intrinsic changes accompany the aged microenvironment to alter migration ability of aged DCs as well.[50] As the migration of DCs to both tissue and draining lymph nodes is crucial for the coordination of innate and adaptive immune response, defects in DC migration with aging is likely a major reason for increased susceptibility to infection and reduced vaccine efficacy in elderly. Adjuvants that can ameliorate this defect, such as the PGD_2 antagonist explored by Zhao *et al.*,[51] may represent a unique way to enhance vaccine efficacy in elderly by enhancing DC migration.

Likely related to altered migratory ability, cytokine production is altered in aged DCs.[52] Basal pro-inflammatory cytokine production is elevated in aged DCs[53] possibly contributing to age-related inflammation. Both pDCs and mDCs secrete IFN-I and IFN-III, staples of antiviral immunity, though in different ratios. While pDCs primarily secrete IFN-I which is important for promoting and enhancing CD4 T cell differentiation, CD8 T Cell and NK cell cytotoxicity, antibody production and antigen cross presentation by DCs, mDCs primarily produce IFN-III, which play a significant role in viral defenses at mucosal surfaces.[43] Aging is associated with decreased IFN-I and IFN-III secretion from pDCs in response to influenza virus and select TLR stimulation.[53,54] Additionally, TLR stimulated TNFα production is impaired in aged pDCs.[53] mDCs also have cytokine secretion impairment, however results vary slightly. TLR stimulated TNFα, IL-6, IL-12_{p40} and IFN-I production was reported as decreased,[53] while others reported increased TNF and IL-6 secretion in response to LPS and ssRNA stimulation in aged mDCs.[47] More recently, diminished IFN-I and IFN-III secretion in mDCs was attributed to histone modification.[55] It is likely that dysregulated cytokine production in aged DCs plays a large role in decreased immune responses in elderly delaying recruitment and activation of other immune cells and prolonging inflammatory responses leading to increased self-damage.

Concordantly, the antigen presenting ability and priming function of DCs also seem to be altered with aging. Though some studies have shown preserved ability of aged DCs to prime allogenic *T* cells,[56] several others report varying impairments with age both *in vitro* and *in vivo*. Monocyte-derived elderly human DCs have impaired ability to phagocytize antigen *via* micropinocytosis and endocytosis *in vitro*.[47] These impairments are also observed *in vivo* as aged murine DCs had decreased uptake of *Listeria monocytogenes* early after infection.[57] Impaired phagocytosis is accompanied by lower levels of costimulatory molecules, MHC-II, CD40, and CD86, and decreased DC accumulation in the spleen early in infection that correlated with reduced CD8 *T* cell priming and expansion.[57] Similarly, aged mucosal DCs have reduced CD80 and CD86 expression and are not able to effectively prime and allow generation of antigen-specific *T* cell responses in response to *Encephalitozoon cuniculi*, an opportunistic intracellular pathogen.[58] Aged mucosal DCs also have reduced IL-15 expression and interestingly, exogenous IL-15 treatment *in vitro* recovered costimulatory molecule expression and the ability to prime *T* cells.[58] Reduced phagocytosis of antigen and CD4 *T* cell priming by aged DCs was also reported in noninfectious murine models.[59] Moreover, human aged pDCs are less efficient inducing CD8 *T* cell cytotoxicity and CD4 *T* cell proliferation *in vitro* compared to young adults.[54]

The ability to present antigen and prime *T* cells is an essential function of DCs linking the innate and adaptive immune systems. Though *T* cell priming was not directly measured, diminished TLR activation and inflammatory responses of elderly mDCs and pDCs *in vitro* correlated to antibody seroconversion after influenza vaccine[53] directly linking impaired DC function to reduced vaccine efficacy. It is likely TLR activation and inflammatory cytokine secretion are not the only reason for decreased vaccine efficacy as impairments in migration, phagocytosis and antigen presentation contribute to DC functional deficits with aging. As DCs are a heterogenous population, some variability in study results are likely due to classification and tissue specificity. Specifically in the lung, DC migration and secretion of inflammatory cytokines is altered.[19,51] Further, impairment in aged DC costimulatory molecule expression and antigen presentation lead to diminished priming and activation of *T* cells during respiratory infection and overall reduced ability to activate the adaptive immune system for better defense.

3. The Aging Adaptive Immune System

Alterations to the adaptive immune system with aging have been studied extensively.[60–65] Both cell-mediated and humoral immunity have age-related deficits, many of which begin with alterations in the hematopoietic stem cells, lymphopoiesis, as well as thymic involution. Indeed, it has been repeatedly shown that aged murine bone marrow hematopoietic stem cells have reduced common lymphoid progenitors, do not generate lymphoid progeny efficiently and have reduced self-renewal potential.[6–8,66,67] Age-related thymic involution is also well described.[61,68,69] These changes, among many others, lead to altered *T* and *B* cell numbers and function with aging. Thus, increased severity of infection and reduced protective effects from vaccination in the elderly are largely attributed to inefficient cell-mediated and humoral immune responses.[1,70]

3.1. *T lymphocytes*

Age-related alterations to *T* cells are multifactorial. Diminished lymphoid progenitors from aged bone marrow and decreased proliferation rates lead to decreased early *T* cell progenitors in the involuted thymus.[69,71] Progressive involution of the thymus, along with other factors, lead to overall decreased production of new naïve *T* cells. This is accompanied by compensatory homeostatic proliferation and continuous exposure to different pathogens leading to overall decreased naïve *T* cells and increased memory *T* cells in the periphery and lymphoid tissue.[72,73] The overall number of *T* cells in the periphery seems to remain stable with age, but there is up to an 80% decrease in peripheral naïve *T* cells.[60] Additionally, naïve *T* cell diversity is diminished and functional deficits including decreased antigen response and proliferation are evident.[60,67,72,73] These age-related decrements occur in both CD4 and CD8 *T* cells, though slight differences exist, and overall lead to the inability to respond efficiently to new antigens and impact both cell-mediated and humoral immunity.

3.1.1. *CD4+ T cells*

CD4 *T* cells, commonly referred to as *T* helper (Th) cells, have multiple functions and aid in many aspects of the immune response. Along with assisting in activation of innate immune cells, CD8 *T* cells, and others, CD4 *T* cells provide cognate help to *B* cells and are essential for germinal center formation and production of high-affinity antibodies.[74,75] Age-associated decreases in naïve CD4 *T* cells are exacerbated by intrinsic age-related defects including reduced *T* cell receptor (TCR) signaling and diminished antigen responses, including decreased IL-2 production and reduced proliferative capacity.[63,76–78] Moreover, exogenous IL-2 can recover proliferative ability *in vitro*.[78] Though the memory CD4 *T* cell population increases, newly formed memory CD4 *T* cells in aged mice have reduced recall responses with decreased cytokine production and proliferation upon restimulation.[74,76]

Upon activation, naïve CD4 *T* cells become effector cells and differentiate into different Th subsets that secrete specific cytokine profiles. With aging there are alterations to Th differentiation with inefficient Th1 and Th2 polarization,[78] as well as reduced *B* cell helper ability.[79] Furthermore, through adoptive CD4 *T* cell transfers it was determined that aged CD4 *T* cells provide inefficient *B* cell help with decreased quantity and quality of the antibody response.[80] While Th1 and Th2 differentiation is poor, aged naïve *T* cells preferentially skew to a Th17 phenotype.[81,82] Additionally, regulatory *T* cells (Treg) are reported to expand in lymphoid tissue with aging,[83,84] though this does not seem to occur in the lung itself.[84] Interestingly, lung-specific changes to other lymphocyte populations also occur with aging. Total *T* cells, as well as the CD4/CD8 *T* cells ratio are increased in the bronchoalveolar lavage of healthy aged humans[85,86] and aged rodents.[36] This correlates with the increased inflammatory environment generated by aged innate immune cells previously discussed. Additionally following influenza infection in aged mice, peak infiltration of CD4 and CD8 *T* cells is delayed and prolonged in the lung similar to the response seen by inflammatory cytokines, lung macrophages and cDCs.[19] Indeed dysregulated cytokine production is also characteristic of aged CD4 *T* cells and postulated to play a role in inflamm-aging,[4] though specific alterations in cytokines vary between studies. While some report IFN-γ production is increased from aged CD4 *T* cells,[87,88] others show decreased production[89] or maintenance.[76] Similarly, discrepancies exist in IL-10 secretion with increased[89] and decreased[90] secretion from aged *T* cells. Differences likely exist in the literature due to cell subtypes, stimulation conditions and subject populations. Despite variance among other cytokines, reduced IL-2 production is consistent and is the hallmark of aged *T* cell cytokine dysfunction where diminished levels reduce proliferative ability and cognate helper function.[74,78] Interestingly, vaccination with attenuated influenza virus genetically altered to express IL-2 restored immune responses in aged mice[91] and may be a potential candidate to increase vaccine efficacy in the elderly.

3.1.2. *CD8+ T cells*

CD8 *T* cells, commonly referred to as cytotoxic *T* lymphocytes, are critical for cell-mediated immunity and viral clearance of infection. Naïve CD8 *T* cells recognize antigen peptides presented on infected cells, become activated, undergo clonal expansion and differentiation into cytotoxic effectors that can induce cell death mainly through granule exocytosis pathways that utilize granzymes and perforins.[92] Resolution of infection triggers contraction of the CD8 *T* cell population and the generation of long-lived memory CD8 *T* cells. While cytotoxic effector function is possible without CD4 *T* cell help, effective long-lived memory CD8 *T* cells formation depends on costimulatory molecules and CD4 *T* cell help, as memory CD8 *T* cells activated independent of CD4 *T* cells respond poorly to secondary challenge.[93] Age-related decreases in naive CD8 *T* cells begin earlier in life and result in severe decreases in naïve CD8 *T* cell number and contraction of the naïve CD8 *T* cell repertoire.[60,94] Additionally, the increased number of memory CD8 *T* cells are more susceptible to increased clonal expansion due to aging and persistent latent infections, overall leading to memory inflation of virus-specific memory CD8 *T* cells and dominance over the memory CD8 *T* cell pool.[60,94,95] Overall this leads to reduced naïve CD8 *T* cells available to respond to new antigens.

Naïve CD8 *T* cells undergo clonal expansion and develop effector function upon activation. Aged CD8 *T* cells proliferate poorly, have altered migration to infection sites and altered cytokine profiles.[96–99] Important for antiviral activity, aged CD8 *T* cells exhibit reduced cytotoxicity.[96,97,100] Following infection, CD8 *T* cells contract to form memory CD8 *T* cell populations. Following respiratory viral infection, virus-specific CD8 *T* cells will remain in the airways.[95,101,102] Interestingly, memory CD8 *T* cell responses in aged mice seem to be less effective at providing protection from secondary challenge.[97,99,103] Moreover these age-related deficits in CD8 *T* cells are evident in the lung. Similar to CD4 *T* cells, there are increased CD8 *T* cells in the lungs of aged mice[36] and a delayed, but prolonged infiltration of CD8 *T* cells in the lung following influenza infection.[19] Additionally, diminished CD8 *T* cell responses, such as infiltration and IFN-γ producing CD8 *T* cells, correlated with delayed viral clearance in the lungs of aged mice infected with respiratory syncytial virus.[96] However, high dose vaccine-induced CD8 *T* cells may be capable of causing further lung damage in aged mice following infection[104] highlighting potential extreme dysregulation in aged CD8 *T* cells effects on the delicate lung tissue. Indeed, the dysregulated CD8 *T* cell responses in aged individuals delay viral clearance and likely exacerbate inflammation leading to greater tissue damage.

3.2. *B lymphocytes*

As previously discussed myeloid skewing of aged hematopoietic stem cells comes at the expense of pro-*B* cells, pre-*B* cells and mature *B* cells in the bone marrow.[66,105,106] This leads to reduced numbers of naïve

B cells in aged individuals and is accompanied by limited naïve *B* cell repertoires.[107] Additionally, trafficking of mature *B* cells into secondary lymphoid tissue is diminished with age, though interestingly, peripheral turnover is reduced and half-life is increased, potentially to compensate for the decreased number naïve *B* cells.[67,106] *B* cells from the bone marrow migrate to the spleen and progress through transitional stages maturing into follicular or marginal zone *B* cells.[67,108] Along with reduced new *B* cells from the bone marrow, the ability to progress through transitional stages is diminished with aging.[106,109] Additionally, exhausted follicular zone *B* cell precursors populate the peripheral blood in aged individuals.[110–112] These cells, termed age-associated *B* cells, are associated with autoimmunity[110] and secrete TNFα,[113] though their specific role in aging is not yet determined.[112]

Neutralizing antibodies are the goal of most vaccines, as the best defense is preventing the infection from occurring or reducing the severity of infection, especially in the susceptible elderly population. With infection or immunization naïve *B* cells that can recognize antigen and have efficient costimulatory signals, specifically CD4 *T* cell help, will be activated, form germinal centers and undergo hypersomatic mutation, class switching and affinity maturation. *B* cells then proliferate and produce both antibody-secreting plasma cells and memory *B* cell populations. Aging results in decreased germinal center formation, somatic hypermutation, and antibody affinity maturation, overall leading to decreased antibody quantity and quality as evident through lower antibody titers and affinity in aged mice and humans.[64,112,114] Though age-related deficits in CD4 *T* cell functions are at least partly responsible for decreased germinal center formation and activation of somatic mutation,[79,114,115] intrinsic alterations in aged *B* cells have substantial impact on antibody production.[62] Indeed aged *B* cells have decreased levels of transcription factor E47, which regulates activation-induced cytidine deaminase and leads to decreased class switch recombination.[62]

Interestingly, increased *B* cells were observed in the lungs of aged mice,[36] but not in the bronchoalveolar lavage from elderly humans[86] though increased IgM, IgA and IgG were noted.[85] It has recently been shown that virus-specific memory *B* cells persist in the lung following influenza infection and are able to rapidly differentiate into plasma cells producing neutralizing antibodies locally that correlate to reduced viral spreading upon reinfection in mice,[116,117] however this cell population has not been evaluated within the context of aging. It is possible that aged *B* cells have reduced ability to form this population in the lung contributing to diminished protection from respiratory infections in the elderly.

4. Aged Lung Immunity and Diminished Vaccine Response

Immunosenescence of both the innate and adaptive immune system result in increased susceptibility to infection, as well as increased severity of infection in the elderly. Moreover, respiratory infections are one of the leading causes of morbidity and mortality in the elderly with hospitalization due to influenza, pneumonia and resultant complications leading to diminished quality of life and disability.[90] Vaccination is considered the most efficient way to prevent infectious disease, however as outlined in this chapter, dysregulated immune responses evident in both innate and adaptive immune cells have vast effects on vaccine efficacy in the elderly. Additionally, as respiratory infections are prevalent in this population, it is important to note that lung-specific immunity is also affected.

Alterations in innate immunity leave the lung particularly vulnerable. Dysregulated cytokine production is evident in aged innate immune cells. Indeed neutrophils, macrophages and DCs are all implicated in inflamm-aging and basal levels of inflammation are evident in the aged lung. Further, infection-induced inflammation is prolonged in the aged lung. It is likely that this persistent inflammation contributes to decrements in lung function in the elderly. Dysregulated cytokine secretion is accompanied by altered migration. Altered chemotaxis results in delayed infiltration into the lung during infection, as well as delayed egress upon resolution. Additionally, diminished migratory ability of respiratory DCs to the draining lymph nodes result in a delay to invoke the adaptive immune system. This is accompanied by reduced upregulation of costimulatory signals and diminished ability to prime and activate *T* cells.

The adaptive immune system also plays a large role in decreased lung immunity with aging. Cell-mediated immunity is primarily responsible for viral clearance. Decreased numbers of naïve *T* cells are accompanied by intrinsic alterations such as diminished antigen responses and reduced proliferation. *T* cell effector functions are also altered. CD4 *T* cells provide inefficient helper functions and CD8 *T* cells have decreased cytotoxicity. Aged *B* cells have decreased germinal center formation, somatic hypermutation and antibody affinity maturation, all leading to decreased antibody quantity and quality. Inefficient adaptive immunity increases severity of respiratory infections in the elderly.

Both innate and adaptive immunity contribute to decreased vaccine efficacy in the elderly. Novel vaccine strategies that can overcome these deficits will increase efficacy and provide protection to the vulnerable aged population. Common vaccine strategies to enhance immunogenicity include increasing antigen dose, adding adjuvants and modifying composition.[118] It is thought that increasing the antigen dose in vaccines will overcome the deficits in APC function and increase antigen presentation. Indeed, high-dose trivalent influenza vaccine is able to increase antibody titers and seroconversion rates in older subjects.[119] Adjuvants are similarly able to modulate the immune response and enhance vaccine efficacy. Different adjuvants are able to differentially skew immune responses to a particular antigen and modulate immune responses to vaccines. While TLR agonist adjuvants, such as CpG or Poly I:C, can induce a Th1 response, other adjuvants, such as aluminum salts or oil in water emulsions, can skew immune responses to favor Th2.[120] Thus particular adjuvants need to be optimized for particular antigens and desired immune responses.

Modifying the composition of the vaccine is another mode to enhance vaccine efficacy. This can be achieved in multiple ways. Inactivated and live attenuated vaccines can induce different immune responses, specifically productive infections from live attenuated influenza vaccines can enhance CD8 *T* cell response in elderly.[118]

Additionally, specific proteins can be targeted in vaccine development to enhance generation of specific neutralizing antibodies. With technological advances, vaccine composition can be further enhanced *via* reverse engineering and epitope-focused immunogen design.[121] Additionally, vector-based vaccines that utilize molecular adjuvants are also particularly appealing. Exploiting CD40L may be particularly useful to recover aged deficits in costimulatory molecules, as the expression of influenza hemagglutinin protein fused with CD40L induced greater antigen-specific *T* cells and serum IgG levels in mice.[122] Further, engineered expression of IL-2 in influenza vaccines similarly overcame *T* cell deficits in aged mice.[91] It is important to note that though numerous animal trials have been performed to determine ways to enhance vaccine efficacy, translation to humans is not always successful and side effects are possible. Continued research illuminating mechanisms of immunosenescence will prove useful in addressing particular deficits and enhancing vaccine efficacy in the elderly.

References

1. Haq K, McElhaney JE. (2014) Immunosenescence: Influenza vaccination and the elderly. *Curr Opin Immunol* **29**: 38–42.
2. Solana R, Tarazona R, Gayoso I *et al.* (2012) Innate immunosenescence: Effect of aging on cells and receptors of the innate immune system in humans. *Semin Immunol* **24**(5): 331–341.
3. Heron M. (2013) Deaths: Leading causes for 2010. *Natl Vital Stat Rep* **62**(6): 1–96.
4. Franceschi C, Bonafe M, Valensin S *et al.* (2000) Inflamm-aging. An evolutionary perspective on immunosenescence. *Ann NY Acad Sci* **908**: 244–254.
5. Shaw AC, Goldstein DR, Montgomery RR. (2013) Age-dependent dysregulation of innate immunity. *Nat Rev. Immunology* **13**(12): 875–887.
6. Sudo K, Ema H, Morita Y *et al.* (2000) Age-associated characteristics of murine hematopoietic stem cells. *J Exp Med* **192**(9): 1273–1280.
7. Cho RH, Sieburg HB, Muller-Sieburg CE. (2008) A new mechanism for the aging of hematopoietic stem cells: Aging changes the clonal composition of the stem cell compartment but not individual stem cells. *Blood* **111**(12): 5553–5561.

8. Pang WW, Price EA, Sahoo D *et al.* (2011) Human bone marrow hematopoietic stem cells are increased in frequency and myeloid-biased with age. *Proc Natl Acad Sci USA* **108**(50): 20012–20017.
9. Shaw AC, Joshi S, Greenwood H *et al.* (2010) Aging of the innate immune system. *Curr Opin Immunol* **22**(4): 507–513.
10. Born J, Uthgenannt D, Dodt C *et al.* (1995) Cytokine production and lymphocyte subpopulations in aged humans. An assessment during nocturnal sleep. *Mech Ageing Dev* **84**(2): 113–126.
11. De Martinis M, Modesti M, Ginaldi L. (2004) Phenotypic and functional changes of circulating monocytes and polymorphonuclear leucocytes from elderly persons. *Immunol Cell Biol* **82**(4): 415–420.
12. Fortin CF, McDonald PP, Lesur O *et al.* (2008) Aging and neutrophils: There is still much to do. *Rejuv Res* **11**(5): 873–882.
13. Wenisch C, Patruta S, Daxbock F *et al.* (2000) Effect of age on human neutrophil function. *J Leukoc Biol* **67**(1): 40–45.
14. Butcher SK, Chahal H, Nayak L *et al.* (2001) Senescence in innate immune responses: Reduced neutrophil phagocytic capacity and CD16 expression in elderly humans. *J Leukoc Biol* **70**(6): 881–886.
15. Nomellini V, Brubaker AL, Mahbub S *et al.* (2012) Dysregulation of neutrophil CXCR2 and pulmonary endothelial icam-1 promotes age-related pulmonary inflammation. *Aging Dis* **3**(3): 234–247.
16. Nomellini V, Faunce DE, Gomez CR *et al.* (2008) An age-associated increase in pulmonary inflammation after burn injury is abrogated by CXCR2 inhibition. *J Leukoc Biol* **83**(6): 1493–1501.
17. Gomez CR, Hirano S, Cutro BT *et al.* (2007) Advanced age exacerbates the pulmonary inflammatory response after lipopolysaccharide exposure. *Critic Care Med* **35**(1): 246–251.
18. Wen J, Li CM, Gu L *et al.* (2014) Aging reduces the expression of lung CINC and MCP-1 mRNA in a P. aeruginosa rat model of infection. *Inflammation* **37**(3): 933–941.
19. Toapanta FR, Ross TM. (2009) Impaired immune responses in the lungs of aged mice following influenza infection. *Respir Res* **10**: 112.
20. Wessels I, Jansen J, Rink L *et al.* (2010) Immunosenescence of polymorphonuclear neutrophils. *Sci World J* **10**: 145–160.
21. Seidler S, Zimmermann HW, Bartneck M *et al.* (2010) Age-dependent alterations of monocyte subsets and monocyte-related chemokine pathways in healthy adults. *BMC immunology* **11**: 30.
22. Della Bella S, Bierti L, Presicce P *et al.* (2007) Peripheral blood dendritic cells and monocytes are differently regulated in the elderly. *Clin Immunol* **122**(2): 220–228.

23. Nyugen J, Agrawal S, Gollapudi S *et al.* (2010) Impaired functions of peripheral blood monocyte subpopulations in aged humans. *J Clin Immunol* **30**(6): 806–813.
24. Hearps AC, Martin GE, Angelovich TA *et al.* (2012) Aging is associated with chronic innate immune activation and dysregulation of monocyte phenotype and function. *Aging cell* **11**(5): 867–875.
25. Stout RD, Suttles J. (2005) Immunosenescence and macrophage functional plasticity: Dysregulation of macrophage function by age-associated microenvironmental changes. *Immunol Revs* **205**: 60–71.
26. Gomez CR, Nomellini V, Faunce DE *et al.* (2008) Innate immunity and aging. *Exp Gerontol* **43**(8): 718–728.
27. Kohut ML, Senchina DS, Madden KS *et al.* (2004) Age effects on macrophage function vary by tissue site, nature of stimulant, and exercise behavior. *Exp Gerontol* **39**(9): 1347–1360.
28. Ortega E, García JJ, De la Fuente M. (2000) Modulation of adherence and chemotaxis of macrophages by norepinephrine. Influence of ageing. *Mol Cell Biochem* **203**(1–2): 113–117.
29. Renshaw M, Rockwell J, Engleman C *et al.* (2002) Cutting edge: Impaired Toll-like receptor expression and function in aging. *J Immunol* **169**(9): 4697–4701.
30. Salvioli S, Monti D, Lanzarini C *et al.* (2013) Immune system, cell senescence, aging and longevity–inflamm-aging reappraised. *Curr Pharm Design* **19**(9): 1675–1679.
31. Epelman S, Lavine KJ, Randolph GJ. (2014) Origin and functions of tissue macrophages. *Immunity* **41**(1): 21–35.
32. Gautier EL, Shay T, Miller J *et al.* (2012) Gene-expression profiles and transcriptional regulatory pathways that underlie the identity and diversity of mouse tissue macrophages. *Nat Immunol* **13**(11): 1118–1128.
33. Boyd AR, Shivshankar P, Jiang S *et al.* (2012) Age-related defects in TLR2 signaling diminish the cytokine response by alveolar macrophages during murine pneumococcal pneumonia. *Exp Gerontol* **47**(7): 507–518.
34. Meyer KC, Rosenthal NS, Soergel P *et al.* (1998) Neutrophils and low-grade inflammation in the seemingly normal aging human lung. *Mech Ageing Dev* **104**(2): 169–181.
35. Li Z, Li J, Bu X *et al.* (2011) Age-induced augmentation of p38 MAPK phosphorylation in mouse lung. *Exp Gerontol* **46**(8): 694–702.
36. Aoshiba K, Nagai A. (2007) Chronic lung inflammation in aging mice. *FEBS letters* **581**(18): 3512–3516.

37. Plowden J, Renshaw-Hoelscher M, Gangappa S *et al.* (2004) Impaired antigen-induced CD8+ T cell clonal expansion in aging is due to defects in antigen presenting cell function. *Cell Immunol* **229**(2): 86–92.
38. Herrero C, Marqués L, Lloberas J *et al.* (2001) IFN-gamma-dependent transcription of MHC class II IA is impaired in macrophages from aged mice. *J Clin Invest* **107**(4): 485–493.
39. Hayek MG, Mura C, Wu D *et al.* (1997) Enhanced expression of inducible cyclooxygenase with age in murine macrophages. *J Immunol* **159**(5): 2445–2451.
40. Wu D, Meydani SN. (2004) Mechanism of age-associated up-regulation in macrophage PGE2 synthesis. *Brain Behav Immun* **18**(6): 487–494.
41. van Duin D, Allore HG, Mohanty S *et al.* (2007) Prevaccine determination of the expression of costimulatory B7 molecules in activated monocytes predicts influenza vaccine responses in young and older adults. *J Infect Dis* **195**(11): 1590–1597.
42. van Duin D, Mohanty S, Thomas V *et al.* (2007) Age-associated defect in human TLR-1/2 function. *J Immunol* **178**(2): 970–975.
43. Gupta S. (2014) Role of dendritic cells in innate and adaptive immune response in human aging. *Exp Gerontol* **54**: 47–52.
44. Shigematsu H, Reizis B, Iwasaki H *et al.* (2004) Plasmacytoid dendritic cells activate lymphoid-specific genetic programs irrespective of their cellular origin. *Immunity* **21**(1): 43–53.
45. Diebold SS, Montoya M, Unger H *et al.* (2003) Viral infection switches non-plasmacytoid dendritic cells into high interferon producers. *Nature* **424**(6946): 324–328.
46. Jing Y, Shaheen E, Drake RR *et al.* (2009) Aging is associated with a numerical and functional decline in plasmacytoid dendritic cells, whereas myeloid dendritic cells are relatively unaltered in human peripheral blood. *Human Immunol* **70**(10): 777–784.
47. Agrawal A, Agrawal S, Cao JN *et al.* (2007) Altered innate immune functioning of dendritic cells in elderly humans: A role of phosphoinositide 3-kinase-signaling pathway. *J Immunol* **178**(11): 6912–6922.
48. Cao JN, Agrawal A, Sharman E *et al.* (2014) Alterations in gene array patterns in dendritic cells from aged humans. *PloS one* **9**(9): e106471.
49. Aprahamian T, Takemura Y, Goukassian D *et al.* (2008) Ageing is associated with diminished apoptotic cell clearance *in vivo. Clin Exp Immunol* **152**(3): 448–455.
50. Linton PJ, Li SP, Zhang Y *et al.* (2005) Intrinsic versus environmental influences on T-cell responses in aging. *Immunol Rev* **205**: 207–219.

51. Zhao J, Legge K, Perlman S. (2011) Age-related increases in PGD(2) expression impair respiratory DC migration, resulting in diminished T cell responses upon respiratory virus infection in mice. *J Clin Invest* **121**(12): 4921–4930.
52. Agrawal A, Gupta S. (2011) Impact of aging on dendritic cell functions in humans. *Ageing Res Revs* **10**(3): 336–345.
53. Panda A, Qian F, Mohanty S *et al.* (2010) Age-associated decrease in TLR function in primary human dendritic cells predicts influenza vaccine response. *J Immunol* **184**(5): 2518–2527.
54. Sridharan A, Esposo M, Kaushal K *et al.* (2011) Age-associated impaired plasmacytoid dendritic cell functions lead to decreased CD4 and CD8 T cell immunity. *Age* **33**(3): 363–376.
55. Prakash S, Agrawal S, Cao J *et al.* (2013) Impaired secretion of interferons by dendritic cells from aged subjects to influenza: Role of histone modifications. *Age* **35**(5): 1785–1797.
56. Tesar BM, Walker WE, Unternaehrer J *et al.* (2006) Murine [corrected] myeloid dendritic cell-dependent toll-like receptor immunity is preserved with aging. *Aging Cell* **5**(6): 473–486.
57. Li G, Smithey MJ, Rudd BD *et al.* (2012) Age-associated alterations in CD8alpha+ dendritic cells impair CD8 T-cell expansion in response to an intracellular bacterium. *Aging cell* **11**(6): 968–977.
58. Moretto MM, Lawlor EM, Khan IA. (2008) Aging mice exhibit a functional defect in mucosal dendritic cell response against an intracellular pathogen. *J Immunol* **181**(11): 7977–7984.
59. Pereira LF, de Souza AP, Borges TJ *et al.* (2011) Impaired in vivo CD4+ T cell expansion and differentiation in aged mice is not solely due to T cell defects: decreased stimulation by aged dendritic cells. *Mech Ageing Dev* **132**(4): 187–194.
60. Arnold CR, Wolf J, Brunner S *et al.* (2011) Gain and loss of T cell subsets in old age-age-related reshaping of the T cell repertoire. *J Clin Immunol* **31**(2): 137–146.
61. Chinn IK, Blackburn CC, Manley NR *et al.* (2012) Changes in primary lymphoid organs with aging. *Semin Immunol* **24**(5): 309–320.
62. Frasca D, Diaz A, Romero M *et al.* (2011) Age effects on B cells and humoral immunity in humans. *Ageing Res Rev* **10**: 330–335.
63. Haynes L, Lefebvre JS. (2011) Age-related Deficiencies in Antigen-Specific CD4 T cell Responses: Lessons from Mouse Models. *Aging Dis* **2**(5): 374–381.

64. Kogut I, Scholz JL, Cancro MP *et al.* (2012) B cell maintenance and function in aging. *Semin Immunol* **24**(5): 342–349.
65. Nikolich-Zugich J. (2014) Aging of the T cell compartment in mice and humans: From no naive expectations to foggy memories. *J Immunol* **193**(6): 2622–2629.
66. Miller JP, Allman D. (2003) The decline in B lymphopoiesis in aged mice reflects loss of very early B-lineage precursors. *J Immunol* **171**(5): 2326–2330.
67. Linton PJ, Dorshkind K. (2004) Age-related changes in lymphocyte development and function. *Nat Immunol* **5**: 133–139.
68. Li L, Hsu HC, Grizzle WE *et al.* (2003) Cellular mechanism of thymic involution. *Scand J Immunol* **57**(5): 410–422.
69. Lynch HE, Goldberg GL, Chidgey A *et al.* (2009) Thymic involution and immune reconstitution. *Trends Immunol* **30**(7): 366–373.
70. Goronzy JJ, Weyand CM. (2013) Understanding immunosenescence to improve responses to vaccines. *Nat Immunol* **14**(5): 428–436.
71. Min H, Montecino-Rodriguez E, Dorshkind K. (2004) Reduction in the developmental potential of intrathymic T cell progenitors with age. *J Immunol* **173**(1): 245–250.
72. Fagnoni FF, Vescovini R, Passeri G *et al.* (2000) Shortage of circulating naive CD8(+) T cells provides new insights on immunodeficiency in aging. *Blood* **95**(9): 2860–2868.
73. Lazuardi L, Jenewein B, Wolf AM *et al.* (2005) Age-related loss of naive T cells and dysregulation of T-cell/B-cell interactions in human lymph nodes. *Immunol* **114**: 37–43.
74. Lefebvre JS, Haynes L. (2012) Aging of the CD4 T Cell Compartment. *Open Longevity Sci* **6**: 83–91.
75. Foy TM, Aruffo A, Bajorath J *et al.* (1996) Immune regulation by CD40 and its ligand GP39. *Ann Review Immunol* **14**: 591–617.
76. Haynes L, Eaton SM, Burns EM *et al.* (2003) CD4 T cell memory derived from young naive cells functions well into old age, but memory generated from aged naive cells functions poorly. *Proc Natl Acad Sci USA* **100**(25): 15053–15058.
77. Rea IM, Stewart M, Campbell P *et al.* (1996) Changes in lymphocyte subsets, interleukin 2, and soluble interleukin 2 receptor in old and very old age. *Gerontol* **42**(2): 69–78.
78. Haynes L, Linton PJ, Eaton SM *et al.* (1999) Interleukin 2, but not other common gamma chain-binding cytokines, can reverse the defect

in generation of CD4 effector T cells from naive T cells of aged mice. *J Exp Med* **190**(7): 1013–1024.

79. Eaton SM, Burns EM, Kusser K *et al.* (2004) Age-related defects in CD4 T cell cognate helper function lead to reductions in humoral responses. *J Expl Med* **200**(12): 1613–1622.
80. Maue AC, Eaton SM, Lanthier PA *et al.* (2009) Proinflammatory adjuvants enhance the cognate helper activity of aged CD4 T cells. *J Immunol* **182**(10): 6129–6135.
81. Huang MC, Liao JJ, Bonasera S *et al.* (2008) Nuclear factor-kappaB-dependent reversal of aging-induced alterations in T cell cytokines. *FASEB J* **22**(7): 2142–2150.
82. Lee JS, Lee WW, Kim SH *et al.* (2011) Age-associated alteration in naive and memory Th17 cell response in humans. *Clin Immunol* **140**(1): 84–91.
83. Nishioka T, Shimizu J, Iida R *et al.* (2006) CD4+CD25+Foxp3+ T cells and CD4+CD25-Foxp3+ T cells in aged mice. *J Immunol* **176**(11): 6586–6593.
84. Chiu BC, Stolberg VR, Zhang H *et al.* (2007) Increased Foxp3(+) Treg cell activity reduces dendritic cell co-stimulatory molecule expression in aged mice. *Mech Ageing Dev* **128**(11–12): 618–627.
85. Meyer KC, Ershler W, Rosenthal NS *et al.* (1996) Immune dysregulation in the aging human lung. *Am J Respir Critic Care Med* **153**(3): 1072–1079.
86. Meyer KC, Soergel P. (1999) Variation of bronchoalveolar lymphocyte phenotypes with age in the physiologically normal human lung. *Thorax* **54**(8): 697–700.
87. Sakata-Kaneko S, Wakatsuki Y, Matsunaga Y *et al.* (2000) Altered Th1/Th2 commitment in human CD4+ T cells with ageing. *Clin Exp Immunol* **120**(2): 267–273.
88. Yen CJ, Lin SL, Huang KT *et al.* (2000) Age-associated changes in interferon-gamma and interleukin-4 secretion by purified human CD4+ and CD8+ T cells. *J Biomed Sci* **7**(4): 317–321.
89. Sharma R, Kapila R, Haq MR *et al.* (2014) Age-associated aberrations in mouse cellular and humoral immune responses. *Aging Clin Exp Res* **26**(4): 353–362.
90. McElhaney JE, Zhou X, Talbot HK *et al.* (2012) The unmet need in the elderly: How immunosenescence, CMV infection, co-morbidities and frailty are a challenge for the development of more effective influenza vaccines. *Vaccine* **30**: 2060–2067.

91. Ferko B, Kittel C, Romanova J *et al.* (2006) Live attenuated influenza virus expressing human interleukin-2 reveals increased immunogenic potential in young and aged hosts. *J Virol* **80**: 11621–11627.
92. Russell JH, Ley TJ. (2002) Lymphocyte-mediated cytotoxicity. *Ann Rev Immunol* **20**: 323–370.
93. Sun JC, Bevan MJ. (2003) Defective CD8 T cell memory following acute infection without CD4 T cell help. *Science* **300**(5617): 339–342.
94. Yager EJ, Ahmed M, Lanzer K *et al.* (2008) Age-associated decline in T cell repertoire diversity leads to holes in the repertoire and impaired immunity to influenza virus. *J Exp Med* **205**: 711–723.
95. Ely KH, Roberts AD, Kohlmeier JE *et al.* (2007) Aging and CD8+ T cell immunity to respiratory virus infections. *Exp Gerontol* **42**(5): 427–431.
96. Fulton RB, Weiss KA, Pewe LL *et al.* (2013) Aged mice exhibit a severely diminished CD8 T cell response following respiratory syncytial virus infection. *J Virol* **87**(23): 12694–12700.
97. Kapasi ZF, Murali-Krishna K, McRae ML *et al.* (2002) Defective generation but normal maintenance of memory T cells in old mice. *Euro J Immunol* **32**(6): 1567–1573.
98. Nikolich-Zugich J, Li G, Uhrlaub JL *et al.* (2012) Age-related changes in CD8 T cell homeostasis and immunity to infection. *Semin Immunol* **24**(5): 356–364.
99. Smithey MJ, Renkema KR, Rudd BD *et al.* (2011) Increased apoptosis, curtailed expansion and incomplete differentiation of CD8+ T cells combine to decrease clearance of L. monocytogenes in old mice. *Euro J Immunol* **41**(5): 1352–1364.
100. Powers DC. (1993) Influenza A virus-specific cytotoxic T lymphocyte activity declines with advancing age. *J Am Geriatr Soc* **41**(1): 1–5.
101. Piet B, de Bree GJ, Smids-Dierdorp BS *et al.* (2011) CD8(+) T cells with an intraepithelial phenotype upregulate cytotoxic function upon influenza infection in human lung. *J Clin Invest* **121**(6): 2254–2263.
102. Knudson CJ, Weiss KA, Hartwig SM *et al.* (2014) The pulmonary localization of virus-specific T lymphocytes is governed by the tissue tropism of infection. *J Virol* **88**(16): 9010–9016.
103. Roberts AD, Ely KH Woodland DL. (2005) Differential contributions of central and effector memory T cells to recall responses. *J Exp Med* **202**(1): 123–133.
104. Parzych EM, DiMenna LJ, Latimer BP *et al.* (2013) Influenza virus specific CD8(+) T cells exacerbate infection following high dose influenza challenge of aged mice. *Bio Med Res Int* **2013**: 876314.

105. Min H, Montecino-Rodriguez E Dorshkind K. (2006) Effects of aging on the common lymphoid progenitor to pro-B cell transition. *J Immunol* **176**(2): 1007–1012.
106. Kline GH, Hayden TA, Klinman NR. (1999) B cell maintenance in aged mice reflects both increased B cell longevity and decreased B cell generation. *J Immunol* **162**(6): 3342–3349.
107. Gibson KL, Wu YC, Barnett Y *et al.* (2009) B-cell diversity decreases in old age and is correlated with poor health status. *Aging cell* **8**(1):18–25.
108. Chung JB, Silverman M, Monroe JG. (2003) Transitional B cells: Step by step towards immune competence. *Trends Immunol* **24**(6): 343–349.
109. Johnson SA, Rozzo SJ, Cambier JC. (2002) Aging-dependent exclusion of antigen-inexperienced cells from the peripheral B cell repertoire. *J Immunology* **168**(10): 5014–5023.
110. Rubtsov AV, Rubtsova K, Fischer A *et al.* (2011) Toll-like receptor 7 (TLR7)-driven accumulation of a novel CD11c(+) B-cell population is important for the development of autoimmunity. *Blood* **118**(5): 1305–1315.
111. Hao Y, O'Neill P, Naradikian MS *et al.* (2011) A B-cell subset uniquely responsive to innate stimuli accumulates in aged mice. *Blood* **118**(5): 1294–1304.
112. Scholz JL, Diaz A, Riley RL *et al.* (2013) A comparative review of aging and B cell function in mice and humans. *Curr Opin Immunol* **25**(4): 504–510.
113. Ratliff M, Alter S, Frasca D *et al.* (2013) In senescence, age-associated B cells secrete TNFalpha and inhibit survival of B-cell precursors. *Aging cell* **12**(2): 303–311.
114. Zheng B, Han S, Takahashi Y *et al.* (1997) Immunosenescence and germinal center reaction. *Immunol Rev* **160**: 63–77.
115. Haynes L, Eaton SM. (2005) The effect of age on the cognate function of CD4+ T cells. *Immunol Rev* **205**: 220–228.
116. Onodera T, Takahashi Y, Yokoi Y *et al.* (2012) Memory B cells in the lung participate in protective humoral immune responses to pulmonary influenza virus reinfection. *Proc Natl Acad Sci USA* **109**(7): 2485–2490.
117. Boyden AW, Legge KL, Waldschmidt TJ. (2012) Pulmonary infection with influenza A virus induces site-specific germinal center and T follicular helper cell responses. *PloS one* **7**(7): e40733.
118. Lefebvre JS, Haynes L. (2013) Vaccine strategies to enhance immune responses in the aged. *Curr Opin Immunol* **25**(4): 523–528.

119. Tsang P, Gorse GJ, Strout CB *et al.* (2014) Immunogenicity and safety of Fluzone((R)) intradermal and high-dose influenza vaccines in older adults >/=65 years of age: A randomized, controlled, phase II trial. *Vaccine* **32**(21): 2507–2517.
120. Egli A, Santer D, Barakat K *et al.* (2014) Vaccine adjuvants-understanding molecular mechanisms to improve vaccines. *Swiss Med Wkly* **144**: w13940.
121. Correia BE, Bates JT, Loomis RJ *et al.* (2014) Proof of principle for epitope-focused vaccine design. *Nature* **507**(7491): 201–206.
122. Fan X, Hashem AM, Chen Z *et al.* (2015) Targeting the HA2 subunit of influenza A virus hemagglutinin via CD40L provides universal protection against diverse subtypes. *Mucosal Immunol* **8**(1): 211–220.

Chapter 10

Respiratory Infection, Airway Colonization and Chronic Inflammation in Aging

Chad Marion* and Charles S. Dela Cruz†

Lung infection is an important threat to the health of older adults. It can be severely debilitating and can lead to deaths. An important risk factor for pneumonia is increasing age. Lung infections are the leading cause of death due to infection in the elderly.[1,2] Pneumonia has once been called "the old man's friend" because it often brought a swift and painless end to a life given the lack of effective treatments at that time. Respiratory infections, as captured by pneumonia and influenza infection, currently ranks as the eighth leading cause of death in individuals older than age 65 and the seventh leading cause of death in individuals older than 85.[3] Hospitalization rates for pneumonia range from 1 per 1000 individuals in the general

*Instructor, Section of Pulmonary, Critical Care and Sleep Medicine, Department of Internal Medicine, Yale School of Medicine, chad.marion@yale.edu;
†Corresponding author: Assistant Professor, Section of Pulmonary, Critical Care and Sleep Medicine, Department of Internal Medicine, Yale School of Medicine, charles.delacruz@yale.edu

population to 12 per 1000 over age 75 years and 33 per 1000 for residents of chronic care facilities.[4] Hospitalization rates for pneumonia increased by 20% from 1988 to 2002 for patients aged 65 to 84 years.[5] The rates of hospitalization for pneumonia were two-fold higher for patients aged 85 years or older than patients aged 75 to 84 years.[5] Mortality from pneumonia increased with age (65–74 years, 6.9%; 75–84 years, 8.9%; >85 years, 17.1%.[6] The risk of death during a hospitalization for pneumonia was 1.5 when compared with the risk of death for the 10 other most frequent causes of hospitalization.

A US study in hospitalized patients with community acquired pneumonia (CAP) observed that patients ≥65 years of age had a much higher incidence of pneumonia compared with the overall incidence (10.12 versus 2.66 per 1000 persons per year).[7] A huge burden of >900,000 cases/year of elderly patients with CAP were reported in US, with 1/20 elderly persons ≥85 years of age developing pneumonia each year.[8] A special entity is the population of elderly persons residing in nursing homes. An incidence of pneumonia of 1.2 episodes per 1000 patient-days has been reported in these facilities, which is up to 10 times the incidence of pneumonia in non-institutionalized elderly persons.[9,10] Mortality due to CAP in the elderly is 23–40%, increasing to 57% in nursing home acquired pneumonia, whereas the mortality rate of pneumonia in the general population is 1–5%.[11–13] Furthermore, a large epidemiological study showed that the mortality rate in elderly CAP patients remains significantly elevated after 1 year when compared to the control population (41 versus 29%).[14,15] The one-year cumulative mortality rate for elderly patients hospitalized for pneumonia is ~50% and is highest especially for those with significant comorbidities.

This review highlights our recent understanding of the cellular and molecular mechanisms that are dysfunctional with aging and the mechanisms that contribute to the enhanced susceptibility to respiratory tract infection in the elderly. This review will focus on host and pathogen interactions and characteristics that predispose the elderly population to respiratory infections.

1. Clinical Pneumonia and Aging

Pneumonia often has an atypical presentation in the elderly where the pulmonary symptoms could be very subtle or absent which often leads to delay in the correct diagnosis. Frequently absent are prominent respiratory symptoms and accompanying fevers; however, mental status changes can be a common feature in the elderly.[16] This contributes to the increase in morbidity and mortality for such respiratory infections in the elderly. Additional tools such as radiographic imaging and microbiologic culture studies are required to aid in the diagnostic process; therefore, empiric approaches to antibiotic therapy pending diagnostic testing is currently advocated.[17] In general, the elderly population is more likely to be hospitalized, have longer hospital stays and a longer recovery time from infections. The respiratory infections often lead to subsequent debilitation and decline in the patient's functional status despite successful treatment for the infection. Elderly individuals in chronic care facilities are especially prone to develop lung infections because of their physical debilitation. They are also known to be colonized in the upper airway with potential pathogenic bacteria.[18,19] Mortality from pneumonia in the elderly is mainly driven by the presence of comorbidities and the presence of potential multidrug-resistant (MDR) pathogens.[6]

Preventative measures, timely diagnosis of pneumonia and expeditious administration of appropriate antibiotic therapy are key in lessening the adverse impact respiratory infections have on the aging population.[20–22] It is of note that despite current available extensive diagnostic technologies, approximately half or more of patients with CAP fail to reveal a specific microbial etiology. Worse clinical outcomes can be the result of delays in the initiation of appropriate therapy while waiting for diagnostic microbiological studies.[23,24] Diagnostic testing should be done rapidly without delaying the initiation of empiric antibiotic therapy. The possibility of an atypical agent, such as *Mycobacterium tuberculosis* or endemic fungi, as a cause of CAP should be considered in the appropriate and susceptible host.

Antibacterial therapy for CAP is generally similar to that for younger individuals but should also be administered empirically on the basis of the presence of cardiopulmonary disease (COPD, congestive heart failure), the presence of modifying factors (nursing home residence, risk factors for drug-resistant *Streptococcus pneumoniae* (DRSP), risk factors for *Pseudomonas aeruginosa* and place of therapy (outpatient versus hospital ward versus intensive care unit). These important factors contribute to pneumonia severity designations.[17] However, elderly adults are often excluded from randomized controlled trials of bacterial pneumonias.[25] There is certainly a lack of data on the comparative efficacy of antibiotic treatment in elderly adults and the general population.

It is also important to consider recurrent pneumonia in the elderly. Rates of recurrent pneumonia within 3–5-years of an episode of CAP are 9–12% with a median time to recurrence of 123–317 days and mortality ranging from 4–10%.[26] Increased age of ≥65 years old and impaired functional statuses are the only patient characteristics that are independently associated with increased risk of recurrence. Modifiable risk factors which include the use of proton-pump inhibitors and systemic and inhaled corticosteroids are associated with increased risk of recurrent pneumonia.[26] Following recovery from an episode of pneumonia, measures have to be made to improve functional status, address modifiable risk factors and optimize medication in the elderly.

2. Risk Factors: Respiratory Infections with Aging

Infections such as influenza, pneumonia and septicemia are among the top ten most common causes of death in adults in the US aged 55 years and above. The elderly are at increased risk for DRSP as an etiology of CAP especially if other risk factors are present such as alcoholism, multiple medical comorbidities, treatment with a beta-lactam antibiotic within the previous 3 months, or immunosuppression. If infection with influenza virus is a likely cause of infection, anti-neuraminidase drugs, which are effective for both chemoprophylaxis and treatment, should be given, especially if such therapy can be started within 36 to 48 h of the onset of symptoms.[27,28] Interventions to prevent pneumonia are preferable to treatment of pneumonia. Immune enhancement with vaccinations to prevent respiratory infections caused by the common pathogens can be safe, protective and cost-effective. Efforts should be placed on interventions to prevent pneumonia in the elderly that include vaccinations (influenza virus, pneumococcus), prophylaxis and early treatment of viral influenza, optimization of nutritional status, decreasing aspiration risk, adequate therapy of chronic disease states, avoidance of institutionalization (if possible) and smoking cessation. The risk of developing CAP rise when various conditions that are common in the elderly are present such as swallowing disorders and recurrent aspiration, cognitive impairment, malnutrition, alcoholism, obstructive lung disease, congestive heart failure, diabetes, renal disease, or immunosuppressive therapy.[12,29–32] Even elderly individuals with no clear evidence of any underlying medical co-morbidities can be at greater risk for developing pneumonia because of alterations of their microbial clearance and immunity that occur with advanced age.

Numerous risk factors have been identified that predispose the elderly to develop lower respiratory tract infection as mentioned above. Oral clearance with the help of salivation and swallowing is an important protective mechanism. The normal hosts can clear over 90% of microorganisms from the oropharynx. If the salivary flow and swallowing mechanisms are intact and oral clearance well maintained, even in advanced age the oropharynx is often colonized with normal flora.[19,33] However, the appearance of pathogenic bacteria in the oral cavity is associated with significantly diminished oropharyngeal clearance and such colonization is associated with increased leukocyte elastase concentrations and buccal epithelial cell desquamation.[34] There are multiple medications used by the elderly that can disrupt salivary flow (anti-depressants, antihistamines, antihypertensives, diuretics and anti-parkinsonian agents). Other factors that commonly affect the elderly such as depressed functional status, inadequate nutritional state, immunosuppressive therapy and institutionalization are associated with colonization of the upper airway with pathogenic bacteria.[19,34] The lungs rely on protective reflexes to prevent aspiration of upper airway contents and intact mucociliary clearance mechanisms to allow rapid clearance of any foreign material from gaining access to the upper respiratory tract. Aspiration is therefore a major risk factor for lung infections especially in the elderly population where there are many factors that increase the likelihood of aspirations, especially in patients over 70 years of age.[35,36] Oral aerobic and anaerobic are important pathogens in elderly patients with aspirations.[37] Even silent aspiration of small amounts of gastric or oropharyngeal secretions can occur and has been linked to chronic bronchiolar inflammation in the elderly.[38,39] Although small amounts of aspirated gastric secretions may be rapidly neutralized, moderate acid exposure of human tracheal epithelial cells can inhibit the production of bactericidal molecules such as human β-defensin-2 and is associated with reduced bactericidal activity in epithelial surface.[40]

Once aspirated secretions or inhaled pathogens gain access to the lower tract airways due to insufficient glottic protective mechanisms and cough clearance, mucociliary clearance reduces the likelihood of triggering infection by transporting them proximally to the glottis. Abnormal ciliary function can lead to chronic inflammation and colonization of the upper and lower respiratory tracts.[41] Mucociliary clearance function appears to decline with advancing age. Nasal epithelial cells from older individuals have lower ciliary beat frequency and increased microtubular abnormalities in cilia, which are associated with depressed nasal mucociliary clearance times. Because nasal ciliary beat frequency correlates well with that of tracheal epithelium,[42] this study suggests that ciliary abnormalities appear with advancing age and may play a role in increased susceptibility to respiratory infection.

Nutrition plays an important role in resistance to infection. Hypoalbuminemia, which usually reflects malnutrition, has been shown to be a risk factor for pneumonia in the elderly.[43] Increased levels of circulating pro-inflammatory cytokines have been associated with cachexia and the aging process has been associated with increased levels of pro-inflammatory cytokines.[44] Malnutrition, food restriction, or starvation can depress serum leptin levels and a decline in leptin levels in the malnourished may play a role in susceptibility to pneumonia.[45,46] Altered body composition and the decline in muscle mass associated with aging and may account for the decrease in diaphragmatic strength that is observed in clinically normal elderly individuals.[47]

In addition to a decline in respiratory muscle strength, there are other aspects of lung functions that decline in clinically healthy individuals with aging.[48,49] Age-associated alterations of the respiratory system include the loss of lung elastic recoil, elastin loss, altered collagen cross-linking, decreased chest wall compliance, loss of gas exchange surface area, increased ventilator-perfusion mismatches, decline in respiratory muscle strength, diminished response to hypercapnic or hypoxemic stimuli, and lower maximal aerobic capacity.[48,49] Changes in lung structure, the chest wall and ventilatory responses occur as part of the normal aging process in clinically healthy individuals who have no clear evidence of pulmonary disease. Structural changes include alterations in lung tissues, particularly elastin and collagen that support the airways. As a consequence of changes in lung matrix with aging, the diameter of bronchioles decreases due to diminished tethering that would normally maintain patency at a given lung volume, the alveolar ducts increase in diameter and the elastic recoil of the lung declines.[48,49] Airways tend to close prematurely and lead to ventilation-perfusion mismatching, air trapping and increase in the alveolartoarterial gradient for oxygen. In addition, the total gas–exchange surface area declines. Not only do structural and functional changes occur in the lung, but the chest wall becomes less compliant due to altered costovertebral articulations and rib cartilage calcifications, narrowing of intervertebral disc spaces and changing the contour of the chest, which can be greatly exacerbated by the presence of kyphoscoliosis or vertebral compression fractures. Ventilatory responses to hypoxic or hypercapnic stimuli also become blunted and elderly individuals tend to have a decline in their maximal aerobic capacity and require a higher breathing rate to maintain adequate ventilation with exertion. Although these changes tend to be mild, the structural and functional changes may significantly limit an elderly individual's ability to cope with a severe stress such as pneumonia, especially in elderly patients who are in an age-associated "fragile" state.[50]

There are many factors that lead to the increased risk of pneumonia in the elderly. With aging, there is depressed oral and mucociliary clearance. Elderly patients often have swallowing disorders, central nervous system dysfunction, neurological disorders and increased use of pharmacologic depressants, all of which can increase risks for aspirations and subsequent respiratory infections. Declining and suppressed immune functions associated with aging, along with malnutrition, makes the elderly population at particular risk for respiratory infections. Even though modifiable risk factors such as aspiration, swallow difficulties and use of sedatives are associated with the development of lung infections in the elderly, immune dysregulation associated with aging leads to susceptibility and increased severity of lung infections. Aging is associated with decline in immune function (also called immunosenescence).[51] Their relative poor vaccine responses and immune dysfunctional changes results in increased morbidity and mortality from infections.[52]

Infection in the aging population is an important problem as best exemplified by the 37-fold increase incidence of elderly patients hospitalized with *S. pneumoniae*, compared to younger adults.[53] Elderly residents of long-term care facilities have a high incidence of pneumonia with case fatality rates that range up to 40%.[32,54] Outbreaks of pneumonia in nursing home residents are often linked to a point source that can be a patient, a caregiver, or a visitor. When a pathogen is introduced into the facility, it often can rapidly disseminate among both residents and healthcare staff. Approximately 0.42 respiratory tract infections were noted per 1000 resident-days in a study involving five monitored nursing homes over a 3-year study period.[55] These outbreaks frequently involved atypical pathogens, occurred more often during winter months and had a case-fatality rate of 8%. Pathogens associated with various outbreaks include viruses (influenza A and B, parainfluenza, respiratory syncytial virus, rhinovirus), *Chlamydia pneumoniae*, Legionella spp., *S. pneumoniae*, *Bordetella* pertussis, *Haemophilus influenzae* and *M. tuberculosis*.[56] Additionally, when individuals are admitted to hospitals where they frequently have extended stays, they are more likely to become colonized with antibiotic-resistant bacteria such as methicillin-resistant *Staphylococcus aureus* and antibiotic-resistant gram-negative bacilli, which may subsequently cause difficult-to-treat respiratory infections.

Determining the relative importance of the different etiologic agents associated with pneumonia in older adults can be challenging. One important reason is due to the difficulty of frail elderly individuals to produce sputum for microbiological determination. However, studying results from the serological and urine antigen testing has helped shed some epidemiological insights. Using paired serum (incident and convalescent samples) in patients who met criteria of clinical pneumonia, 46% of the study subjects with pneumonia were in patients above age 60 years. Of these patients, *S. pneumoniae* was the etiologic agent, followed by *Chlamydophila* species in 12%, *Mycoplasma pneumoniae* in 10%, *H. influenzae* in 4% and respiratory viruses (which include parainfluenza virus, respiratory syncytial virus, adenovirus and influenza virus) in 10% of the patients studied. The study highlights the importance of *S. pneumoniae* as a cause of CAP in elderly persons. CAP due to *H. influenzae, S. aureus* and enteric gram-negative bacilli occur more frequently in the elderly than in younger age groups.[57] Pneumonia that is associated with aspiration is usually associated with *S. pneumoniae, H. influenzae,* or *S. aureus* unless poor dentition is present, raising the possibility of pneumonia caused by anaerobic bacteria. The elderly are more likely to have colonization with gram-negative bacilli, particularly if they reside in long-term care facilities. The presence of diseases that alter lung structure such as COPD or bronchiectasis, both common in elderly, also increase the likelihood of gram-negative bacilli as a cause of bacterial pneumonia.

Viral pneumonias, although comprising a smaller proportion of lower respiratory tract infections in the elderly, can have significant morbidity and mortality as well as predispose the elderly individual to subsequent serious bacterial pneumonia.[58] The role of viruses in pneumonia in the elderly is likely underappreciated and the literature is scarce on this topic. Viral culture and rapid antigen detection assays are insensitive in elderly patients hospitalized with lower respiratory tract infections.[59] However, the diagnostics of respiratory viral infections has improved in the past ten years with the use of genetic-based technologies.[60] The detection of new respiratory viruses and previously known viruses has improved. This will likely lead to better appreciation and understanding of the role of viruses in lung infections in the elderly.

Residents of long-term care facilities with their distinct populations of elderly patients are at particularly high risk for developing pneumonia. However, there are few trials that focus therapies to reduce respiratory infections in the elderly who live in the community or in a long-term care setting. But there is very good evidence supporting the administration of annual influenza vaccines and, to some degree pneumococcal vaccines, to older adults.[61–65] Immunosenescence contributes to poor vaccine responses in the elderly and vaccine designers are starting to pay more attention to this as noted by a recent study showing that a higher quadruple dosing of the trivalent inactivated influenza vaccine improves antibody responses and better protection in those age 65 years of age or older.[66] A matched case control study with CAP above age 65 years old showed that the 23-valent pneumococcal polysaccharide vaccine reduced hospitalization for pneumonia in the elderly and supports a vaccination program for this age group;[67,68] however, there is still a huge need to further optimize the pneumococcal vaccine in the elderly.

Unfortunately, vaccine responses tend to be attenuated in the elderly due to waning humoral and cell-mediated immune responses.[69–71] Efforts are ongoing and needed to develop novel vaccine approaches to raise protective immunity in the aging population. Some of these approaches include the use of vaccine in higher dosages, booster vaccines, different immunization routes and the use of novel adjuvants.[72,73] Understanding the underlying mechanisms of immunosenescence through biological, cellular and molecular approaches will result in a rational approach to developing more effective vaccines for protecting the elderly. Nonetheless, vaccination of patients at risk for respiratory infections with both the influenza and pneumococcal vaccines has been demonstrated to be both safe and effective.[74] Other interventions such as cessation of cigarette smoking are also very important.

Pneumococcal vaccine diminishes the risk of bacteremia in elderly patients,[75] and efficacy has been demonstrated in immunocompetent individuals over age 65 years as well as in populations with increased risks (COPD, diabetes, congestive heart failure, anatomic asplenia) for pneumococcal pneumonia.[76,77] However, vaccine-induced antibodies to pneumococcal capsular polysaccharides tend to wane with time, particularly in the elderly[74] and revaccination with polysaccharide pneumococcal vaccine, which appears to be safe, has been advocated 5 years after the first dose for elderly individuals.[78] The influenza vaccine has also been demonstrated to be effective in attenuating or preventing illness in both the elderly and younger populations and can prevent illness in up to 90% of individuals under 65 years of age when the vaccine and circulating influenza virus strain are matched.[79,80] Although somewhat less effective in the elderly, particularly those with chronic illness, the influenza vaccine can still attenuate influenza infection and prevent severe illness and death caused by influenza infection itself or subsequent bacterial lower respiratory tract infections.

3. Altered Host Defense and Lung Immunity with Aging

Aging is associated with altered and dysfunctional immunity. There are a number of mechanisms to explain this increased incidence and susceptibility to infection. Age-associated immunological responses and regulation wane or change over time and vary between individuals. Such immunological changes also take place in the lung due to the natural aging process and with time lead to lung function decline. Mucociliary clearance becomes impaired. Elastic recoil properties decline with age leading to functional decline of the lung as exemplified by emphysema.[81,82] These changes in lung structure and function and immunosenescence increase the risk of lung infections in the elderly. It is important to study how pulmonary host defense mechanisms against infectious pathogens decline with age that may foster insights and strategies to reduce susceptibility of elderly to lung infections.

3.1. *Innate immunity*

The innate immune system is the highly conserved arm of the immune system made up of immune and structural cells such as the epithelial cells. The innate immunity is relatively non-specific with respect to its response to a broad array of exogenous antigenic stimuli. On the other hand, the adaptive immune system takes more time to develop its antigen specificity. However, both non-immune and immune defenses tend to decline with advancing age, although many aspects of immunity can remain fairly robust even in centenarians.[83,84] Pattern-recognition receptors bind to various determinants (e.g. lipopolysaccharide, lipoteichoic acids, mannans, peptidoglycans, glucans or bacterial DNA) found on microbial agents and provide the innate immune system with its ability to immediately respond to a microbial challenge. Stimulation of innate immune receptors triggers the production and release of cytokines and co-stimulatory molecules. Pathogen-associated molecular patterns (PAMPs) are highly conserved, absent from mammalian tissues, are shared by large classes of microorganisms and are recognized by innate immune receptors.[85] Innate immune responses may be able to adequately deal with a microbial challenge without significant activation of adaptive immunity.

The innate immune responses trigger and augment adaptive immune responses (e.g. *via* co-stimulatory molecules) as needed to meet an invading pathogen and heighten responses needed to prepare for future challenges. Other important components of innate immune responses include dendritic cells, phagocytic cells, the alternate complement pathway and antimicrobial molecules such as nitric oxide, defensins and collectins. Dendritic cells and macrophages play a major immunoregulatory role and provide the key link between innate and adaptive immune responses. As antigen-presenting cells, dendritic cells and macrophages stimulate primary *T* cell responses and *T* cell differentiation *via* production of co-stimulatory molecules and cytokine production.

Neutrophils are usually recruited very early into inflamed tissues. Many neutrophil functions, including adhesion, migration into inflamed tissue and phagocytosis, are unchanged with aging. However, the ability of neutrophils to kill phagocytosed organisms is diminished in the elderly compared with younger individuals and the defect has been linked to a decrease in the production of reactive oxygen species (ROS).[86] Neutrophils are important for early responses to injured and inflamed tissues. Aged neutrophils are also more susceptible to cell death. Neutrophils in the aging lung have less anti-microbial activity. Because cytokine-mediated signaling pathways that protect neutrophils are dysfunctional, neutrophils from elderly individuals are more prone to apoptosis. Increased neutrophil apoptosis and diminished antibacterial activity as a consequence of advanced age may contribute to more frequent and more severe respiratory infections in the elderly.[87]

Dendritic cells serve as "professional" antigen presenting cells and interact with both *T* cells and *B* cells to facilitate their activation, enhance cytolytic *T* cell activity and drive the production of antibodies. Dendritic cells provide a key link between the innate and adaptive arms of the immune system. Dendritic cells localized to non-lymphoid tissues have diminished antigen-presenting activity, which may be related to decreased major histocompatibility complex (MHC) II expression. Dendritic cells are known for their potent antigen presenting ability to interact with *T* and *B* cells for their activation. Studies show variability in the number and nature of dendritic cells with aging. Recent study show that circulating levels of plasmacytoid dendritic cells, a subset of dendritic cells important for antiviral response, are 50% lower in elderly compared to younger subjects.[88]

Macrophages can also act as antigen-presenting cells and efficiently phagocytose microbes and foreign particles. Macrophages kill bacteria intracellularly *via* production of superoxide anion with its downstream reactive oxygen intermediates as well as the production of reactive nitrogen intermediates. Cytokine production by macrophages stimulated *in vitro* has been shown to decline with age and *in vivo* assays of macrophage function have shown altered recruitment to sites of injury and areas of wound healing. Decreased macrophage infiltration has been observed in elderly humans. Collectively, experimental observations suggest that age-related changes in macrophage function may impair the ability to eradicate infection, which can contribute to more frequent and more severe respiratory infections.

Natural killer (NK) cells are important for the destruction of tumor cells as well as cells that harbor intracellular pathogens, such as viruses. Absolute numbers of NK cells increase with aging. However, the functional activities of these cells appear to diminish and correlate with a tendency for NK cells to become more agranular in appearance and less capable of cytolytic activity toward tumor cells.[89,90]

3.2. *Adaptive immunity*

Adaptive immunity responds to specific antigens and these responses to specific molecular moieties are mediated and coordinated by *T* and *B* lymphocytes derived from fetal liver and bone marrow precursors in the developing embryo, the thymus gland and other lymphoid tissues (spleen, lymph nodes, and mucosa-associated lymphoid tissue), which play key roles in generating adaptive immune responses. Adaptive immunity is considered a more sophisticated form of host defense that has a component of memory allowing responses to a repeat invader (e.g. virus or bacterium) to occur more quickly and more effectively. *T* cell antigen specificity is localized to the *T* cell receptor (TCR) and *T* cells undergo selective expansion of appropriate *T* cell clones with a specific antigen upon stimulation. *B* cell antigen specificity is localized to cell surface antibody receptors and secreted antibodies. *B* cells contribute to antigen specificity by selective activation of *B* cell clones that have antibody specificity for the target pathogen and *B* cells display "editing" of the antibody upon repeat exposures to enhance future specificity.

Age-associated changes in *T* lymphocyte populations have been extensively examined. The thymus gland clearly begins to gradually involute shortly after birth and undergoes replacement by fatty tissue that is nearly complete by the age of 60 years in humans. Consequently, the numbers of CD3+, CD4+ and CD8+ T cells decrease with advancing age.[91] Naïve *T* cell populations gradually decline and memory *T* cells (CD45RO+) eventually predominate. However, memory cell responses also gradually wane with aging. TCR repertoire diversity declines and *T* helper cell activity diminishes. Reduced proliferative responses, a shift of Th1 to Th2 cytokine profiles, a decline in Fas-mediated *T* cell apoptosis and increased HLA-DR expression on *T* cells have also been observed.[91] Some observations suggest that as many components of immunity decline with advanced age due to sustained antigenic stress over an individual's lifespan. There is a shift to a chronic, pro-inflammatory state as effector and memory cells gradually replace naïve cells and expanded effector and memory *T* cells secrete increased amounts of pro-inflammatory cytokines.

Decreased *B* cell production with aging has been described for humans. More specifically, a transition from the presence of naïve *B* cells to "antigen-experienced" *B* cells appears to occur and it is suspected that the distribution of *B* cell subsets present in the elderly differs from that of younger individuals. The functional ability to produce antibody remains intact with aging; however, the quality of antibody produced with aging is lower with the antibodies exhibiting lower affinity and avidity for antigen. This observation is likely explained by deficient somatic hypermutation that is the typical mechanism to enhance antibody specificity for antigen. Interestingly, prolonged survival appears to correlate with fairly well preserved immune responses in the very old, whereas decreased survival in a longitudinal study in a Swedish population was associated with the "immune cluster parameter" of impaired *T* cell proliferative response to mitogenic stimulation, increased numbers of CD8+ cytotoxic/suppressor cells and low numbers of CD4+ *T* cells and CD19+ *B* cells. Additionally, other important modulators of immune function that can have a significant effect on the elderly include the neuroendocrine system responses to stress. Elderly individuals display a gradual increase in endogenous glucocorticoids with age and a hypothalamus–pituitary–adrenal axis can impair immune function yet cause an exaggerated response to stressors such as infection.

3.3. *Low-grade inflammation in the aging lung*

The term "inflammaging" has been coined to describe the persistent low-grade tissue inflammation that is often associated with advanced aging.[83,84] While the acquired immune system shows functional decline in its ability to respond to new pathogens during aging, increased circulating levels of inflammatory cytokines are increased with age. Inflammaging denotes increase in the inflammatory response that happens with age resulting in a low-grade chronic systemic and pro-inflammatory state, which is characterized by increased levels of pro-inflammatory cytokines (interleukin-6 [IL-6], tumor necrosis factor-alpha [TNF-α] and interleukin-1 beta [IL-1β]). All of these have been shown to increase with aging and be involved in the pathogenesis of many age-associated lung diseases.

Low-grade lung inflammation can occur as a result of waning tissue defenses against oxygen and free radical stresses and as a result of decline in endogenous anti-aging factors such as sirtuins. The source of chronic inflammation that comes with aging has been largely attributed to progressive activation of immune cells.[92] However, the process of cellular senescence, whereby the cells cease to divide, telomeres shorten, and trigger a DNA damage response, is an important contributor to chronic inflammation or inflammaging. The "aged" or senescent cells remain metabolically active, adopt a flattened cell morphology and exhibit a more promiscuous expression of pro-inflammatory and secretory modulators, a phenotyped that has been termed senescence-associated secretory phenotype (SASP).[93–95] Some have posit that the PAMP receptors, such as the Toll-like receptors (TLRs) that are important in innate immunity, are dysfunctional with aging and are interconnected with the phenomenon of cellular senescence and SASP.[96,97] All this contributes to lung senescence. Animal models have suggested that elevated cytokine levels can result in increased susceptibility to infection. For example, young mice (4–5 months) infused with aging-relevant physiological levels of TNF-α resulted in 100-fold more *S. pneumoniae* in the lung, compared with similar mice that received saline only.[98] The potential link between such low-grade inflammation and susceptibility to infections is supported by a positive correlation between pro-inflammatory cytokines and the higher incidence of pneumonia in healthy elderly population. They found that in well-functioning elderly subjects, pre-infection systemic levels of these cytokines were associated with higher risk of community acquired pneumonia requiring hospitalization.[99] More studies are needed to define the underlying mechanisms how low-grade inflammation in aging contribute to increased incidence and worse outcomes of lung infections.

4. Bacterial Colonization, Chronic Lung Diseases and Aging

It is well recognized that aging adults commonly have diseases that involve the lungs. Some of these aging-associated lung diseases include: Chronic obstructive lung disease (COPD), non-cystic fibrosis related bronchiectasis (BCT), interstitial lung disease (ILD) and lung cancer. Cystic fibrosis (CF) itself could be considered as an aging disease given patients are now surviving longer into their fourth decades. Each of these diseases is associated with various microorganisms that colonize, infect and potentially lead to progression of the underlying primary lung disorder. Here we consider the microbial population that forms the airway microenvironment in several chronic lung diseases and the potential role these organisms play in pathogenesis during aging.[19]

4.1. *Chronic obstructive pulmonary disease (COPD)*

One of the most common lung diseases in the aging population is COPD, which is characterized by a limited reversibility of airflow obstruction. The risk of developing COPD increases with age, which is why COPD is especially prevalent in the elderly affecting 25% of those aged more than 75 years of age. The alteration in airflow not only leads to symptoms of shortness of breath and cough, but also leads to physiologic alterations in gas exchange and clearance of inhaled environmental irritants, including bacteria. In fact, given COPD has been attributed to a dysregulation of innate immunity in response to oxidants and microbes, some have described the disease to have features of accelerated aging.[100] Bacteria and viruses become more important in more severe COPD.[101] In addition, physiologic aging, independent from smoking exposure, has been associated with physiological and anatomical changes similar to emphysema. Although patients with COPD are exposed to all types of inhaled bacteria, there is a preference for certain bacteria to colonize the airways of COPD patients. For community dwellers with stable COPD, the most common airway colonizers include *Haemophilus spp., S. pneumoniae, S. aureus, P. aeruginosa* and *M. catarrhalis.*[102] The frequency of each microbe varies from study to study, likely due to differences in sample collection and possibly due to seasonal and regional variations in microbial population as well as recent history of antibiotic exposure. However, this microbial population may not hold true in patients with frequent (>3) COPD exacerbation per year or in patients who have COPD that live in long-term healthcare facilities.[103] Little is known about how bacterial colonization changes with age in COPD and requires further investigations.

Microorganisms not only colonize the airways of COPD patients but they also contribute to the progression of disease and worsening of symptoms. A common measure of COPD severity is the progressive decline in FEV1. Several factors are known to lead to the decline in FEV1 including normal aging and continued exposure to tobacco smoke. Research demonstrates that bacterial colonization also play a role in FEV1 decline in patients with COPD when compared to non-smokers and ex-smokers. COPD patients with bacterial colonization have lower FEV1 at baseline when compared to COPD patients without colonization, ex-smokers or non-smokers.[104–107] The decline in FEV1 correlates with the quantitative bacterial load recovered from sputum of stable COPD patients.[106] Interestingly, not only does the bacterial load seem to play a role in FEV1 decline, but a change in the microbial species in a patient's sputum many also lead to more rapid decline in FEV1 and more frequent COPD exacerbations.[103,106] It is unknown if there is a particular change in microbial pattern that leads to a more rapid decline in FEV1 or if a decline in FEV1 predisposes COPD patients to more virulent pathogenic colonization. This relationship deserves further investigation especially in the aging lung.

A cornerstone of COPD pathogenesis is the presence of airway inflammation. The degree of airway inflammation is known to positively correlate with the progression of airway disease and decline in FEV1.[108–110] Increasing airway inflammation induces a neutrophil predominant inflammatory cell recruitment to the airway that, in turn, leads to further airway damage and inflammation.[111,112] The mechanism by which bacterial colonization leads to more rapid FEV1 decline is beginning to be understood. The presence of microbial determinants leads to the expression of various inflammatory cytokine. COPD patients with colonization of potentially pathogen-associated bacteria have higher levels of interleukin-8 in both bronchoalveolar lavage and sputum and likely higher levels of TNF-α and IL-6. Bacterial colonization that induces higher levels of TNF-α, IL-8 and matrix metalloproteinase activity are associated with neutrophil recruitment and more frequent COPD exacerbations.[111,112] This suggests that the presence of bacterial colonization may play a role in the progression of FEV1 decline in COPD through activation of inflammation. The exact bacterial determinants and the deleterious host response that induces progression of COPD deserve further studying. It has been reported that there are specific dysfunction of TLR activations (TLR4, TLR1) in models of COPD and aging;[113,114] such changes in the innate immunity will likely contribute to the quantity and quality of the microbial species that colonizes the airways of the COPD patients.

4.2. *Cystic fibrosis (CF)*

CF is the most common life-shortening autosomal recessive disease caused by the mutation of the CF transmembrane receptor (CFTR) gene.[115] The CFTR functions as a cAMP-regulated chloride channel in the apical membrane of epithelial cells. The CF patients can be seen as an aging population as a result of the improved centralized medical care, aggressive antimicrobial management and new therapies. Microbial lung infections are the major cause of morbidity and mortality in the hereditary metabolic disorder CF. The bacterial growth, colonization and its persistence, in addition to the accompanying inflammation, eventually can affect lung function. These changes result in a vicious cycle of tissue damage, microbial alterations and lung inflammation. Patients with CF disease die primarily as a result of chronic lung infection and or exacerbation with a respiratory pathogen. *S. aureus* and mucoid *P. aeruginosa* continue to be the key pulmonary pathogens. Recent microbiome studies have identified 2 groups of bacteria that may play a role in chronic CF lung infections: Anaerobic bacteria and *Streptococcus angionsus* group organisms. Microbiome studies also show that the diversity of organisms decline over time, possibly as a result of aggressive antimicrobial therapy. There is a question whether *P. aeruginosa* is the "apex predator" pathogen in the CF airway microbiome that eliminates other bacterial competitors while it adapts itself for chronic survival in the lung.[116] There are a few studies using mouse model of CF showing that older mice have impaired defense of bacterial clearance compared to younger mice.[117] A study suggests that CFTR-deficient mice suffered from age-dependent pulmonary inflammation, respiratory epithelial cell death and susceptibility to *P. aeruginosa* infection as a result of increased ceramide accumulation.[117] However, another study found that the clinical course of acute gram-negative infectious such as with *P. aeruginosa* infection in CF mice was age-independent.[118]

4.3. *Non-Cystic fibrosis bronchiectasis (BCT)*

Non-cystic fibrosis BCT is a chronic lung disease that leads to permanent widening of the airways.[119] It is associated with altered mucociliary function that decreases airway clearance mechanisms and leads to increased bacterial colonization. BCT is also present in other chronic lung disease, such as COPD and ILD, but it can also be an independent disease in select patients with previous pneumonia, immunodeficiencies, genetic disorders, chronic aspiration and other lung disorders.

BCT is less common than COPD, therefore less is known about bacterial colonization in BCT during aging and the role potential pathogen-associated microbial colonizers play in disease progression. In the limited studies available, many of the colonizers do not differ from the microbes seen in COPD. Again, *Haemophilus spp.*, *S. pneumoniae*, *S. aureus*, *P. aeruginosa* and *M. catarrhalis* are frequently cultured from the sputum or bronchoalveolar lavage from BCT patients. Notable exceptions that differ in the organisms cultured in COPD do exist. BCT patients tend to also be colonized by *Streptococcus viridans*, *Neisseria spp. and coagulase-negative Staphylococcus.*[120,121] The pathogenic consequences of these differences are not known; however, the presence of bacterial colonization in BCT patients is associated with BCT exacerbations, an FEV1 <80% predicted and the presence of cystic BCT changes in CT scan.[122] Although the presence of bacterial colonization is associated with FEV1 less than 80% predicted, there is no direct correlation between FEV1 with the predicted pathogenicity of the colonizing bacteria. This suggests that the presence of any pathogen worsens FEV1 and that the decline in lung function is independent of the particular bacterial determinants but could be dependent on host immune factors. A over-exuberant host immune response to pathogen in BCT patients has been described.[123] As seen in colonized COPD patients, the presence of bacterial colonization in clinically stable BCT patients leads to more neutrophil recruitment, IL-8, TNF-α, IL-6 and matrix metalloproteinase.[124]

4.4. *Interstitial lung disease (ILD)*

ILD is a large, heterogeneous group of inflammatory lung diseases with a common endpoint of parenchymal fibrosis and with incidence that increases with aging. ILD can be associated with connective tissue disease but idiopathic ILD, known as idiopathic pulmonary fibrosis (IPF), is known to occur with no clear etiology and patients with IPF have overall poor prognosis. The use of certain ILD therapeutics, that are immune suppressing, has been associated with increased infection and number of isolated pathogens. Several theories have been proposed suggesting that pathogens are involved in the pathogenesis of ILD; however, there is limited data available on bacterial colonization in ILD. Of the limited data, there appears to be about 1 in 5 patients with a diagnosis of ILD who have bacterial isolation by sputum or bronchoalveolar lavage. In the ILD patients who have positive cultures, there appears to be a gram-negative predominance; this differs from the colonization seen with patients with COPD and BCT. The three most common organisms seen in hospitalized ILD patients include *Klebsiella pneumoniae, P. aeruginosa* and *Acinetobacter* spp.[125] The most common gram-positive bacteria are *S. aureus* and *coagulase-negative* Staphylococcus.[125] The role of bacterial colonization in the progression of ILD needs additional exploration. Overt respiratory infection and immunosuppression carry a high morbidity and mortality and polymorphisms in genes related to epithelial integrity and host defense have been identified that predispose individuals to IPF. A prospective study of IPF patients found that baseline bacterial burden based on 16S ribosomal RNA quantitative polymerase chain reaction and pyrosequencing predicted increased rate of lung volume decline and risk of death.[126] This bacterial burden was associated with a MUC5b mucin gene polymorphism, an important IPF host susceptibility gene. Bacteria such as *Haemophilus, Streptococcus, Neisseria* and *Veillonella* spp. are found to be more abundant in IPF patients than control patients. However, change of the microbiome with aging in IPF is not well-characterized. Another IPF study found that disease progression was significantly associated with increased relative abundance of Streptococcus and Staphylococcus, suggesting possible contribution of these organisms to IPF pathogenesis.[127]

4.5. *Lung cancer*

Lung cancer remains a leading cause of cancer-related death worldwide with tobacco smoking as the leading etiology.[128] With the high prevalence of disease and the ubiquitous nature of bacteria, bacterial colonization in lung cancer has gained some attention. It has been postulated that bacterial colonization may play a role in lung cancer progression by increasing pulmonary inflammation and delaying the prescription of immunosuppressive chemotherapy in actively infected patients.[129] Lung cancer is frequently associated with other chronic lung diseases, such as COPD and ILD. With the overlap and not surprisingly, many of the bacterial colonizers are shared between COPD, ILD and lung cancer, but lung cancer patients tend to have larger variation of bacterial colonizers. Both gram-positive and gram-negative organisms are described as colonizers in lung cancer. Some of the more common gram-positives include *S. pneumoniae, S. aureus, Streptococcus viridans and coagulase negative Staphylococcus.* Common gram-negative organism includes *Haemophilus spp., P. aeruginosa, M. catarrhalis, Neisseria spp., Escherichia coli, Enterobacter spp., Stenotrophomonas maltophilia and Klebsiella spp.*[130–132] In patients with lung cancer, the presence of bacterial colonization was associated with older age and COPD co-morbidity.[131] Bacterial colonization is not influenced by cancer type, cancer stage or smoking status; however, patients with body mass index >25 and/or centrally located tumors have a higher incidence of bacterial colonization.[130,132]

It is possible that lung cancer survival can be influenced by the presence of bacterial colonization. The overall patient survival was shortened by about four months in colonized patients when compared to non-colonized patients.[131] Surgical resection is considered in certain patients with lung cancer, but colonization increases the risk of death. Pneumonia is a common cause of peri-operative death in lung cancer patients and bacterial colonization may play a role in post-operative mortality.[132] Up to 30 % of patients have an infection complication post resection with tracheobronchitis being the most common complication, followed by pneumonia, although there is only about 50% concordance with the colonizer and the post-operative infectious etiology.[132] Clinical risk factors for post-operative infections, in addition to bacterial colonization, include moderate to severe COPD and poorly controlled pain post-operatively.[130,132] Therefore, a holistic approach must be taken to limit perioperative infections in lung cancer patients.

Bacterial colonization is common in multiple chronic pulmonary diseases. The presence of both gram-negative and gram-positive bacteria is well described but the mechanisms by which bacterial colonization induces the development and progression of lung diseases with aging is not fully understood. Understanding colonization in chronic lung disease may help improve management of these diseases, prevent progression of these diseases and improve the quality of life of the aging patients who suffer from these often debilitating lung disorders.

5. Conclusions

The aging process is associated with physiological and immune alterations in the lung that compromises the ability of the aging host to deal with external stresses (respiratory infections) causing fragility and age-related lung diseases. Immune cells important for lung homeostasis and during host defense are relatively activated during the aging process. The inflamed lung seen in aging likely contribute to changes in the microbes in the local lung environment and contribute to many pulmonary disorders that are characterized by chronic inflammation. Currently there still exist many knowledge gaps of the underlying process that leads to immune senescence and the pathways that define the important host cell and microbe interaction in the aging lung. Understanding of these critical host immune-microbe interactions by comparing the young and the old lung in many pulmonary disease processes will lead to better diagnosis, treatment and prevention of age-related lung diseases that will continue to increase in numbers in our rapidly aging population.

References

1. Chong CP, Street PR. (2008) Pneumonia in the elderly: A review of the epidemiology, pathogenesis, microbiology, and clinical features. *South Med J* **101**: 1141–1145.
2. Rello J, Rodriguez R, Juber P *et al.* (1996) Severe community-acquired pneumonia in the elderly: Epidemiology and prognosis. Study Group for Severe Community-Acquired Pneumonia. *Clin Infect Dis* **23**: 723–728.
3. Heron M. (2013) Deaths: Leading causes for 2010. *Natl Vital Stat Rep* **62**: 1–96.

4. Fein AM. (1999) Pneumonia in the elderly: Overview of diagnostic and therapeutic approaches. *Clin Infect Dis* **28**: 726–729.
5. Fry AM, Shay DK, Holman RC *et al.* (2005) Trends in hospitalizations for pneumonia among persons aged 65 years or older in the United States, 1988–2002. *JAMA* **294**: 2712–2719.
6. Cillóniz C, Polverino E, Ewig S *et al.* (2013) Impact of age and comorbidity on cause and outcome in community-acquired pneumonia. *Chest* **144**: 999–1007.
7. Marston BJ, Plouffe JF, File TM *et al.* (1997) Incidence of community-acquired pneumonia requiring hospitalization. Results of a population-based active surveillance Study in Ohio. The Community-Based Pneumonia Incidence Study Group. *Arch Intern Med* **157**: 1709–1718.
8. Jackson ML, Neuzil KM, Thompson WW *et al.* (2004) The burden of community-acquired pneumonia in seniors: results of a population-based study. *Clin Infect Dis* **39**: 1642–1650.
9. Marrie TJ. (2002) Pneumonia in the long-term-care facility. *Infect Control Hosp Epidemiol* **23**: 159–164.
10. Mortensen EM, Coley CM, Singer DE *et al.* (2002) Causes of death for patients with community-acquired pneumonia: Results from the Pneumonia Patient Outcomes Research Team cohort study. *Arch Intern Med* **162**: 1059–1064.
11. Arnold FW, LaJoie AS, Brock GN *et al.* (2009) Improving outcomes in elderly patients with community-acquired pneumonia by adhering to national guidelines: Community-Acquired Pneumonia Organization International cohort study results. *Arch Intern Med* **169**: 1515–1524.
12. Torres A, El-Ebiary M, Riquelme R *et al.* (1999) Community-acquired pneumonia in the elderly. *Semin Respir Infect* **14**: 173–183.
13. Zalacain R, Torres A, Celis R *et al.* (2003) Community-acquired pneumonia in the elderly: Spanish multicentre study. *Eur Respir J* **21**: 294–302.
14. Kaplan V, Angus DC, Griffin MF *et al.* (2002) Hospitalized community-acquired pneumonia in the elderly: Age- and sex-related patterns of care and outcome in the United States. *Am J Respir Crit Care Med* **165**: 766–772.
15. Kaplan V, Clermont G, Griffin MF *et al.* (2003) Pneumonia: Still the old man's friend? *Arch Intern Med* **163**: 317–323.
16. Metlay JP., Schulz R, Li YH *et al.* (1997) Influence of age on symptoms at presentation in patients with community-acquired pneumonia. *Arch Intern Med* **157**: 1453–1459.

17. Mandell LA, Wunderink RG, Anzueto A *et al.* (2007) Infectious Diseases Society of America/American Thoracic Society consensus guidelines on the management of community-acquired pneumonia in adults. *Clin Infect Dis* **44**: S27–S72.
18. Mojon P. (2002) Oral health and respiratory infection. *J Can Dent Assoc* **68**: 340–345.
19. Smaldone GC. (2001) Deposition and clearance: Unique problems in the proximal airways and oral cavity in the young and elderly. *Respir Physiol* **128**: 33–38.
20. Schmidt-Ioanas M, Lode H. (2006) Treatment of pneumonia in elderly patients. *Expert Opin Pharmacother* **7**: 499–507.
21. Chong CP, Street PR. (2008) Pneumonia in the elderly: A review of severity assessment, prognosis, mortality, prevention, and treatment. *South Med J* **101**: 1134–1140.
22. ThiemU, Heppner HJ, Pientka L. (2011) Elderly patients with community acquired pneumonia: Optimal treatment strategies. *Drugs Aging* **28**: 519–537.
23. Waterer GW, Kessler LA, Wunderink RG. (2006) Delayed administration of antibiotics and atypical presentation in community-acquired pneumonia. *Chest* **130**: 11–15.
24. Luna CM, Aruj P, Niederman MS *et al.* (2006) Appropriateness and delay to initiate therapy in ventilator-associated pneumonia. *Eur Respir J* **27**: 158–164.
25. Avni T, Shiver-Ofer S, Leibovici L *et al.* (2015) Participation of elderly adults in randomized controlled trials addressing antibiotic treatment of pneumonia. *J Am Geriatr Soc* **63**: 233–243.
26. Dang TT, Majumdar SR, Marrie TJ *et al.* (2015) Recurrent pneumonia: A review with focus on clinical epidemiology and modifiable risk factors in elderly patients. *Drugs Aging* **32**: 13–19.
27. Treanor JJ, Hayden FG, Vrooman PS *et al.* (2000) Efficacy and safety of the oral neuraminidase inhibitor oseltamivir in treating acute influenza: A randomized controlled trial. US Oral Neuraminidase Study Group. *JAMA* **283**: 1016–1024.
28. Gillissen A, Höffken G. (2002) Early therapy with the neuraminidase inhibitor oseltamivir maximizes its efficacy in influenza treatment. *Med Microbiol Immunol* **191**: 165–168.
29. Ruiz M, Ewig S, Marcos M A *et al.* (1999) Etiology of community-acquired pneumonia: Impact of age, comorbidity, and severity. *Am J Respir Crit Care Med* **160**: 397–405.

30. Ruiz M, Ewig S, Torres A *et al.* (1999) Severe community-acquired pneumonia. Risk factors and follow-up epidemiology. *Am J Respir Crit Care Med* **160**: 923–929.
31. Baik I, Curhan GC, Rimm EB *et al.* (2000) A prospective study of age and lifestyle factors in relation to community-acquired pneumonia in US men and women. *Arch Intern Med* **160**: 3082–3088.
32. Loeb M, McGeer A, McArthur M *et al.* (1999) Risk factors for pneumonia and other lower respiratory tract infections in elderly residents of long-term care facilities. *Arch Intern Med* **159**: 2058–2064.
33. Laforce FM, Hopkins J, Trow R *et al.* (1976) Human oral defenses against gram-negative rods. *Am Rev Respir Dis* **114**: 929–935.
34. Palmer LB, Albulak K, Fields S *et al.* (2001) Oral clearance and pathogenic oropharyngeal colonization in the elderly. *Am J Respir Crit Care Med* **164**: 464–468.
35. Teramoto S, Fukuchi Y, Sasaki H *et al.* (2008) High incidence of aspiration pneumonia in community- and hospital-acquired pneumonia in hospitalized patients: A multicenter, prospective study in Japan. *J Am Geriatr Soc* **56**: 577–579.
36. Teramoto S, Kawashima M, Komiya K *et al.* (2009) Health-care-associated pneumonia is primarily due to aspiration pneumonia. *Chest* **136**: 1702–1703.
37. El-Solh AA, Pietrantoni C, Bhat A *et al.* (2003) Microbiology of severe aspiration pneumonia in institutionalized elderly. *Am J Respir Crit Care Med* **167**: 1650–1654.
38. Kikuchi R, Watabe N, Konno T *et al.* (1994) High incidence of silent aspiration in elderly patients with community-acquired pneumonia. *Am J Respir Crit Care Med* **150**: 251–253.
39. Matsuse T, Oka T, Kida K *et al.* (1996) Importance of diffuse aspiration bronchiolitis caused by chronic occult aspiration in the elderly. *Chest* **110**: 1289–1293.
40. Nakayama K, Jia YX, Hirai H *et al.* (2002) Acid stimulation reduces bactericidal activity of surface liquid in cultured human airway epithelial cells. *Am J Respir Cell Mol Biol* **26**: 105–113.
41. Puchelle E, Zahm JM, Bertrand A. (1979) Influence of age on bronchial mucociliary transport. *Scand J Respir Dis* **60**: 307–313.
42. Ho JC, Chan KN, Hu WH *et al.* (2001) The effect of aging on nasal mucociliary clearance, beat frequency, and ultrastructure of respiratory cilia. *Am J Respir Crit Care Med* **163**: 983–988.

43. Riquelme R, Torres A, El-Ebiary M *et al.* (1996) Community-acquired pneumonia in the elderly: A multivariate analysis of risk and prognostic factors. *Am J Respir Crit Care Med* **154**: 1450–1455.
44. Yeh SS, Schuster MW. (1999) Geriatric cachexia: The role of cytokines. *Am J Clin Nutr* **70**: 183–197.
45. Khan S, Kolls JK. (2006) Malnutrition in the critically ill: Don't hold the leptin. *Am J Respir Crit Care Med* **173**: 140–141.
46. Mancuso P, Huffnagle GB, Olszewski MA *et al.* (2006) Leptin corrects host defense defects after acute starvation in murine pneumococcal pneumonia. *Am J Respir Crit Care Med* **173**: 212–218.
47. Polkey MI, Harris ML, Hughes PD *et al.* (1997) The contractile properties of the elderly human diaphragm. *Am J Respir Crit Care Med* **155**: 1560–1564.
48. Dyer C. (2012) The interaction of ageing and lung disease. *Chron Respir Dis* **9**: 63–67.
49. Sharma G, Goodwin J. (2006) Effect of aging on respiratory system physiology and immunology. *Clin Interv Aging* **1**: 253–260.
50. Stiesmeyer JK. (1992) Care of the elderly mechanically ventilated patient: Preserving the fragile environment. *AACN Clin Issues Crit Care Nurs* **3**: 129–136.
51. Kumar R, Burns EA. (2008) Age-related decline in immunity: Implications for vaccine responsiveness. *Expert Rev Vaccines* **7**: 467–479.
52. Dorrington MG, Bowdish DM. (2013) Immunosenescence and novel vaccination strategies for the elderly. *Front Immunol* **4**: 171.
53. van der Poll T, Opal SM. (2009) Pathogenesis, treatment, and prevention of pneumococcal pneumonia. *Lancet* **374**: 1543–1556.
54. Starczewski AR, Allen SC, Vargas E *et al.* (1988) Clinical prognostic indices of fatality in elderly patients admitted to hospital with acute pneumonia. *Age Ageing* **17**: 181–186.
55. Loeb M, McGeer, A, McArthurM *et al.* (2000) Surveillance for outbreaks of respiratory tract infections in nursing homes. *CMAJ* **162**: 1133–1137.
56. Strausbaugh LJ, Sukumar SR, Joseph CL. (2003) Infectious disease outbreaks in nursing homes: An unappreciated hazard for frail elderly persons. *Clin Infect Dis* **36**: 870–876.
57. Woodhead M. (1994) Pneumonia in the elderly. *J Antimicrob Chemother* **34**: 85–92.
58. Treanor J, Falsey A. (1999) Respiratory viral infections in the elderly. *Antiviral Res* **44**: 79–102.

59. Flamaing J, Engelmann I, Joosten E *et al.* (2003) Viral lower respiratory tract infection in the elderly: A prospective in-hospital study. *Eur J Clin Microbiol Infect Dis* **22**: 720–725.
60. Jartti L, Langen H, Söderlund-Venermo M *et al.* (2011) New respiratory viruses and the elderly. *Open Respir Med J* **5**: 61–69.
61. Monto AS, Hornbuckle K, Ohmit SE. (2001) Influenza vaccine effectiveness among elderly nursing home residents: A cohort study. *Am J Epidemiol* **154**: 155–160.
62. Fukushima W, Hayashi Y, Mizuno Y *et al.* (2008) Selection bias in evaluating of influenza vaccine effectiveness: A lesson from an observational study of elderly nursing home residents. *Vaccine* **26**: 6466–6469.
63. Muszkat M, Friedman G, Dannenberg HD *et al.* (2003) Response to influenza vaccination in community and in nursing home residing elderly: Relation to clinical factors. *Exp Gerontol* **38**: 1199–1203.
64. Namkoong H, Funatsu Y, Oishi K *et al.* (2015) Comparison of the immunogenicity and safety of polysaccharide and protein-conjugated pneumococcal vaccines among the elderly aged 80 years or older in Japan: An open-labeled randomized study. *Vaccine* **33**: 327–332.
65. Valenzuela MT, Altuzarra RH, Trucco OA *et al.* (2007) Immunogenicity of a 23-valent pneumococcal polysaccharide vaccine in elderly residents of a long-term care facility. *Braz J Infect Dis* **11**: 322–326.
66. DiazGranados CA, Dunning AJ, Kimmel M *et al.* (2014) Efficacy of high-dose versus standard-dose influenza vaccine in older adults. *N Engl J Med* **371**: 635–645.
67. Weinberger B, Grubeck-Loebenstein B. (2012) Vaccines for the elderly. *Clin Microbiol Infect* **18**: 100–108.
68. Domínguez A, Izquierdo C, Salleras L *et al.* (2010) Effectiveness of the pneumococcal polysaccharide vaccine in preventing pneumonia in the elderly. *Eur Respir J* **36**: 608–614.
69. Boraschi D, Italiani P. (2014) Immunosenescence and vaccine failure in the elderly: Strategies for improving response. *Immunol Lett* **162**: 346–353.
70. Targonski PV, Jacobson RM, Poland GA. (2007) Immunosenescence: Role and measurement in influenza vaccine response among the elderly. *Vaccine* **25**: 3066–3069.
71. Ong R, Kwa AL, Lee W. (2011) Dual pneumococcal and influenza vaccination in elderly patients with chronic illnesses: Protective benefits overestimated? *Clin Infect Dis* **52**: 558–559.

72. Aspinall R, Lang PO. (2014) Vaccine responsiveness in the elderly: Best practice for the clinic. *Expert Rev Vaccines* **13**: 885–894.
73. Oviedo-Orta E, Li CK, Rappuoli R. (2013) Perspectives on vaccine development for the elderly. *Curr Opin Immunol* **25**: 529–534.
74. Artz AS, Ershler WB, Longo DL. (2003) Pneumococcal vaccination and revaccination of older adults. *Clin Microbiol Rev* **16**: 308–318.
75. Sisk JE, Moskowitz AJ, Whang W *et al.* (1997) Cost-effectiveness of vaccination against pneumococcal bacteremia among elderly people. *JAMA* **278**: 1333–1339.
76. Butler JC, Breiman RF, Campbell JF *et al.* (1993) Pneumococcal polysaccharide vaccine efficacy. An evaluation of current recommendations. *JAMA* **270**: 1826–1831.
77. Simberkoff MS, Cross AP, Al-Ibrahim M *et al.* (1986) Efficacy of pneumococcal vaccine in high-risk patients. Results of a Veterans Administration Cooperative Study. *N Engl J Med* **315**: 1318–1327.
78. Ortqvist A. (2001) Pneumococcal vaccination: Current and future issues. *Eur Respir J* **18**: 184–195.
79. Nichol KL, Margolis KL, Wuorenma J *et al.* (1994) The efficacy and cost effectiveness of vaccination against influenza among elderly persons living in the community. *N Engl J Med* **331**: 778–784.
80. Gross PA, Hermogenes AW, Sacks HS *et al.* (1995) The efficacy of influenza vaccine in elderly persons. A meta-analysis and review of the literature. *Ann Intern Med* **123**: 518–527.
81. Pawelec G, Larbi A. (2008) Immunity and ageing in man: Annual Review 2006/2007. *Exp Gerontol* **43**: 34–38.
82. Meyer KC. (2010) The role of immunity and inflammation in lung senescence and susceptibility to infection in the elderly. *Semin Respir Crit Care Med* **31**: 561–574.
83. Franceschi C, Valensin S, Bonafè M *et al.* (2000) The network and the remodeling theories of aging: Historical background and new perspectives. *Exp Gerontol* **35**: 879–896.
84. Franceschi C. (2007) Inflammaging as a major characteristic of old people: Can it be prevented or cured? *Nutr Rev* **65**: S173–S176.
85. Takeda, K, Akira S. (2005) Toll-like receptors in innate immunity. *Int Immunol* **17**: 1–14.
86. Lee A, Whyte MK, Haslett C. (1993) Inhibition of apoptosis and prolongation of neutrophil functional longevity by inflammatory mediators. *J Leukoc Biol* **54**: 283–288.

87. Esparza B, Sanchez H, Ruiz M *et al.* (1996) Neutrophil function in elderly persons assessed by flow cytometry. *Immunol Invest* **25**: 185–190.
88. Shodell M, Siegal FP. (2002) Circulating, interferon-producing plasmacytoid dendritic cells decline during human ageing. *Scand J Immunol* **56**: 518–521.
89. Strauss-Albee DM, Horowitz A, Parham P *et al.* (2014) Coordinated regulation of NK receptor expression in the maturing human immune system. *J Immunol* **193**: 4871–4879.
90. Solana, R, Campos C, Pera A *et al.* (2014) Shaping of NK cell subsets by aging. *Curr Opin Immunol* **29**: 56–61.
91. Hakim FT, Gress RE. (2007) Immunosenescence: Deficits in adaptive immunity in the elderly. *Tissue Antigens* **70**: 179–189.
92. Franceschi C, Capri M, Monti D *et al.* (2007) Inflammaging and anti-inflammaging: A systemic perspective on aging and longevity emerged from studies in humans. *Mech Ageing Dev* **128**: 92–105.
93. Franceschi C, Campisi J. (2014) Chronic inflammation (inflammaging) and its potential contribution to age-associated diseases. *J Gerontol A Biol Sci Med Sci*: S4–S9.
94. Campisi J. (2013) Aging, cellular senescence, and cancer. *Annu Rev Physiol* **75**: 685–705.
95. Campisi J, Andersen JK, Kapahi P *et al.* (2011) Cellular senescence: A link between cancer and age-related degenerative disease? *Semin Cancer Biol* **21**: 354–359.
96. Volkova M, Zhang Y, Shaw AC *et al.* (2012) The role of Toll-like receptors in age-associated lung diseases. *J Gerontol A Biol Sci Med Sci* **67**: 247–253.
97. Shaw AC, Goldstein DR, Montgomery RR. (2013) Age-dependent dysregulation of innate immunity. *Nat Rev Immunol* **13**: 875–887.
98. Hinojosa E, Boyd AR, Orihuela CJ. (2009) Age-associated inflammation and toll-like receptor dysfunction prime the lungs for pneumococcal pneumonia. *J Infect Dis* **200**: 546–554.
99. Yende S, Tuomanen EI, Wunderink R *et al.* (2005) Preinfection systemic inflammatory markers and risk of hospitalization due to pneumonia. *Am J Respir Crit Care Med* **172**: 1440–1446.
100. Lee J, Sandford A, Man P *et al.* (2011) Is the aging process accelerated in chronic obstructive pulmonary disease? *Curr Opin Pulm Med* **17**: 90–97.

101. Brusselle GG, Joos GF, Bracke KR. (2011) New insights into the immunology of chronic obstructive pulmonary disease. *Lancet* **378**: 1015–1026.
102. Cabrera-Rubio R, Garcia-Núñez M, Setó L *et al.* (2012) Microbiome diversity in the bronchial tracts of patients with chronic obstructive pulmonary disease. *J Clin Microbiol* **50**: 3562–3568.
103. Tumkaya M, Atis S, Ozge C *et al.* (2007) Relationship between airway colonization, inflammation and exacerbation frequency in COPD. *Respir Med* **101**: 729–737.
104. Khurana S, Ravi A, Sutula J *et al.* (2014) Clinical characteristics and airway inflammation profile of COPD persistent sputum producers. *Respir Med* **108**: 1761–1770.
105. Sibila O, Garcia-Bellmunt L, Giner J *et al.* (2014) Identification of airway bacterial colonization by an electronic nose in Chronic Obstructive Pulmonary Disease. *Respir Med* **108**: 1608–1614.
106. Wilkinson TM, Patel IS, Wilks M, *et al.* (2003) Airway bacterial load and FEV1 decline in patients with chronic obstructive pulmonary disease. *Am J Respir Crit Care Med* **167**: 1090–1095.
107. Soler N, Ewig S, Torres A *et al.* (1999) Airway inflammation and bronchial microbial patterns in patients with stable chronic obstructive pulmonary disease. *Eur Respir J* **14**: 1015–1022.
108. Yende S, Waterer GW, Tolley E A *et al.* (2006) Inflammatory markers are associated with ventilatory limitation and muscle dysfunction in obstructive lung disease in well functioning elderly subjects. *Thorax* **61**: 10–16.
109. Miller J, Edwards LD, Agustí A *et al.* (2013) Comorbidity, systemic inflammation and outcomes in the ECLIPSE cohort. *Respir Med* **107**: 1376–1384.
110. Agustí A, Edwards LD, Rennard SI *et al.* (2012) Persistent systemic inflammation is associated with poor clinical outcomes in COPD: A novel phenotype. *PLoS One* **7**: e37483.
111. Sethi S, Maloney J, Grove L *et al.* (2006) Airway inflammation and bronchial bacterial colonization in chronic obstructive pulmonary disease. *Am J Respir Crit Care Med* **173**: 991–998.
112. Sethi S, Wrona C, Eschberger K *et al.* (2008) Inflammatory profile of new bacterial strain exacerbations of chronic obstructive pulmonary disease. *Am J Respir Crit Care Med* **177**: 491–497.
113. Zhang X, Shan P, Jiang G *et al.* (2006) Toll-like receptor 4 deficiency causes pulmonary emphysema. *J Clin Invest* **116**: 3050–3059.
114. Lee C, Link H, Baluk P *et al.* (2004) Vascular endothelial growth factor (VEGF) induces remodeling and enhances TH2-mediated sensitization and inflammation in the lung. *Nat Med* **10**: 1095–1103.

115. Stoltz DA, Meyerholz DK, Welsh MJ. (2015) Origins of cystic fibrosis lung disease. *N Engl J Med* **372**: 351–362.
116. Gilligan PH. (2014) Infections in patients with cystic fibrosis: Diagnostic microbiology update. *Clin Lab Med* **34**: 197–217.
117. Teichgräber V, Ulrich M, Endlich N *et al.* (2008) Ceramide accumulation mediates inflammation, cell death and infection susceptibility in cystic fibrosis. *Nat Med* **14**: 382–391.
118. Munder A, Wölbeling F, Kerber-Momot T *et al.* (2011) Acute intratracheal Pseudomonas aeruginosa infection in cystic fibrosis mice is age-independent. *Respir Res* **12**: 148.
119. Chen Y, Vaccarino V, Williams C *et al.* (1999) Risk factors for heart failure in the elderly: A prospective community-based study. *Am J Med* **106**: 605–612.
120. Klingman KL, Pye A, Murphy TF *et al.* (1995) Dynamics of respiratory tract colonization by Branhamella catarrhalis in bronchiectasis. *Am J Respir Crit Care Med* **152**: 1072–1078.
121. Cabello H, Torres A, Celis R. (1997) Bacterial colonization of distal airways in healthy subjects and chronic lung disease: A bronchoscopic study. *Eur Respir J* **10**: 1137–1144.
122. Lee JH, Kim YK, Kwag HJ *et al.* (2004) Relationships between high-resolution computed tomography, lung function and bacteriology in stable bronchiectasis. *J Korean Med Sci* **19**: 62–68.
123. Atamas SP, Chapoval SP, Keegan AD. (2013) Cytokines in chronic respiratory diseases. *F1000 Biol Rep* **5**: 3.
124. RosellA, Monsó E, Soler N *et al.* (2005) Microbiologic determinants of exacerbation in chronic obstructive pulmonary disease. *Arch Intern Med* **165**: 891–897.
125. Lu HW, Ji XB, Liang S *et al.* (2014) Pathogen characteristics reveal novel antibacterial approaches for interstitial lung disease. *Pulm Pharmacol Ther* **29**: 250–254.
126. Molyneaux PL, Cox MJ, Willis-Owen SA *et al.* (2014) The role of bacteria in the pathogenesis and progression of idiopathic pulmonary fibrosis. *Am J Respir Crit Care Med* **190**: 906–913.
127. Han MK, Zhou Y, Murray S *et al.* (2014) Lung microbiome and disease progression in idiopathic pulmonary fibrosis: An analysis of the COMET study. *Lancet Respir Med* **2**: 548–556.
128. Dela Cruz CS, Tanoue LT, Matthay RA. (2011) Lung cancer: Epidemiology, etiology, and prevention. *Clin Chest Med* **32**: 605–644.
129. Gomes M, Teixeira AL, Coelho A *et al.* (2014) The role of inflammation in lung cancer. *Adv Exp Med Biol* **816**: 1–23.

130. Ioanas M, Angrill J, Baldo X *et al.* (2002) Bronchial bacterial colonization in patients with resectable lung carcinoma. *Eur Respir J* **19**: 326–332.
131. Laroumagne S, Lepage B, Hermant C *et al.* (2013) Bronchial colonisation in patients with lung cancer: A prospective study. *Eur Respir J* **42**: 220–229.
132. Belda J, Cavalcanti M, Ferrer M *et al.* (2005) Bronchial colonization and postoperative respiratory infections in patients undergoing lung cancer surgery. *Chest* **128**: 1571–1579.

Chapter 11

HIV, the Lung and Aging

Lynn M. Schnapp*,† and Kristina Crothers‡

1. Introduction

By 2020, adults age 50 and older are estimated to constitute the majority of HIV infected patients living in the United States (US).[1] Life expectancies are into the 60's and beyond,[2] and among HIV infected patients who initiate therapy early and demonstrate a robust response, life expectancy approaches that of uninfected individuals.[2–4] Aging of the HIV infected population can be attributed to substantially improved survival resulting from potent combinations of antiretroviral therapy (ART). Adults age 50 and older, defined as elderly amongst those with HIV, also account for approximately 10% of new HIV infections.[1,5]

The aging of the HIV infected population has resulted in a changing spectrum of disease. Comorbid diseases contribute substantially to morbidity and mortality in this aging population.[6–10] Mortality related to AIDS-defining conditions has decreased markedly among those on

* Corresponding Author.

† Division of Pulmonary, Critical Care, Allergy and Sleep Medicine, Department of Medicine, Medical University of South Carolina, 96 Jonathan Lucas Street, Suite 812 - CSB, MSC 630, Charleston, SC 29425, Phone: 843-792-3067, Fax: 843-876-2057, E-mail: Schnapp@musc.edu

‡ Division of Pulmonary and Critical Care Medicine, Department of Medicine, University of Washington, Harborview Medical Center, 325 9th Avenue, PO Box 359762, Seattle, WA 98104, Phone: 206-744-9874, Fax: 206-744-8584.

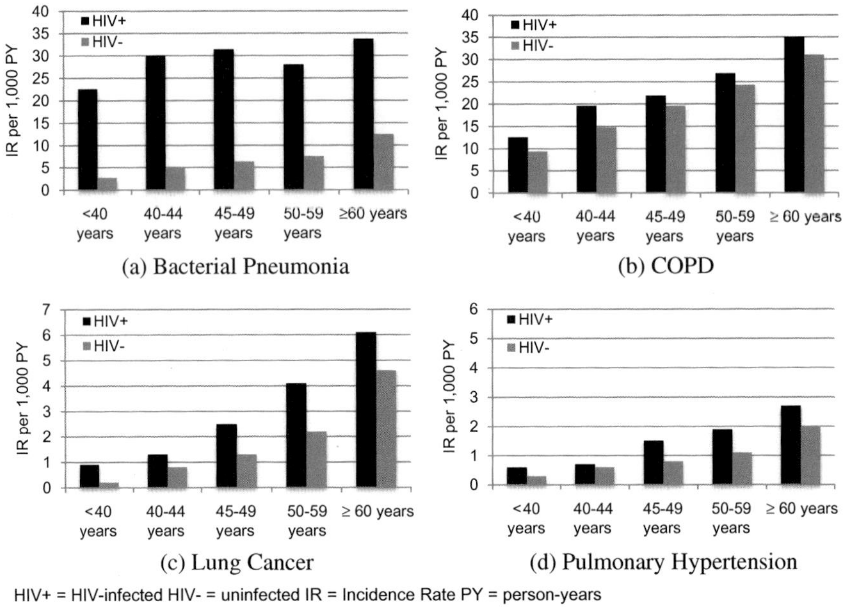

Fig. 1. Incidence Rate Per 1,000 Person-Years of Pulmonary Diagnoses Stratified by Age and HIV Status. Based on Data from the Veterans Aging Cohort Study.[12]

effective ART.[6,11] Serious non-AIDS conditions account for the majority of deaths in recent studies and are expected to increase.[6–10]

HIV is an independent risk factor for many lung diseases of aging. The most commonly encountered lung diseases in HIV infected patients that also increase in frequency with age include bacterial community-acquired pneumonia, chronic obstructive pulmonary disease (COPD), and lung cancer (Fig. 1).[12] Notably, these diseases are also related to smoking. This is particularly important given that the prevalence of smoking among HIV infected populations is substantially higher than in the general US population (~40–50% of HIV infected are current smokers versus 20% in the general population).[13] Although results were conflicting prior to combination ART (likely from competing risks of AIDS-related mortality),[14–16] cigarette smoking is now clearly associated with considerably increased morbidity and mortality in HIV infected persons.[17,18]

Thus, smoking-related comorbidities with a long latency of onset, such as COPD and lung cancer, are expected to become increasingly common as HIV infected persons age. Indeed, COPD is now one of the most prevalent comorbidities in HIV infected patients — diagnosed in 12–15% [19,20] and is substantially more common in older HIV infected patients.[12,21] Smoking also contributes to persistent risk of bacterial pneumonia, one of the most frequent infectious complications in those with HIV, despite ART. Further, while the types of cancer have shifted such that AIDS-defining cancers related to immunosuppression have declined in the current era with widespread use of ART,[22,23] lung cancer is now the most common non-AIDS defining cancer (NADC) and leading source of NADC mortality amongst HIV infected individuals.[24,25] Thus, a better understanding of the impact of aging and lung complications in those with HIV infection is of increasing importance to improve clinical care and to develop novel preventative and therapeutic strategies.[26]

2. HIV, Aging, and Immunosenescence

HIV infection shares many features that are characteristic of premature tissue aging and accelerated replicative senescence. Tissue aging refers to the decrease in the capacity of an organ to repair and regenerate tissues. Cellular senescence is characterized by cell growth arrest in the setting of cell stress and is characterized by a distinct morphological and biochemical phenotype. Increasing evidence suggests that HIV infected individuals experience increased incidence and earlier age of onset of many of the co-morbidities associated with aging including osteoporosis, atherosclerosis, chronic renal insufficiency, and neurocognitive decline,[27,28] as well as specific pulmonary diseases discussed in this chapter. Together, the immune alterations and associated co-morbidities suggest that HIV infection causes accelerated aging.[28]

While many studies have demonstrated that HIV infected patients have higher rates of cardiovascular disease compared to age-matched HIV uninfected individuals,[29,30] the impact of HIV on development of age-related lung diseases is just beginning to be understood. It is likely many of the same mechanisms that contribute to cardiovascular disease in HIV infected persons contribute to lung diseases. This includes the increased prevalence of smoking, which induces oxidative stress and is a known risk factor for premature aging. The lung may be particularly vulnerable to the dual effects of aging and HIV infection, given the deleterious effects of smoking and its role as an immune surveillance organ combined. Furthermore, HIV infection causes significant alterations in the immune response and host defense, which recapitulate many features found in immunosenescence, described below.

Both HIV and aging have profound effects on the immune system (Table 1, Fig. 2). Immunosenescence can be broadly defined as a functional limitation of immunity due to age-related changes to both innate and adaptive immunity systems. Chronic activation of the innate immune system, with changes in both cell surface receptors, increased T cell activation and impaired function of immune cells are observed with aging, as well as with HIV infection. The number of naïve $CD4^+$ and $CD8^+$ T cells decreases with normal aging and with HIV infection, and HIV-1 infection causes premature aging of naïve $CD4^+$ T cells and memory $CD4^+$ and $CD8^+$ T cells.[29] Loss of the

Table 1. Changes in adaptive immunity in HIV infection and aging.[26,29,46]

Major category	HIV infection	Aged uninfected patients
Cell-mediated immunity		
Thymus function	Decreased	Decreased
$CD4^+/CD8^+$ ratio	Decreased	Decreased
Naïve T cell number	Decreased	Decreased
Memory T cell number	Decreased	Normal to increased
T cell repertoire	Decreased	Decreased
T cell proliferative responses	Decreased	Decreased
CD28– CD8+ T cells	Increased	Increased
CD8+CD57+	Increased	Increased
Humoral immunity		
Naïve B cell number	Normal–low	Normal-low
Memory B cell number	Increased	Increased
Total IgA and IgG level	Polyclonal increase	Normal to increased
Memory response	Low–normal	Normal

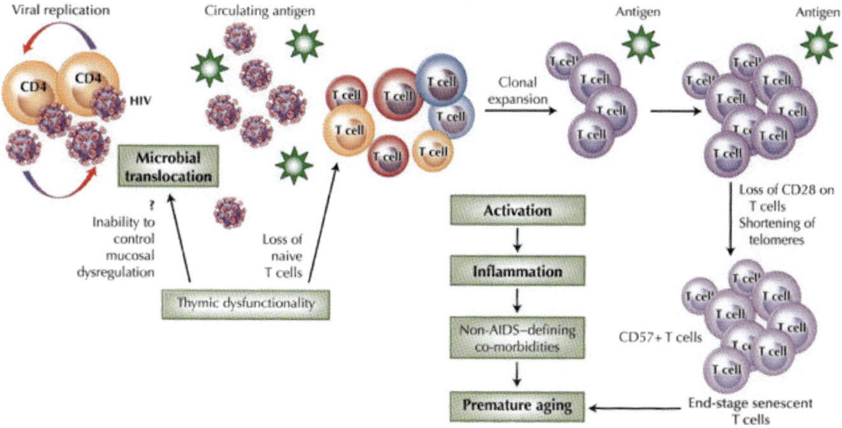

Fig. 2. Accelerated Aging Model in HIV Infection. Viral replication results in release of virions (infectious and noninfectious HIV) into circulation. Residual ongoing replication continues to activate immune cells despite highly active antiretroviral therapy. Microbial translocation adds to the antigenic burden. Loss of thymic function alters T cell homeostasis. Immune activation due to circulating antigen is the central event in the senescent pathway. Activated cells undergo clonal expansion in response to the persistent antigen, resulting in differentiation and accumulation of nonfunctional end stage senescent cells. Activated cells release inflammatory mediators, causing optimal and suboptimal inflammation associated with non-AIDS-defining co-morbidities and premature aging.[28]

co-stimulatory molecule CD28 on T cells, with excessive secretion of proinflammatory cytokines is a critical feature of immune senescence. With down regulation of CD28 on T effector cells, these so-called senescent cells are proinflammatory and may have a viable effector function, but their expansion can contribute to heightened systemic inflammation and collateral harm. Chronic viral infection and inflammation are associated with increased number of CD28- T cells, which is particularly relevant to HIV infection, given the prevalence of co-infection with cytomegalovirus (CMV) in this population. In addition, phagocytic capacity, synthesis of reactive oxygen intermediaries and the intracellular killing efficiency of neutrophils are impaired in the elderly, and similarly impaired in HIV infection. Many of the features of immune senescence appear to persist in chronic HIV infection despite ART.[29]

A number of other factors may contribute to accelerated aging and a greater burden of age-related comorbid diseases in HIV infected patients. Chronic HIV infection is characterized by a state of chronic inflammation and immune activation. Leakiness of the gastrointestinal and genital mucosa,[31,32] due to dysregulated mucosal lymphocytes,[33] is thought to be a major underlying cause of persistent immune activation during suppressive ART, allowing microbial products including lipopolysaccharide (LPS) to leak into the systemic circulation and activate the immune system.[34] In addition, associated co-infections such as with CMV and hepatitis C are also thought to be important drivers of chronic immune activation in HIV. This sustained inflammatory environment is reflected by increased markers of inflammation in the systemic circulation (including IL-6, C-reactive protein (CRP), soluble CD14 (sCD14) and D-dimer), which remain elevated in HIV infected individuals despite suppressive ART.[33,35,36]

Age of HIV infection is also important in a patient's immune and virologic response. Acquisition of HIV at an older age is associated with accelerated HIV progression, and older age appears to accentuate HIV related alterations in immune function.[37] Age may also impact immunological response to ART, although older HIV infected patients appear to have less treatment failure than younger patients, possibly due to better adherence and socio-economic stability of older patients. Older patients treated with ART experience a lower absolute $CD4^+$ cell gain and a longer time to maximum response independent of baseline $CD4^+$ cell and plasma HIV RNA levels.[37–39] Additional mechanisms relevant to HIV and senescence for the development of different lung diseases are discussed in further detail below.

3. HIV and Bacterial Pneumonia

Recurrent bacterial pneumonia, defined as two or more episodes within 12 months, is an AIDS-defining illness. Despite a significant decrease in incidence, bacterial pneumonia remains more frequent in HIV infected compared to uninfected individuals and this elevated risk persists in the combination ART era.[40,41] Bacterial pneumonia is a common cause of morbidity and is associated with increased short and long-term mortality in HIV infected patients in the combination ART era.[42] The most common cause of bacterial pneumonia in both HIV infected and elderly patients is *Streptococcus pneumoniae.*

Numerous factors contribute to increased risk for pneumonia in HIV infected persons, particularly $CD4^+$ lymphocyte count. Bacterial pneumonia can occur throughout the course of HIV infection and at any $CD4^+$ lymphocyte count, although the incidence increases as the $CD4^+$ lymphocyte count declines. Additional behavioral risk factors for bacterial pneumonia include injection drug use and cigarette smoking.

Advancing age is a recognized risk factor for pneumonia in HIV infected as in uninfected populations.[12,43] Altered function of monocytes and alveolar macrophages (AM), as well as toll-like receptor 4 (TLR4) signaling in HIV infected individuals may confer susceptibility to lung infections.[44,45] Age-related changes in macrophage function can include impaired cytokine production, recruitment, and phagocytic ability, and dendritic cells may be decreased in number and function.[46] B cell dysfunction is also found in both HIV infected patients and aged patients, which can be clinically manifested by the increased risk of serious pulmonary infections such as pneumococcal pneumonia in the HIV population.[43] Additional changes reflective of immunosenescence in HIV infected compared to uninfected patients are summarized in Table 1.

Changes in lung structure and function with aging, decreased compliance of the chest wall, and impaired mucociliary clearance may also confer greater risk of pneumonia with age.[46] A greater risk of osteoporosis and fragility fractures in HIV,[47] including of the vertebral bodies, could also contribute to anatomic changes in chest wall structure and lung function. The extent to which these factors contribute to risk for pneumonia in HIV infected persons is not well understood. Finally, underlying comorbidities, particularly COPD, are additional important risk factors for pneumonia in aging HIV infected patients.

4. HIV and COPD

The high prevalence of COPD among HIV infected patients is not only because of greater rates of smoking in HIV infected patients, but HIV infection confers an independent risk for COPD, even without prior AIDS related pulmonary complications.[48,49] We demonstrated increased COPD diagnoses in HIV infected compared to uninfected veterans in the ART era,[12,50] and found that HIV infection was an independent risk factor for COPD, by ICD-9 codes or patient self-report. HIV infected subjects were 50–60% more likely to have COPD than HIV uninfected subjects.[50] Furthermore, COPD appears to present at earlier ages in HIV infected patients (Fig. 1).[12] When comparing pulmonary function test results by HIV status, HIV infection is an independent risk factor for a low diffusing capacity of the lung for carbon monoxide (DLCO).[51] This is most likely explained by emphysema, as HIV infected patients appear more likely to have emphysema that is more severe and that tends to be more diffuse when compared to HIV uninfected patients.[52]

The complex pathogenesis of COPD in HIV remains unclear, and likely involves multiple pathways, including immune, apoptotic, proteolytic, and oxidative stress mechanisms.[53–55] Chronic innate immune activation may be involved, as we found that elevated levels of soluble CD14, the LPS co-receptor, were associated with emphysema in HIV infected patients in a cross-sectional study.[52] Furthermore, HIV infection appears to confer a phenotype of premature frailty,[56] and has been associated with senescence-related changes in the immune system and other organ systems.[57–61] As a result, HIV infection may render the lung more susceptible to the earlier presentation of diseases such as COPD, which has been suggested as a disease of accelerated lung senescence.[62–67] We discuss a number of potential biologically plausible pathways that are linked to senescence and that may contribute to the development of a unique signature of COPD in the setting of HIV.

Cellular senescence is characterized by irreversible cell cycle arrest, which can be induced by cellular damage caused by oxidative stress, DNA damage, telomerase shortening and other triggers.[68,69] Although senescent cells do not proliferate, they are metabolically active and upregulate a number of secreted proteins that define a senescence-associated secretory phenotype (SASP).[68] These include a number of pro-inflammatory cytokines including IL-8, IL-6, IL-1, and growth regulatory factors that can contribute to the development of COPD. Senescent cells also alter the extracellular matrix directly through changes in structural proteins (e.g. collagens, laminins) and enzymes involved in matrix remodeling (e.g. MMPs, TIMPs).[70] Thus, senescent cells are not merely passive bystanders, as their "secretome" affects the neighboring cells and extracellular environment. Senescent cells are identified in culture and *in vivo* by a number of characteristics including senescence-associated β-galactosidase (SA-βgal) expression, impaired proliferation, increased expression of the cell cycle inhibitors p16 and p21, and increased expression of senescence-associated secreted proteins. Collectively, these markers have been used to show that senescent cells exist and accumulate with age *in vivo* in a variety of mammalian tissues.[68,69,71]

There is a growing body of literature suggesting a causative role of cellular senescence in the pathogenesis of COPD. Several studies have demonstrated increased markers of cellular senescence, including SA-βgal, and cyclin kinase inhibitors p21, and p16 in epithelium of COPD patients.[63,65,66] Cellular senescence is also accelerated by smoking.[72] Cigarette smoke increases senescent markers in epithelial cells and fibroblasts.[72] A global analysis of COPD gene expression demonstrated significant enrichment of cellular senescent markers, and concomitant suppression of anti-senescent mediators.[73]

While there is increasing interest in determining the role of HIV infection in premature cellular senescence, few studies have been published to date specifically in HIV related COPD. We previously demonstrated that HIV infected lymphocytes increase secretion of TGFβ1, which caused increased fibronectin secretion by fibroblasts.[74] Of interest, TGFβ1 is a known inducer of epithelial cell

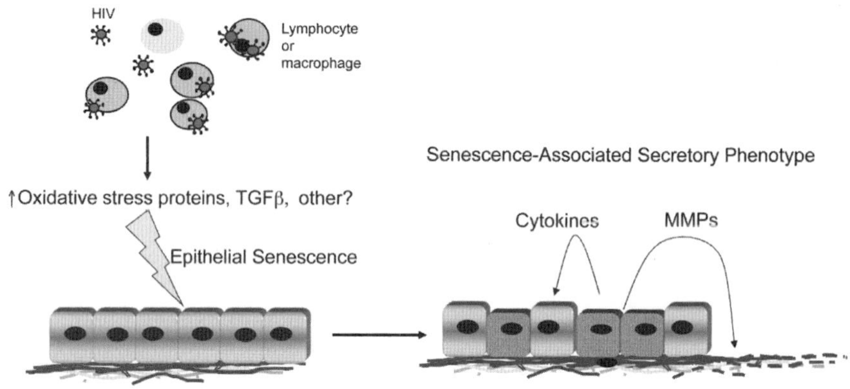

Fig. 3. Potential Mechanism: HIV Infection Accelerates Epithelial Senescence, which Contributes to the Premature Development of COPD. MMP: matrix metalloproteinase

senescence.[75,76] Possible mechanisms by which epithelial cell senescence may cause COPD in HIV infection are shown in Fig. 3.

T cell function and telomere length may also be associated with COPD. In a recent study, 147 HIV infected patients underwent pulmonary function testing and analysis of peripheral markers of inflammation, T cell activation and senescence.[77] The majority of patients were men (67%), and current or former smokers (83%). Approximately 29% of patients had evidence of airflow obstruction (FEV1/FVC <0.7) and 34% had DLCO <60% predicted. Both airflow obstruction and low DLCO were correlated with increased markers of immune activation and inflammation (CD25, CD69 expression on T cells, and IL-6). Airflow obstruction was also associated with shorter telomeres in PBMC, a marker of replicative senescence. In contrast, the number of T cells expressing markers of senescence correlated with less airflow obstruction. Thus, the study shows evidence of peripheral immune activation and alterations in senescent markers that correlate with pulmonary function. Unanswered questions include whether these findings are unique to HIV associated airflow obstruction and given the cross-sectional nature of the study, do not prove causality. Nonetheless, the results provide intriguing data on the role of senescence and T cell function in HIV associated COPD.

Macrophages also play a critical role in the pathogenesis of COPD. HIV can be detected and recovered from AM and lymphocytes; cigarette smoke may enhance susceptibility of AM to HIV infection.[78–82] The number of macrophages is about 10-fold higher in the lungs of smokers than non-smokers,[83–86] and emphysema develops coincident with increased macrophage influx in several mouse models.[87–92] Macrophages produce a variety of proteinases that can cause extracellular matrix damage that leads to emphysema. In HIV infected smokers, upregulation of metalloproteinases by macrophages appears to play an important role in pathogenesis of emphysema.[55] Interestingly, a report that examined AIDS lung autopsy specimens detected HIV infected macrophages associated with areas of emphysema, with adjacent, uninfected (possibly epithelial) cells positive for MMP-9.[93] HIV infected immune cells may release additional factors that accelerate the development of senescence.

Finally, whether and the degree to which persistence of the HIV virus within the lung contributes to the development and progression of COPD is uncertain. Genetic compartmentalization between lung and blood has demonstrated clonal expansion of the virus in the lung of select individuals[94] and HIV DNA sequences in induced sputa during suppressive ART can have greater accumulation of resistance mutations when compared to PBMC, with divergence of HIV *env* in sputa-derived viruses.[78] We speculate that low-level expression of viral proteins and of virions by HIV infected alveolar $CD4^+$ cells despite suppressive ART may contribute to lung epithelial damage. This may be in part due to immune activation in the lung, fueled by the local production of HIV RNA and proteins from persisting proviruses as seen in other sites,[95–97] or low-level but full cycles of viral replication due to insufficient ART concentrations in the lung compartment.[98] A recent study demonstrated that direct interaction of HIV or the envelope glycoprotein of HIV-1 (but not Tat) with epithelial cells caused impairment of barrier function and upregulation of inflammatory cytokines such as TNFα.[32] Alternatively, other microbes causing persistent antigenic stimulus and immune activation, such as CMV or *Pneumocystis jirovecii*, could also be important drivers of COPD.[99] Further studies are needed to determine the role of HIV and other infections in perpetuating inflammation and lung damage.

5. HIV and Lung Cancer

With increased use of ART, AIDS-defining cancers related to immunosuppression have declined.[22,23,100,101] In contrast, NADC have increased primarily among HIV infected persons ≥50 years of age.[100,101] Lung cancer is the most common infection-unrelated NADC and a leading cause of mortality in HIV infected persons.[24,100–105] Increased lung cancer in HIV infected patients has been demonstrated in multiple studies with incidence rate ratios ranging from 1.7 to 4.7.[24,104,106–113] HIV infected patients develop lung cancer at younger ages compared to uninfected patients, (age 50 versus 54 years).[104]

Reasons for the increased risk of lung cancer in HIV infection are not fully understood. As in HIV uninfected persons, cigarette smoking and age are strong risk factors for disease, but these factors incompletely explain the association between HIV infection and lung cancer. Chronic pulmonary inflammation as a result of underlying structural lung disease such as COPD,[12,49,50] an established lung cancer risk factor,[114–116] may be a particularly important driver of lung cancer risk among HIV infected persons irrespective of $CD4^+$ cell count. Prior lung disease and infections, particularly bacterial pneumonia and tuberculosis, are also purported risk factors;[117–121] these are increased in HIV[12] and may partially explain the risk for lung cancer.[122]

Immunodeficiency appears to be important in risk for lung cancer. Although several studies have not demonstrated an association with lung cancer and various markers of immunosuppression or control of HIV such as baseline $CD4^+$ cell count, nadir $CD4^+$ count, or baseline ART exposure,[108,111,123] a meta-analysis by Grulich *et al.* comparing cancer incidence in studies of HIV/AIDS patients and solid organ transplant recipients found similar risk increases for lung cancer in both groups, suggesting a causal role for immunosuppression.[124]

Furthermore, in the large French Hospital Database cohort[125] and the EuroSIDA cohort,[103] current $CD4^+$ count was inversely related to lung cancer incidence.

Cellular senescence may be linked to increased risk for lung cancer in the setting of HIV. By inducing cell growth arrest in the setting of stress, cellular senescence is thought to be a protective mechanism against the development of cancer. Yet, over the long term, senescent cells may create an environment that is permissive for cancer growth. Although senescent cells lack regenerative ability, they are resistant to apoptosis and accumulate over the lifespan of an organism. Furthermore, their secretome has been postulated to induce preneoplastic changes in adjacent stromal cells. Additional studies are needed to better understand the pathogenesis and role of immmunosenescence in the development of lung cancer in HIV infection.

6. HIV and Pulmonary Hypertension

HIV infection is an established risk factor for the development of pulmonary hypertension (PH), also specified as World Health Organization (WHO) Group 1 pulmonary arterial hypertension (PAH), with an incidence of approximately 0.5% in HIV infected patients,[126,127] which has persisted despite ART. Although not classically considered a disease of aging, the mean age at PH diagnosis and prevalence of PH in the elderly has increased significantly over the past two decades.[128] Similarly, in the Veterans Aging Cohort Study, diagnoses of PH increased with age in both HIV infected and uninfected persons (Fig. 1).

It is not clear if the pathogenesis of HIV associated Group 1 PH is distinct. Possible causes of PH in HIV include effects of HIV proteins, interactions with opiates, and inflammation.[129–131] HIV proteins such as gp120, Nef and Tat may interact with pulmonary endothelial cells to contribute to disease pathogenesis.[132] Chronic immune activation may also contribute to pulmonary endothelial dysfunction.

HIV infection increases the incidence of disorders such as COPD, cardiovascular disease and chronic thromboembolic disease,[133] which contribute to development of secondary PH (WHO Groups 2-5). HIV infected individuals with elevated echocardiographic pulmonary artery pressures have more respiratory complaints, more advanced HIV disease, airway obstruction, lower DLCO, and systemic and pulmonary inflammation.[134] These findings suggest that PH may co-exist with COPD in this population and share similar inflammatory mechanisms. As a result, the prevalence of secondary causes of PH may increase as HIV infected patients age.

7. Conclusion

In summary, given greater longevity of HIV infected patients, the interaction of chronic HIV infection and aging will influence an increasing burden and spectrum of lung diseases in those with HIV. HIV infection and aging have many similar impacts on immune function, contributing to a younger presentation and increased prevalence of pulmonary diseases related to aging in the HIV population. Additional studies are needed to improve our understanding of unique mechanisms by which HIV may cause lung disease via mechanisms that include accelerated cellular senescence. Future work should include identifying novel ways of preventing or ameliorating disease, such as by decreasing microbial translocation or mitigating the effects of chronic antigenic stimulus such as from CMV infection to decrease chronic immune activation and inflammation. Given the high prevalence and strong association of lung and multiple other comorbidities and mortality with cigarette smoking, additional efforts should also focus on improving smoking cessation rates amongst HIV infected persons.

References

1. Brooks JT, Buchacz K, Gebo KA, Mermin J. (2012) HIV infection and older Americans: The public health perspective. *Am J Public Health* **102(8)**: 1516–1526.
2. CDC (2011) HIV surveillance–United States, 1981–2008. *MMWR Morb Mortal Wkly Rep* **60(21)**: 689–693.
3. van Sighem AI, Gras LA, Reiss P *et al.* (2010) Life expectancy of recently diagnosed asymptomatic HIV infected patients approaches that of uninfected individuals. *AIDS* **24(10)**: 1527–1535.

4. Zwahlen M *et al.* (2009) Mortality of HIV infected patients starting potent antiretroviral therapy: Comparison with the general population in nine industrialized countries. *Int J Epidemiol* **38(6)**: 1624–1633.
5. Centers for Disease Control and Prevention. (2011) HIV Surveillance Report, vol. 23. Available at http://www.cdc.gov/hiv/topics/surveillance/resources/reports/. Accessed February 2015.
6. Mocroft A, *et al.* (2002) Changes in the cause of death among HIV positive subjects across Europe: results from the EuroSIDA study. *AIDS* **16(12)**: 1663–1671.
7. Braithwaite RS *et al.* (2005) Estimating the proportion of patients infected with HIV who will die of comorbid diseases. *Am J Med* **118(8)**: 890–898.
8. Crum NF *et al.* (2006) Comparisons of causes of death and mortality rates among HIV infected persons: Analysis of the pre-, early, and late HAART (highly active antiretroviral therapy) eras. *J Acquir Immune Defic Syndr* **41(2)**: 194–200.
9. Lau B, Gange SJ, Moore RD. (2007) Risk of non-AIDS-related mortality may exceed risk of AIDS-related mortality among individuals enrolling into care with CD4+ counts greater than 200 cells/mm3. *J Acquir Immune Defic Syndr* **44(2)**: 179–187.
10. Marin B *et al.* (2009) Non-AIDS-defining deaths and immunodeficiency in the era of combination antiretroviral therapy. *AIDS* **23(13)**: 1743–1753.
11. Palella FJ. Jr, *et al.* (1998) Declining morbidity and mortality among patients with advanced human immunodeficiency virus infection. HIV Outpatient Study Investigators. *N Engl J Med* **338(13)**: 853–860.
12. Crothers K, Huang L, Goulet JL *et al.* (2011) HIV Infection and risk for incident pulmonary diseases in the combination antiretroviral therapy era. *Am J Respir Crit Care Med* **183(3)**: 388–395.
13. CDC (2010) Vital signs: Current cigarette smoking among adults aged >or=18 years — United States, 2009. *MMWR Morb Mortal Wkly Rep* **59(35)**: 1135–1140.
14. Burns DN, Hillman D, Neaton JD *et al.* (1996) Cigarette smoking, bacterial pneumonia, and other clinical outcomes in HIV-1 infection. Terry Beirn Community Programs for Clinical Research on AIDS. *J Acquir Immune Defic Syndr Hum Retrovirol* **13(4)**: 374–383.
15. Page-Shafer K, Delorenze GN, Satariano WA *et al.* (1996) Comorbidity and survival in HIV infected men in the San Francisco Men's Health Survey. *Ann Epidemiol* **6(5)**: 420–430.

16. Galai N, Park LP, Wesch J *et al.* (1997) Effect of smoking on the clinical progression of HIV-1 infection. *J Acquir Immune Defic Syndr Hum Retrovirol* **14(5)**: 451–458.
17. Crothers K, Griffith TA, McGinnis KA *et al.* (2005) The impact of cigarette smoking on mortality, quality of life, and comorbid illness among HIV-positive veterans. *J Gen Inter Med* **20(12)**: 1142–1145.
18. Crothers K, Goulet JL, Rodriguez-Barradas MC *et al.* (2009) Impact of cigarette smoking on mortality in HIV-positive and HIV-negative veterans. *AIDS Educ Preven* **21(3 Suppl)**: 40–53.
19. Crothers K, Huang L, Goulet JL *et al.* (2006) Increased infectious and non-infectious pulmonary diseases among HIV positive compared to HIV negative veterans. *Proc Am Thorac Soc* **3**: A477.
20. Hull MW, Phillips P, Montaner JS. (2008) Changing global epidemiology of pulmonary manifestations of HIV/AIDS. *Chest* **134(6)**: 1287–1298.
21. Justice AC, Lasky E, McGinnis KA *et al.* (2006) Medical disease and alcohol use among veterans with human immunodeficiency infection: A comparison of disease measurement strategies. *Med Care* **44(8 Suppl 2)**: S52–S60.
22. Engels EA, Biggar RJ, Hall HI *et al.* (2008) Cancer risk in people infected with human immunodeficiency virus in the United States. *Int J Cancer* **123(1)**: 187–194.
23. Seaberg EC, Wiley D, Martinez Maza O *et al.* (2010) Cancer incidence in the multicenter AIDS Cohort Study before and during the HAART era: 1984–2007. *Cancer* **116(23)**: 5507–5516.
24. Engels EA, Brock MV, Chen J *et al.* (2006) Elevated incidence of lung cancer among HIV infected individuals. *J Clin Oncol* **24(9)**: 1383–1388.
25. Simard EP, Engels EA. (2010) Cancer as a cause of death among people with AIDS in the United States. *Clin Infect Dis* **51(8)**: 957–962.
26. Effros RB, Fletcher CV, Gebo K *et al.* (2008) Aging and infectious diseases: Workshop on HIV infection and aging: What is known and future research directions. *Clin Infect Dis* **47(4)**: 542–553.
27. Pathai S, Bajillan H, Landay AL *et al.* (2014) Is HIV a model of accelerated or accentuated aging? *J Gerontol A Biol Sci Med Sci* **69(7)**: 833–842.
28. Desai S, Landay A. (2010) Early immune senescence in HIV disease. *Curr HIV/AIDS Rep* **7(1)**: 4–10.
29. Deeks SG. (2011) HIV infection, inflammation, immunosenescence, and aging. *Annu Rev Med* **62**: 141–155.

30. Freiberg MS, Chang CC, Kuller H *et al.* (2013) HIV infection and the risk of acute myocardial infarction. *JAMA Intern Med* **173(8)**: 614–622.
31. Chege D, Sheth P, Kain T *et al.* (2011) Sigmoid Th17 populations, the HIV latent reservoir and microbial translocation in men on long-term antiretroviral therapy. *AIDS* **25(6)**: 741–749.
32. Nazli A, Chan O, Dobson-Belaire WN *et al.* (2010) Exposure to HIV-1 directly impairs mucosal epithelial barrier integrity allowing microbial translocation. *PLoS Pathog* **6(4)**:e1000852.
33. Mehandru S, Poles MA, Tenner Racz, K *et al.* (2006) Lack of mucosal immune reconstitution during prolonged treatment of acute and early HIV-1 infection. *PLoS Med* **3(12)**:e484.
34. Brenchley JM, Price DA, Asher TE *et al.* (2006) Microbial translocation is a cause of systemic immune activation in chronic HIV infection. *Nat Med* **12(12)**: 1365–1371.
35. Kuller LH, Tracy R, Belloso W *et al.* (2008) Inflammatory and coagulation biomarkers and mortality in patients with HIV infection. *PLoS Med* **5(10)**:e203.
36. Nixon DE, Landay AL. (2010) Biomarkers of immune dysfunction in HIV. *Curr Opin HIV AIDS* **5(6)**: 498–503.
37. Kalayjian RC, Landay A, Pollard RB *et al.* (2003) Age-related immune dysfunction in health and in human immunodeficiency virus (HIV) disease: Association of age and HIV infection with naive CD8+ cell depletion, reduced expression of CD28 on CD8+ cells, and reduced thymic volumes. *J Infect Dis* **187(12)**: 1924–1933.
38. Gandhi RT, Spritzler J, Chan E *et al.* (2006) Effect of baseline- and treatment-related factors on immunologic recovery after initiation of antiretroviral therapy in HIV-1-positive subjects: Results from ACTG 384. *J Acquir Immune Defic Syndr* **42(4)**: 426–434.
39. Viard JP, Mocorft A, Chiesi A *et al.* (2001) Influence of age on CD4 cell recovery in human immunodeficiency virus-infected patients receiving highly active antiretroviral therapy: Evidence from the EuroSIDA study. *J Infect Dis* **183(8)**: 1290–1294.
40. Sogaard OS, Lohse N, Gerstoft J *et al.* (2008) Hospitalization for pneumonia among individuals with and without HIV infection, 1995–2007: A Danish population-based, nationwide cohort study. *Clin Infect Dis* **47(10)**: 1345–1353.
41. Segal LN, Methe BA, Nolan A *et al.* (2011) HIV-1 and bacterial pneumonia in the era of antiretroviral therapy. *Proc Am Thorac Soc* **8(3)**: 282–287.

42. Sogaard OS, Lohse N, Gerstoft J *et al.* (2009) Mortality after hospitalization for pneumonia among individuals with HIV, 1995–2008: A Danish cohort study. *PLoS One* **4(9)**:e7022.
43. Krone CL, van de Groep K, Trzcinski K *et al.* (2014) Immunosenescence and pneumococcal disease: An imbalance in host-pathogen interactions. *Lancet Respir Med* **2(2)**: 141–153.
44. Tachado SD, Li X, Bole M *et al.* (2010) MyD88-dependent TLR4 signaling is selectively impaired in alveolar macrophages from asymptomatic HIV+ persons. *Blood* **115(17)**: 3606–3615.
45. Patel NR, Zhu J, Tachado SD *et al.* (2007) HIV impairs TNF-alpha mediated macrophage apoptotic response to Mycobacterium tuberculosis. *J Immunol* **179(10)**: 6973–6980.
46. Meyer KC. (2010) The role of immunity and inflammation in lung senescence and susceptibility to infection in the elderly. *Semin Respir Crit Care Med* **31(5)**: 561–574.
47. Shiau S, Broun EC, Arpadi SM *et al.* (2013) Incident fractures in HIV infected individuals: A systematic review and meta-analysis. *AIDS* **27(12)**: 1949–1957.
48. Diaz PT, Clanton TL, Pacht ER. (1992) Emphysema-like pulmonary disease associated with human immunodeficiency virus infection. *Ann Intern Med* **116(2)**: 124–128.
49. Diaz PT, King MA, Pacht ER *et al.* (2000) Increased susceptibility to pulmonary emphysema among HIV-seropositive smokers. *Ann Intern Med* **132(5)**: 369–372.
50. Crothers K, Butt AA, Gilbert CL *et al.* (2006) Increased COPD among HIV-positive compared to HIV-negative veterans. *Chest* **130(5)**: 1326–1333.
51. Crothers K, McGinnis K, Kleerup E *et al.* (2013) HIV Infection is associated with reduced pulmonary diffusing capacity. *J Acquir Immune Defic Syndr.* **64(3)**: 217–218.
52. Attia EF, Akqun KM, Wongtrakool C *et al.* (2014) Increased risk of radiographic emphysema in HIV is associated with elevated soluble CD14 and nadir CD4. *Chest* **146(6)**: 1543–1553.
53. Crothers K. (2007) Chronic obstructive pulmonary disease in patients who have HIV infection. *Clin Chest Med* **28(3)**: 575–587.
54. Petrache I, Diab K, Knox KS *et al.* (2008) HIV associated pulmonary emphysema: A review of the literature and inquiry into its mechanism. *Thorax* **63(5)**: 463–469.

55. Kaner RJ, Santiago F, Crystal RG. (2009) Up-regulation of alveolar macrophage matrix metalloproteinases in HIV1(+) smokers with early emphysema. *J Leukoc Biol* **86(4)**: 913–922.
56. Desquilbet L, Jacobson LP, Fried LP *et al.* (2007) HIV-1 infection is associated with an earlier occurrence of a phenotype related to frailty. *J Gerontol A Biol Sci Med Sci* **62(11)**: 1279–1286.
57. Appay V, Almeida JR, Sauce D *et al.* (2007) Accelerated immune senescence and HIV-1 infection. *Exp Gerontol* **42(5)**: 432–437.
58. Deeks SG. (2009) Immune dysfunction, inflammation, and accelerated aging in patients on antiretroviral therapy. *Top HIV Med* **17(4)**: 118–123.
59. Deeks SG, Phillips AN. (2009) HIV infection, antiretroviral treatment, ageing, and non-AIDS related morbidity. *BMJ* **338**: a3172.
60. Cao W, Jamieson BD, Hulton LE *et al.* (2009) Premature aging of T cells is associated with faster HIV-1 disease progression. *J Acquir Immune Defic Syndr* **50(2)**: 137–147.
61. Tenorio AR, Spritzler J, Martinson J *et al.* (2009) The effect of aging on T-regulatory cell frequency in HIV infection. *Clin Immunol* **130(3)**: 298–303.
62. Aoshiba K, Nagai A. (2009) Senescence hypothesis for the pathogenetic mechanism of chronic obstructive pulmonary disease. *Proc Am Thorac Soc* **6(7)**: 596–601.
63. MacNee W. (2009) Accelerated lung aging: A novel pathogenic mechanism of chronic obstructive pulmonary disease (COPD). *Biochem Soc Trans* **37(Pt 4)**: 819–823.
64. MacNee W, Tuder RM. (2009) New paradigms in the pathogenesis of chronic obstructive pulmonary disease I. *Proc Am Thorac Soc* **6(6)**: 527–531.
65. Tsuji T, Aoshiba K, Nagai A. (2006) Alveolar cell senescence in patients with pulmonary emphysema. *Am J Respir Crit Care Med* **174(8)**: 886–893.
66. Tsuji T, Aoshiba K, Nagai A. (2010) Alveolar cell senescence exacerbates pulmonary inflammation in patients with chronic obstructive pulmonary disease. *Respiration* **80(1)**: 59–70.
67. Ito K, Barnes PJ. (2009) COPD as a disease of accelerated lung aging. *Chest* **135(1)**: 173–180.
68. Campisi J, d'Adda di Fagagna F. (2007) Cellular senescence: When bad things happen to good cells. *Nat Rev Mol Cell Biol* **8(9)**: 729–740.

69. Rodier F, Campisi J. (2011) Four faces of cellular senescence. *J Cell Biol.* **192(4)**: 547–556.
70. Sprenger CC, Plymate SR, Reed MJ. (2010) Aging-related alterations in the extracellular matrix modulate the microenvironment and influence tumor progression. *Int J Cancer* **127(12)**: 2739–2748.
71. Narita M. (2009) SASP reflects senescence. *EMBO Rep* **10(3)**: 228–230.
72. Nyunoya T, Monick MM, Klingelhutz A *et al.* (2006) Cigarette smoke induces cellular senescence. *Am J Respir Cell Mol Biol* **35(6)**: 681–688.
73. Acquaah-Mensah GK, Malhotra D, Vulimiri M *et al.* (2012) Suppressed expression of T-box transcription factors is involved in senescence in chronic obstructive pulmonary disease. *PLoS Comput Biol* **8(7)**: e1002597.
74. Pal S, Schnapp LM. (2004) HIV infected lymphocytes regulate fibronectin synthesis by TGF beta 1 secretion. *J Immunol* **172(5)**: 3189–3195.
75. Katakura Y, Nakata E, Miura T *et al.* (1999) Transforming growth factor beta triggers two independent-senescence programs in cancer cells. *Biochem Biophys Res Commun* **255(1)**: 110–115.
76. Minagawa S, Araya J, Numata, T *et al.* (2011) Accelerated epithelial cell senescence in IPF and the inhibitory role of SIRT6 in TGF-{beta}-induced senescence of human bronchial epithelial cells. *Am J Physiol Lung Cell Mol Physiol* **300(3)**:L391–L401.
77. Fitzpatrick ME, Singh V, Bertolet M *et al.* (2014) Relationships of pulmonary function, inflammation, and T-cell activation and senescence in an HIV infected cohort. *AIDS* **28(17)**: 2505–2515.
78. Wagner TA, Tobin NH, McKernan JL *et al.* (2009) Increased mutations in Env and Pol suggest greater HIV-1 replication in sputum-derived viruses compared with blood-derived viruses. *AIDS* **23(8)**:923–928.
79. Salahuddin SZ, Rose RM, Groopman JE *et al.* (1986) Human T lymphotropic virus type III infection of human alveolar macrophages. *Blood* **68(1)**: 281–284.
80. Abbud RA, Finegan CK, Guay LA *et al.* (1995) Enhanced production of human immunodeficiency virus type 1 by in vitro-infected alveolar macrophages from otherwise healthy cigarette smokers. *J Infect Dis* **172(3)**: 859–863.
81. Semenzato G, Agostini C, Ometto L *et al.* (1995) CD8+ T lymphocytes in the lung of acquired immunodeficiency syndrome patients harbor human immunodeficiency virus type 1. *Blood* **85(9)**: 2308–2314.

82. Twigg HL, Weiden M, Valentine F *et al.* (2008) Effect of Highly Active Antiretroviral Therapy on Viral Burden in the Lungs of HIV infected Subjects. *J Infect Dis* **197(1)**: 109–116.
83. Retamales I, Elliott WM, Meshi B *et al.* (2001) Amplification of inflammation in emphysema and its association with latent adenoviral infection. *Am J Respir Crit Care Med* **164(3)**: 469–473.
84. Russell RE, Thorley A, Culpitt SV *et al.* (2002) Alveolar macrophage-mediated elastolysis: Roles of matrix metalloproteinases, cysteine, and serine proteases. *Am J Physiol Lung Cell Mol Physiol* **283(4)**:L867–L873.
85. Eidelman D, Saetta MP, Ghezzo H *et al.* (1990) Cellularity of the alveolar walls in smokers and its relation to alveolar destruction. Functional implications. *Am Rev Respir Dis* **141(6)**: 1547–1552.
86. Finkelstein R, Fraser RS, Ghezzo H *et al* (1995) Alveolar inflammation and its relation to emphysema in smokers. *Am J Respir Crit Care Med* **152(5 Pt 1)**: 1666–1672.
87. Glasser SW, Detmer EA, Ikegami M *et al.* (2003) Pneumonitis and emphysema in sp-C gene targeted mice. *J Biol Chem* **278(16)**: 14291–14298.
88. Wert SE, *et al.* (2000) Increased metalloproteinase activity, oxidant production, and emphysema in surfactant protein D gene-inactivated mice. *Proc Natl Acad Sci USA* **97(11)**: 5972–5977.
89. Zheng T, Zhu Z, Wang Z *et al.* (2000) Inducible targeting of IL-13 to the adult lung causes matrix metalloproteinase- and cathepsin-dependent emphysema. *J Clin Invest* **106(9)**: 1081–1093.
90. Wang Z, Zheng T, Zhu Z *et al.* (2000) Interferon gamma induction of pulmonary emphysema in the adult murine lung. *J Exp Med* **192(11)**: 1587–1600.
91. Hautamaki RD, Kobayashi DK, Senior RM *et al.* (1997) Requirement for macrophage elastase for cigarette smoke-induced emphysema. *Science* **277**: 2002–2004.
92. Kassim SY, Fu X, Liles WC *et al.* (2005) NADPH oxidase restrains the matrix metalloproteinase activity of macrophages. *J Biol Chem* **280**: 30201–30205.
93. Yearsley MM, Diaz PT, Knoell D *et al.* (2005) Correlation of HIV-1 Detection and Histology in AIDS-Associated Emphysema. *Diagn Mol Pathol* **14(1)**: 48–52.
94. Heath L, Fox A, McClure J *et al.* (2009) Evidence for limited genetic compartmentalization of HIV-1 between lung and blood. *PLoS One* **4(9)**:e6949.

95. Hatano H, Delwart EL, Norris PJ *et al.* (2010) Evidence of persistent low-level viremia in long-term HAART-suppressed, HIV infected individuals. *AIDS* **24(16)**: 2535–2539.
96. Yukl SA, Gianella S, Sinclaire E *et al.* (2010) Differences in HIV burden and immune activation within the gut of HIV-positive patients receiving suppressive antiretroviral therapy. *J Infect Dis* **202(10)**: 1553–1561.
97. Yukl SA, Shergill AK, McQuaid K *et al.* (2010) Effect of raltegravir-containing intensification on HIV burden and T-cell activation in multiple gut sites of HIV-positive adults on suppressive antiretroviral therapy. *AIDS* **24(16)**: 2451–2460.
98. Sigal A, Kim JT, Balazs AB *et al.* (2011) Cell-to-cell spread of HIV permits ongoing replication despite antiretroviral therapy. *Nature* **477(7362)**: 95–98.
99. Morris A, Sciurba FC, Lebadeva IP *et al.* (2004) Association of chronic obstructive pulmonary disease severity and Pneumocystis colonization. *Am J Respir Crit Care Med* **170(4)**: 408–413.
100. Simard EP, Pfeiffer RM, Engels EA. (2011) Cumulative incidence of cancer among individuals with acquired immunodeficiency syndrome in the United States. *Cancer* **117(5)**: 1089–1096.
101. Shiels MS, Pfeiffer RM, Gail MH *et al.* (2011) Cancer burden in the HIV infected population in the United States. *J Natl Cancer Inst* **103(9)**: 753–762.
102. Achenbach CJ, Cole SR, Kitahata MM *et al.* (2011) Mortality after cancer diagnosis in HIV infected individuals treated with antiretroviral therapy. *AIDS* **25(5)**: 691–700.
103. Reekie J, Kosa C, Engsig F *et al.* (2010) Relationship between current level of immunodeficiency and non-acquired immunodeficiency syndrome-defining malignancies. *Cancer* **116(22)**: 5306–5315.
104. Shiels MS, Pfeiffer RM, Engels EA. (2010) Age at cancer diagnosis among persons with AIDS in the United States. *Ann Intern Med* **153(7)**: 452–460.
105. Petoumenos K, Hui E, Kumarasamy N *et al.* (2010) Cancers in the TREAT Asia HIV Observational Database (TAHOD): A retrospective analysis of risk factors. *J Int AIDS Soc* **13**: 51.
106. Cadranel J, Garfield D, Lavole A *et al.* (2006) Lung cancer in HIV infected patients: Facts, questions and challenges. *Thorax* **61(11)**: 1000–1008.

107. Chaturvedi AK, Pfeiffer RM, Chang L *et al.* (2007) Elevated risk of lung cancer among people with AIDS. *AIDS* **21(2)**: 207–213.
108. Clifford GM, Polesel J, Rickenbach M *et al.* (2005) Cancer risk in the Swiss HIV Cohort Study: Associations with immunodeficiency, smoking, and highly active antiretroviral therapy. *J Natl Cancer Inst* **97(6)**: 425–432.
109. Hakimian R, Fang H, Thomas L *et al.* (2007) Lung cancer in HIV infected patients in the era of highly active antiretroviral therapy. *J Thorac Oncol* **2(4)**: 268–272.
110. Hessol NA, Seaberg EC, Preston Martin S *et al.* (2004) Cancer risk among participants in the women's interagency HIV study. *J Acquir Immune Defic Syndr* **36(4)**: 978–985.
111. Kirk GD, Merlo C, O'Driscoll P *et al.* (2007) HIV infection is associated with an increased risk for lung cancer, independent of smoking. *Clin Infect Dis* **45(1)**: 103–110.
112. Shiels MS, Cole SR, Mehta SH *et al.* (2010) Lung cancer incidence and mortality among HIV infected and HIV-uninfected injection drug users. *J Acquir Immune Defic Syndr* **55(4)**: 510–515.
113. Sigel K, Wisnevesky J, Gordon K *et al.* (2012) HIV is an Independent Risk Factor for Incident Lung Cancer Among HIV infected Veterans. *AIDS* **26(8)**: 1017–1025.
114. Turner MC, Chen Y, Krewski D *et al.* (2007) Chronic obstructive pulmonary disease is associated with lung cancer mortality in a prospective study of never smokers. *Am J Respir Crit Care Med* **176(3)**: 285–290.
115. Koshiol J, Rotunno M, Consonni D *et al.* (2009) Chronic obstructive pulmonary disease and altered risk of lung cancer in a population-based case-control study. *PLoS One* **4(10)**:e7380.
116. Wilson DO, Weissfeld JL, Balkan A *et al.* (2008) Association of radiographic emphysema and airflow obstruction with lung cancer. *Am J Respir Crit Care Med* **178(7)**: 738–744.
117. Wu AH, Elizabeth TH, Fontham H *et al.* (1995) Previous lung disease and risk of lung cancer among lifetime nonsmoking women in the United States. *Am J Epidemiol* **141(11)**: 1023–1032.
118. Liang HY, Li XL, Yu XS *et al.* (2009) Facts and fiction of the relationship between preexisting tuberculosis and lung cancer risk: a systematic review. *Int J Cancer* **125(12)**: 2936–2944.

119. Mayne ST, Buenconsejo J, Janerich DT. (1999) Previous lung disease and risk of lung cancer among men and women nonsmokers. *Am J Epidemiol* **149(1)**: 13–20.
120. Littman AJ, Thornquist MD, White E *et al.* (2004) Prior lung disease and risk of lung cancer in a large prospective study. *Cancer Causes Control* **15(8)**: 819–827.
121. Ramanakumar AV, Parent ME, Menzies D *et al.* (2006) Risk of lung cancer following nonmalignant respiratory conditions: evidence from two case-control studies in Montreal, Canada. *Lung Cancer* **53(1)**: 5–12.
122. Shebl FM, Engels EA, Goedert JJ *et al.* (2010) Pulmonary infections and risk of lung cancer among persons with AIDS. *J Acquir Immune Defic Syndr* **55(3)**: 375–379.
123. Lavole A, Wislez M, Antoine M *et al.* (2006) Lung cancer, a new challenge in the HIV infected population. *Lung Cancer* **51(1)**: 1–11.
124. Grulich AE, van Leeuwen MT, Falster MO *et al.* (2007) Incidence of cancers in people with HIV/AIDS compared with immunosuppressed transplant recipients: A meta-analysis. *Lancet* **370(9581)**: 59–67.
125. Guiguet M, Boue, F, Cadranel J *et al.* (2009) Effect of immunodeficiency, HIV viral load, and antiretroviral therapy on the risk of individual malignancies (FHDH-ANRS CO4): A prospective cohort study. *Lancet Oncol* **10(12)**: 1152–1159.
126. Mondy KE, Gottdiener J, Overton EH *et al.* (2011) High prevalence of echocardiographic abnormalities among HIV infected persons in the era of highly active antiretroviral therapy. *Clin Infect Dis* **52(3)**: 378–386.
127. Barnett CF, Hsue PY. (2013) Human immunodeficiency virus-associated pulmonary arterial hypertension. *Clin Chest Med* **34(2)**: 283–292.
128. Lador F, Herve P. (2013) A practical approach of pulmonary hypertension in the elderly. *Semin Respir Crit Care Med* **34(5)**: 654–664.
129. Almodovar S, Knight R, Amanda A *et al.* (2012) Human Immunodeficiency Virus nef signature sequences are associated with pulmonary hypertension. *AIDS Res Human Retroviruses* **28(6)**: 607–618.
130. Spikes L, Dalvi P, Tawfik O *et al.* (2012) Enhanced pulmonary arteriopathy in simian immunodeficiency virus-infected macaques exposed to morphine. *Am J Respir Crit Care Med* **185(11)**: 1235–1243.
131. Porter KM, Walp ER, Elms SC *et al.* (2013) Human immunodeficiency virus-1 transgene expression increases pulmonary vascular resistance and exacerbates hypoxia-induced pulmonary hypertension development. *Pulmonary Circulation* **3(1)**: 58–67.

132. Almodovar S, Hsue PY, Morelli J *et al.* (2011) Pathogenesis of HIV-associated pulmonary hypertension: Potential role of HIV-1 Nef. *Proc Am Thorac Soc* **8(3)**: 308–312.
133. Malek J, Rogers R, Kufera J *et al.* (2011) Venous thromboembolic disease in the HIV infected patient. *Am J Emerg Med* **29(3)**: 278–282.
134. Morris A, Gingo MR, George MP *et al.* (2012) Cardiopulmonary function in individuals with HIV infection in the antiretroviral therapy era. *AIDS* **26(6)**: 731–740.

Chapter 12

Geriatric Pulmonary Hypertension: Recent Epidemiologic Trends and Treatment Update

Vanessa Yap*, George A. Kuchel[†,§], and Raymond J. Foley[‡,§]

1. Introduction

Pulmonary hypertension (PH) is a hemodynamic and pathophysiological condition that refers to the presence of abnormally high pulmonary vascular pressure.[1] The first classification of PH was proposed in 1973, which designated only two categories- primary or secondary PH, depending on the presence or absence of identifiable causes or risk factors.[2,3] The second world symposium on pulmonary hypertension (WSPH) held in Evian, France in 1998 attempted to create categories of PH that shared similar pathogenesis, clinical

*Division of Pulmonary/Critical Care, UConn Health, 263 Farmington Avenue, Farmington, CT 06030-1321 USA, Tel: 860-679-3585; Fax: 860-679-1103; Email: yap@uchu.edu

†UConn Center on Aging, UConn Health, 263 Farmington Avenue, Farmington, CT 06030-5215 USA, Tel: 860-679-3956; Fax: 860-679-1307; Email: kuchel@uchc.edu

‡Division of Pulmonary/Critical Care, UConn Health, 263 Farmington Avenue, Farmington, CT 06030-1321 USA, Tel: 860-679-3585; Fax: 860-679-1103; Email: rfoley@uchc.edu

§Corresponding authors.

features and therapeutic options, which allowed defining homogenous groups of patients to conduct clinical trials and to obtain approval for specific pulmonary arterial hypertension (PAH) therapies worldwide. Further revisions were made at the third WSPH in 2003 in Venice, Italy. The terms idiopathic pulmonary arterial hypertension (IPAH), familial PAH and associated-PAH were introduced and pulmonary veno-occlusive disease (PVOD) and pulmonary capillary hemangiomatosis (PCH) were also moved into a single subcategory of PAH. In 2008, the fourth WSPH held in Dana Point (California, USA) revised previous classifications into the subgroups as they exist today, categorizing a homogenous group of patients with similar pathogenesis, hemodynamic characteristics,[4] clinical features and therapeutic options, as shown in Table 1.[2] In 2013, the fifth WSPH met in Nice, France where modifications in the classification of PH include shifting of PH associated with chronic hemolytic anemias from group 1 to group 5; congenital diseases related to pediatric PH were added to groups 2 and 5. There were no changes for groups 3 and 4.[5]

PAH is a chronic and progressive pulmonary vascular disease that leads to right heart failure[1] and ultimately death if untreated.[6] It is a syndrome resulting from restricted flow through the pulmonary arterial circulation, which leads to pathological increases in pulmonary vascular resistance (PVR).[1] It is hallmarked by an intense and characteristic remodeling of small caliber pulmonary arteries due to the proliferation of endothelial and smooth muscle cells and medial hypertrophy[7] and reduced rates of apoptosis, although excessive vasoconstriction plays a significant role in approximately 20% of patients.[1] In the previous and current diagnostic paradigm, it is categorized in Group I pulmonary hypertension.

2. Recent Epidemiologic Trends in PAH

PAH may occur in association with various diseases including congenital heart disease, connective tissue disease, portal hypertension and infection with human immunodeficiency virus. Some cases are related to the use of appetite-suppressants, some are heritable, but the majority is idiopathic in origin (IPAH).[8] PAH was previously

Table 1. PH WHO groups.[1]

1. Pulmonary arterial hypertension (PAH)
1.1 Idiopathic (IPAH)
1.2 Familial (FPAH)
1.3 Associated with (APAH):
1.3.1 Connective tissue disorder
1.3.2 Congenital systemic-to-pulmonary shunts
1.3.3 Portal hypertension
1.3.4 HIV infection
1.3.5 Drugs and toxins
1.3.6 Other (thyroid disorders, glycogen storage disease, Gaucher's disease, hereditary hemorrhagic telangiectasia, hemoglobinopathies, chronic myeloproliferative disorders, splenectomy)
1.4 Associated with significant venous or capillary involvement
1.4.1 PVOD
1.4.2 PCH
1.5 Persistent PH of the newborn
2. Pulmonary hypertension with left heart disease
2.1 Left-sided atrial or ventricular heart disease
2.2 Left-sided valvular heart disease
3. Pulmonary hypertension associated with lung diseases and/or hypoxemia
3.1 Chronic obstructive pulmonary disease
3.2 Interstitial lung disease
3.3 Sleep disordered breathing
3.4 Alveolar hypoventilation disorders
3.5 Chronic exposure to high altitude
3.6 Developmental abnormalities
4. Pulmonary hypertension due to chronic thrombotic and/or embolic disease (CTEPH)
4.1 Thromboembolic obstruction of proximal pulmonary arteries
4.2 Thromboembolic obstruction of distal pulmonary arteries
4.3 Nonthrombotic pulmonary embolism (tumor, parasites, foreign material)
5. Miscellaneous
Sarcoidosis, histiocytosis X, lymphangiomatosis, compression of pulmonary vessels (adenopathy, tumor, fibrosing mediastinitis)

considered as an illness that affects mostly the young but has been increasingly recognized in the elderly.[6,7]

IPAH is considered a rare condition and registries have made important contributions to our current understanding of this disease

(Table 2).[7,8] One of the first was the National Institutes of Health (NIH) registry of primary PH.[3] This registry collected data from 32 centers diagnosed by uniform criteria as having primary PH. The mean age was 36 and less than 10% of patients were older than 60 years.[7] Survival rates at 1 and 3 years were 68% and 48% respectively.[3,8] The 5-year survival rate was reported at 34%.[3,9] With the emergence of effective therapies, the awareness of PAH has increased among patients and physicians.[8] More recent registries from the US and Europe have demonstrated the changing demographics in patients diagnosed with PAH. The REVEAL (Registry to Evaluate Early and Long-term PAH Disease Management) registry, a multicenter, observational US-based registry whose purpose is to provide information about current demographic and treatment practices for patients diagnosed with PAH, demonstrated the mean age at diagnosis was 50 years old and 5% of the patients were diagnosed at ≥75 years of age.[8,10,11] Comparably, the French National PAH registry revealed an average age at diagnosis of 52 years, 12.8% patients older than 65 years.[12] In June 2007, COMPERA (Comparative, Prospective Registry of Newly Initiated Therapies for PH), a European-based registry on medical therapies for PH was launched, recruiting patients from PH centers in Austria, Belgium, Germany, Italy, Netherlands, Switzerland and the United Kingdom. In the first interim analysis, the mean age of enrolled patients was 65 years.[8] In the largest series so far on incident, treatment naïve, idiopathic, heritable and anorexigen-associated patients with PAH in the UK and Ireland diagnosed between 2001–2009, the median age was 50 years and 13.5% of the patients were older than 70 years at the time of diagnosis.[13] With the aging of the population in western countries, the increase in life expectancy, the growing awareness of physician and patients to PAH and availability of potential treatments, it is not that uncommon to see geriatric patients being diagnosed with PAH today.[7]

There has been a marked female preponderance, which has increased over time in the United States. The NIH registry reported a 1.7:1 female-to-male ratio in the total cohort and a 4.3:1 ratio among blacks.[3] The Surveillance of Pulmonary Hypertension in America registry, conducted from 1998 to 2001 in the US, reported a 4.3:1 ratio.[14]

Table 2. Baseline characteristics of PAH at the time of diagnosis from different registries.[7]

Registry	NIH[9]	French[7]	United States[6]	REVEAL[8]	United Kingdom/ Ireland[4]	ASPIRE[11,a]	COMPERA[5]
Year	1987	2006	2007	2010	2012	2012	2013
Subjects, *n*	187	674	578	2,525	482	175	587
Age, years	36 ± 15	50 ± 15	48 ± 14	50.1 ± 14.4	50.1 ± 17.1	55 ± 16	71 ± 16
Women, %	63	65.3	77	55.6	69.9	67	60.3
mPAP, mmHg	60 ± 18	55 ± 15	52 ± 14	50.7 ± 13.6	54.1 ± 13.9	53 ± 13	44 ± 12
PAWP, mmHg	[b]	8 ± 3	10 ± 4	9.1 ± 3.5	9.2 ± 3.5	10 ± 3	10 ± 3
RAP, mmHg	9.7 ± 6	8 ± 5	11 ± 7	9.3 ± 5.6	10.1 ± 6.0	11 ± 6	8 ± 5
CI, $L/min/m^2$	2.27 ± 0.9	2.50 ± 0.8	2.3 ± 0.9	2.4 ± 0.8	2.1 ± 0.7	2.3 ± 0.8	2.2 ± 0.7
PVRi (WU/m^2)	26 ± 14	20.5 ± 10.2	—	21.1 ± 12.5	23.1 ± 10.3	—	—
PVR (WU)	—	—	12.5 ± 7.3	—	12.8 ± 6.3	12.0 ± 5.8	9.6 ± 5.5

Abbreviations: CI, cardiac index; mPAP, mean pulmonary artery pressure; PAH, pulmonary arterial hypertension; PAWP, pulmonary artery wedge pressure; PVRi, pulmonary vascular resistance index; PVR, pulmonary vascular resistance; RAP, right atrial pressure.
Note: Data are expressed as mean ± SD or % unless otherwise stated.
(a) Patients diagnosed with idiopathic PAH.
(b) PAWP was 8.69 ± 3.9 in males and 7.94 ± 3.7 in females.

The REVEAL Registry demonstrated a 4.1:1 female-to-male ratio among patients with IPAH and a 3.8:1 ratio among those with APAH (associated PAH). A 5.4:1 ratio among 312 (12%) blacks supports the previous finding of higher female predominance. However, the French Registry, conducted from October 2002 to October 2003, reported a 1.9:1 ratio[12] while the national study from UK and Ireland did not report statistically significant difference in sex ratio.[13] The reason for this demographic variability over time and between countries is unclear. A role for hormonal influences (particularly estrogens) in the pathogenesis of PAH has been considered.[15]

3. Clinical Features of PAH in the Elderly

PAH has been increasingly recognized in older patients in recent years, to some extent changing the clinical features and landscape of this illness. As recently as 1987, a national US registry described PAH as a disease mostly of young women with a mean age at entry of 36 ± 15 years and diagnosis after the age of 60 taking place in less than 10% of subjects.[3] The subsequent decades have witnessed a major and sustained increase in this diagnosis later in life. In the United States, the diagnosis of PAH increased more than 3-fold between 1990 and 2002.[16] The impact on age-specific hospitalization rates was even more striking with a 6-fold increase among individuals 85 years and older taking place between 1980 and 2002.[16] Moreover, the percentage of male patients diagnosed with PAH is also increasing. These US findings have increasingly been replicated in other countries including France[12], the UK[13] and Ireland.[13]

These truly dramatic changes with the growing emergence of a geriatric form of PAH,[17] may be attributed to a number of different considerations starting with a demographic expansion of numbers of older adults in western societies[18] and an increasing degree of multiple morbidity in later life[19] to increased case finding related to the growing use of echocardiography and right heart catheterization (RHC) in elderly patients with improved physicians' awareness and rigorous evaluations for PAH as a potential explanation for older patients' symptoms.[18]

The first population-based data defining the relationship between pulmonary arterial systolic pressure (PASP) and age showed that pulmonary artery pressures increase with age in subjects from the general community. The increase in pulmonary artery pressure was coupled with increases in pulse pressure and estimated left heart filling pressures; suggesting that age-associated blood vessel stiffening and diastolic dysfunction contribute to changes in pulmonary artery pressure.[7,20] A study by Ling, *et al.* concluded that although there were significant differences between the younger and older subgroups in the study cohort, these are likely to represent the two ends of a continuous spectrum of the same disease.[13] Thus, recent data from international registries and specialized PH centers have demonstrated that PAH in the elderly is an emerging demographic of PAH.[7] Delay in diagnosis however persists, likely because the non-specific PH symptoms were more commonly attributed to old age or other more common illnesses before PAH was suspected.[13]

Nevertheless, in spite of a growing literature characterizing the nature of the physiological considerations in the geriatric form of PAH, surprisingly little has been learned in regards to a description of these individuals from the perspective of non-cardiopulmonary functional performance, frailty, associated co-morbid conditions and patient-relevant clinical outcomes. Further compounding this challenge is the fact that there are currently no Quality of Life or Disability Measurement tools which have been specifically designed or validated for use in the context of PAH.[21] Nevertheless, in the only such assessment, Lin *et al.*[13] have used PAH data from the United Kingdom and Ireland to describe important age-related and temporal associations with significant comorbid conditions. In this cohort younger subjects appeared to have more significant hemodynamic impairments while older individuals exhibited many more comorbidities.[13] Furthermore, in comparison with earlier cohorts, subjects diagnosed in 2007–2009 were older, more obese, had lower percent diffusing capacity of carbon monoxide and had many more comorbidities, paradoxically with better survival.[13] These findings must be replicated across different cohorts. Nevertheless, an interesting analogy may be emerging with geriatric congestive heart failure in which associated frailty and comorbidities together with a diastolic as opposed to a systolic cardiac etiology assume a far greater role in determining patient-relevant outcomes than is the case for the traditional measures of ventricular contractility.[22]

In addition to the need for further observational studies of late onset PAH in which non-cardiopulmonary factors such as associated comorbidities and frailty are considered, geriatric factors will also need to be incorporated into the design and selection of relevant outcome measures in the context of clinical trials.[23,24] Although physical performance measures such as the 6 minute walk are used in both PAH[10,11] and geriatric CHF research,[25] the validity of this and other outcome measures in PAH trials remains unknown.

4. Interactions with Normative Aging: Physiologic Considerations

A broad range of clinical and translational literature has succeeded in increasingly defining the impact of aging on the respiratory system,[26–28] with a progressive decline in most aspects of lung function.[28,29] Decreases in the elasticity of lungs and the chest wall, together with declines in respiratory muscle strength contribute to what appear to be mostly inevitable declines in forced expiratory volume in 1 second.[28,29] At the same time, air trapping increases, vital capacity declines and total capillary lung volume is also lower.[30]

In contrast to the above changes, age-related increases in vascular stiffness have been attributed to systemic systolic hypertension rather than intrinsic aging.[31] Older adults are also more likely to demonstrate an unusual degree of stiffness in their pulmonary arteries with increased collagen and elastin deposition.[32–34] Aging is also associated with declines in left heart compliance resulting in a growing burden of diastolic dysfunction in old age with as many as one-half of individuals over the age of 75 showing evidence of subclinical mild diastolic dysfunction on echocardiography.[22,35] Given the common and progressive nature of these changes involving left ventricular compliance. It is possible that they contribute to an age-related increase in systolic pulmonary artery pressure of approximately 1 mmHg per decade.[20] It remains to be seen to what extent these age-associated increases can be considered to remain normative.[36] Moreover, alternative validation of these echocardiographic findings may be needed in some cases.

In contrast to these relatively mild increases in basal PA pressure with aging, exercising older adults demonstrate a dramatically exaggerated increase on this Doppler echocardiographic measurement. For example, healthy elderly subjects were shown to essentially double their mean sPAP during exercise increasing from approximately 30 mmHg to nearly 60 mmHg.[37,38] These findings are in keeping with evidence of homeostatic dysregulation in other aging systems where basal values may remain relatively unchanged or are slightly increased, while a homeostatic challenge uncovers evidence of "homeostatic failure" with exaggerated and often less effective responses, increased vulnerability (frailty) and a lengthened period required for the system to return to a previous basal state.[39] Nevertheless, it remains to be seen to what extent these findings influence overall function in older adults and how they should influence the determination of normative findings on echocardiography or angiography.

5. Interactions with Normative Aging: Biologic Considerations

Since aging represents the most important risk factor for many chronic conditions and since biological underpinnings of aging are increasingly well understood, it has been proposed that strategies designed to address these aging-related pathways could also help prevent or slow the progression of aging-related chronic diseases and conditions.[40,41] With these considerations in mind, it is important to note that the pro-inflammatory senescent secretory phenotype[42] demonstrates a number of features which are relevant and could contribute to the development or onset of PAH. A number of factors from reactive oxidative species, inflammation and deficits in cellular remodeling and proliferation are believed to contribute to the vasculopathy which is central to PAH[43,44] and are at the same time key features of many senescent cells.[42] Moreover, senescent cells often shift their activities towards the production and secretion of components of the extracellular matrix such as collagen and elastin[42] which in turn contribute to the decreased elasticity of the aging lung.[32–34] Finally, age-related changes in apoptosis, proliferative capacity and differentiation[42] could similarly interact with and influence comparable changes associated with PAH.[45,46]

6. Heart Failure with Preserved Ejection Fraction as A Confounder in PAH

There is concern that PH-HFpEF may often be misclassified as having category I PAH because both patient groups can have a normal LVEF.[47] Hemodynamic values are important in distinguishing patients with PAH as PAH-specific therapies are ineffective, potentially harmful and costly for pulmonary venous hypertension[48] but at the same time, misclassification will deprive PAH patients from beneficial therapy. Left sided heart failure with preserved ejection fraction (HFpEF) is defined as symptomatic heart failure occurring in the setting of a LVEF ≥50% and accounts for about one-half of all hospitalizations for heart failure in the US.[49] PH is frequently present in HFpEF because of both elevated pulmonary venous pressure and some element of pulmonary vasoconstriction.[50] Once pulmonary vascular disease progresses the cardiac output is reduced from right ventricular dysfunction and decreased venous return to the left heart with normalization of the left ventricular filling pressure (LVFP). These patients then have normal left heart filling pressures but significantly elevated pulmonary pressures that can be misdiagnosed as PAH.[6,51] There is a growing belief that elderly patients are more susceptible to the development of PH possibly due to age-related vascular stiffening.[52] Most HFpEF patients with PH have elevated pulmonary arterial pressure (PAP) because of increased left-side filling pressure with normal PVR or transpulmonary gradient (TPG). However, a subset of HFpEF patients develop intrinsic pulmonary vascular disease in addition to elevated filling pressures, leading to not only elevated PAP, but also increased PVR and TPG.[49]

Compared with PAH, patients with PH-HFpEF have been found to be older and with increased prevalence of co-morbid conditions including hypertension, diabetes mellitus, obesity and cardiovascular disease.[47,49,53] A cross-sectional study suggested that PAH and PH-HFpEF could be more accurately differentiated using predictive modeling. Old age, presence of hypertension and coronary artery disease, the absence of right atrial enlargement, higher aortic systolic pressure, higher mean right atrial pressure and higher cardiac output best differentiated PAH from PH-HFpEF.[7,49] The differences are shown in Table 3. Female preponderance has also been reported in PH-HFpEF suggesting potential genetic or hormonal predisposition. There also may be a link between the metabolic syndrome and PH suggesting a possible inflammatory component.[4] Patients with PH-HFpEF have clinical, echocardiographic and hemodynamic characteristics distinct from PAH and from HFpEF without pulmonary vascular disease. These distinctions place them in a separate diagnostic group from PAH.[49]

Table 3. Distinguishing clinical features among patients with PAH, HFpEF and PH-HFpEF.[49]

Characteristics	HFpEF	PAH	PH-HFpEF
Age	Older	Younger	Older
Comorbidities	Frequent	Rare	More frequent
Right atrial enlargement	Absent	More frequent	Less frequent
Left atrial enlargement	Frequent	Absent	Frequent
Aortic systolic pressure	Elevated	Normal	Elevated
Mean right atrial pressure	Normal	Normal-High	High
Cardiac output	Normal	Low	Normal
PVR	Normal	Markedly elevated	Moderately elevated

Comorbidities include hypertension, diabetes mellitus, obesity, and coronary artery disease. PAH indicate mean pulmonary artery pressure; PH-HFpEF, pulmonary hypertension because of pulmonary vascular disease associated with heart failure and preserved ejection fraction; HFpEF, heart failure with preserved ejection fraction without pulmonary vascular disease.

7. Controversies

7.1. *Echocardiography*

Doppler echocardiography is the best first screening test in evaluating a patient with suspected PH. Pulmonary artery systolic pressure (PASP) can be measured non-invasively using the Bernoulli equation and correlates relatively well with PASP measured invasively.[54] It however has intrinsic and operator dependent limitations that make early diagnosis and screening challenging. Reported false-positive results seen with PH screening by echocardiography has been as high as 45%.[15]

7.2. *Pulmonary capillary wedge pressure*

Pulmonary capillary wedge pressure (PCWP) represents an alternative measure to left ventricular end diastolic pressure (LVEDP), which is the gold standard for determining Left Ventricular Filling Pressure. Many factors can interfere with the accurate measurement of PCWP, including factors related to the measurement techniques themselves and patient-specific factors, such as obesity, hypoxemia and ventilation.[48] Recent studies have shown that, in PAH patients, PCWP can lead to erroneous PH classification compared with a diagnosis based on LVEDP. In a large study of PH patients ($n = 4{,}320$) undergoing both right and left heart catheterizations, it was found that PCWP frequently underestimates LVEDP, that it is poorly calibrated to LVEDP and that it has a moderate ability to discriminate between patients with normal or elevated LVEDP.[55] Perhaps most importantly, these results suggest that approximately half of all patients who meet the hemodynamic criteria for PAH on the basis of PCWP measurements may, in fact, have elevated PCWPs. Measuring LVEDP routinely among all patients referred for evaluation for PH carries increased risks and inconveniences for patients as well as increased costs and resource utilization. Halpern *et al.* therefore suggest a more conservative approach in routine practice in which clinicians obtain left-heart hemodynamic measurements whenever there are reasons to suspect left-heart disease based on the patient's history or physical examination or whenever the diagnosis is uncertain following RHC and when patients do not show favorable responses to initial therapy.[55]

8. Diagnosis

Patients suspected of having PH based on history, physical examination, chest radiography and electrocardiogram should have an echocardiogram performed. Evaluation for other potential etiologies is appropriate in all patients suspected of having PAH as etiology dictates treatment of PH. Patients with a known bone morphogenetic protein receptor 2 (BMPR2) mutation, scleroderma spectrum of diseases and portal hypertension who are undergoing evaluation for liver transplantation are at sufficient risk for the development of PAH to warrant periodic screening.[1]

In general, pivotal tests are required for a definitive diagnosis and baseline characterization. These are tests that are essential to establishing a diagnosis of any type of PAH either by identification of criteria of associated disease or exclusion of diagnoses other than IPAH. An abnormality of one assessment does not preclude that another abnormality is contributing or predominant. Contingent tests are recommended to elucidate or confirm results of the pivotal tests and need only be performed in the appropriate clinical context. The combination of pivotal and appropriate contingent tests contributes to assessment of the differential diagnoses, as demonstrated in Fig. 1.[1]

The diagnosis of PAH requires confirmation with a complete right heart catheterization (RHC). The current hemodynamic definition of PAH is a mean pulmonary artery pressure (mPAP) ≥25 mmHg; a pulmonary capillary wedge pressure (PCWP), left atrial pressure, or left ventricular end-diastolic pressure (LVEDP) ≤15 mmHg; and a PVR >3 Wood units. Acute vasodilator testing, which involves the administration of inhaled nitric oxide(NO), intravenous epoprostenol or intravenous adenosine to test the presence of pulmonary vasoreactivity, defined as a reduction in mPAP of at least 10 mmHg to an absolute mPAP of <40 mmHg without a decrease in cardiac output, has prognostic value and should be performed in all IPAH

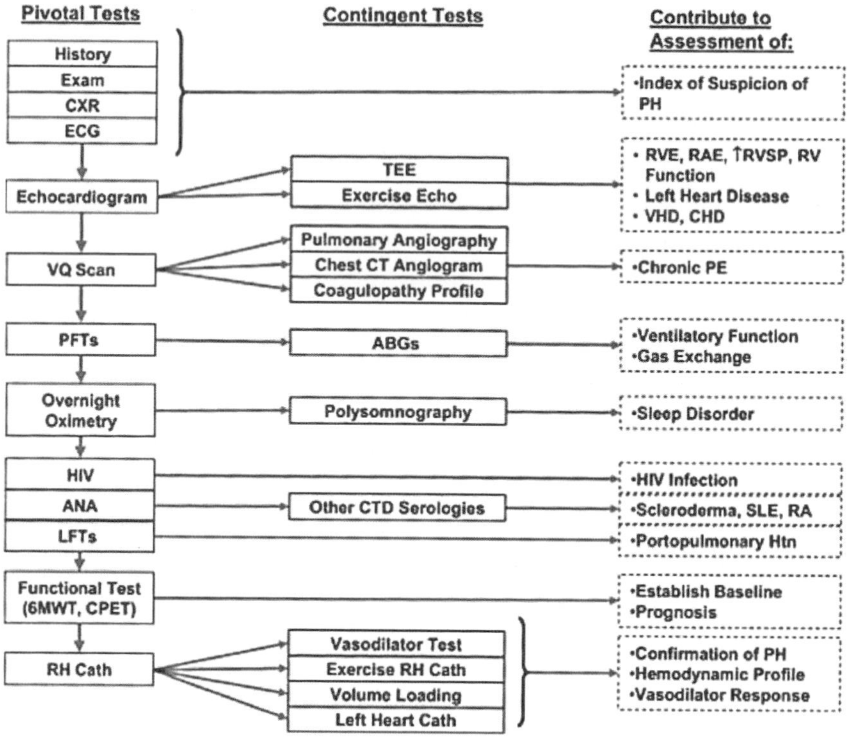

Fig. 1. Diagnostic Approach to PAH.[1]

patients who might be considered potential candidates for long-term calcium-channel blocker therapy.[1]

9. Management

The complexity of the treatment algorithm for PAH has progressively increased with the advent of new drug therapies, different routes of administration and advances in other areas of PAH treatment. The current treatment algorithm was updated at the 5th WSPH in 2013 and may be divided into 3 main areas: (1) general measures, (2) initial therapy and (3) clinical response to the initial therapy.[56] The treatment algorithm is shown in Fig. 2.

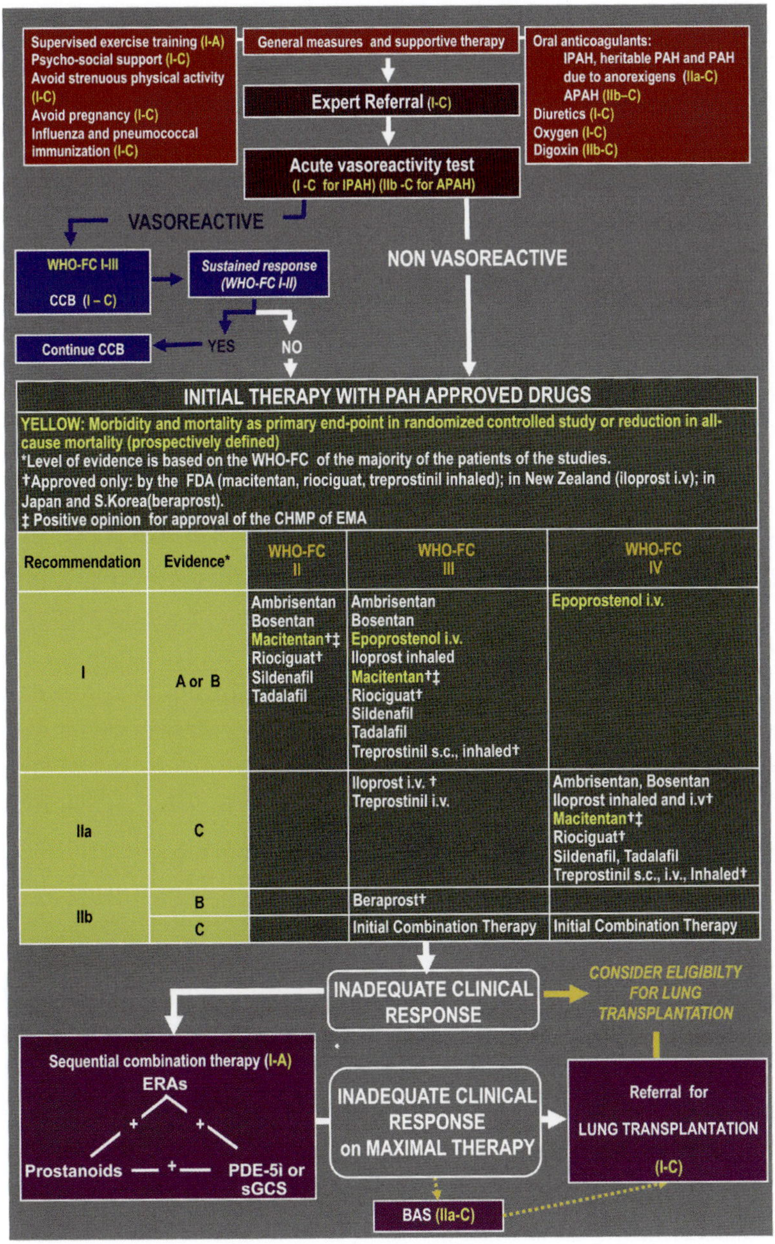

Fig. 2. Treatment Algorithm.[56]

The suggested initial approach for the treatment of PAH is the adoption of general measures, the initiation of the supportive therapy and referral to an expert center. Vasoreactive patients should be treated with optimal doses of calcium channel blockers (CCB) and assessed for adequate response after 3 to 4 months of treatment.[56]

9.1. *General measures*

Recommendation for rehabilitation and exercise training has been upgraded to Class I with a level of evidence A with the concordant results of 3 randomized controlled trials (RCTs). Patients should be encouraged to be active within symptom limits and should avoid excessive physical activity that leads to distressing symptoms, but when physically deconditioned, may undertake supervised exercise rehabilitation.[56]

Consensus from the 2009 American College of Cardiology/American Heart Association (ACC/AHA) recommends warfarin in IPAH patients titrated to an international normalized ratio of 1.5 to 2.5. Diuretics are indicated to manage right ventricular volume overload, which is commonly manifest as elevated jugular venous pressure, lower extremity edema, and abdominal distention. As hypoxemia is a potent pulmonary vasoconstrictor, long-term oxygen therapy is suggested to maintain arterial blood O_2 pressure ≥60 mmHg.[56] Digoxin is sometimes used in those patients with right heart failure and a low cardiac output and in patients with atrial arrhythmias.[1]

High-volume specialized centers have been shown to obtain improved outcomes for patients while maintaining patient satisfaction, lower complication rates, shorter length of hospital stay and best values for healthcare payers. For patients diagnosed with PAH, referral to a center specializing in pulmonary vascular disease is recommended.

9.2. *PAH specific therapy*

Treatment with PAH-approved drugs needs to be initiated in PAH patients who are not vasoreactive or are vasoreactive but not respond-

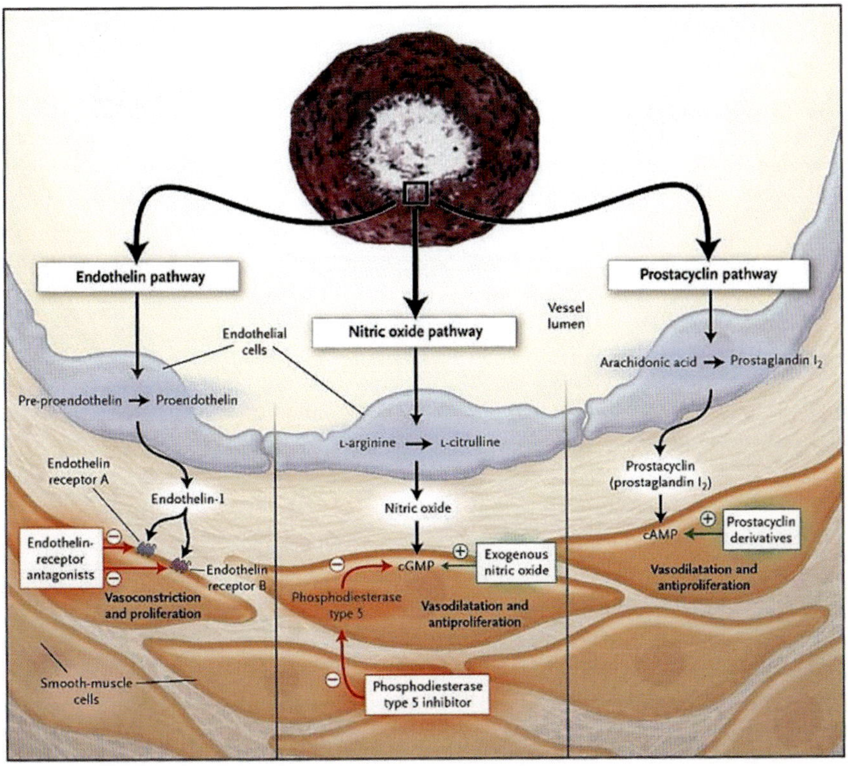

Fig. 3. Targets for Current or Emerging Therapies in PAH.[66]

ing to the appropriate calcium channel blocker. The approved therapies for PAH target separate signaling pathways known to be involved in the disease pathogenesis (Fig. 3): the prostacyclin pathway, endothelin pathway, and NO pathway (including phosphodiesterase 5 inhibitors and soluble guanylate cyclase stimulator agents).

Prostacyclin is the main product of the metabolism of arachidonic acid in the pulmonary vascular endothelium. It induces relaxation of vascular smooth muscle by stimulating the production of cyclic AMP (cAMP) and inhibits the growth of smooth-muscle cells and is a powerful inhibitor of platelet aggregation.[12] In patients with PAH, there is a deficiency of prostacyclin in the pulmonary vascular circulation. The list of pivotal trials of the prostacyclin analogues are listed in Table 4.

Table 4. List of pivotal trials for PAH specific therapy.

	Study Name/Drug	N/Etiol/ Class	Design	Positive Results
Prostacyclin analogues	AIR Inhaled iloprost versus placebo[58]	203 PH III, IV	Double-blind 12-week	• Composite end point • 6MWD • Symptoms • Hemodynamics • 6MWD
	TRIUMPH 1 Inhaled treprostinil versus placebo[60]	235 PAH III, IV*	Double-blind 12-week on background oral Rx	
	SQ treprostinil versus SQ placebo[59]	470 PAH II–IV	Double-blind 12-week	• 6MWD • Symptoms • Hemodynamics
	IV epoprostenol versus conventional Rx[57]	81 IPAH/FPAH III,IV	Open-label 12-week	• 6MWD • Symptoms • Hemodynamics • Survival
Endothelin receptor antagonists	BREATHE-1 Oral bosentan versus placebo[62]	213 PAH III, IV	Double-blind 16-week	• 6MWD • Delay clinical worsening • Symptoms
	EARLY Oral bosentan versus placebo[63]	185 PAH II	Double-blind 6-month	• Delay clinical worsening • Hemodynamics
	ARIES-1&2 Oral ambrisentan versus placebo[64]	394 PAH II, III	Double-blind 12-week	• 6MWD • Delay clinical worsening
	SERAPHIN Oral macitentan versus placebo[65]	742 PAH II, III		• Delay disease progression • 6MWD • Symptoms
sGC stimulator	PATENT-1 Oral riociguat versus placebo[67]	278 PAH I–IV	Double-blind 12-week	• 6MWD • Symptoms • Hemodynamics • Delay clinical worsening
	CHEST-1 Oral riociguat versus placebo[68]	261 CTEPH I–IV	Double-blind 16-week	• 6MWD • Symptoms • Hemodynamics

(*Continued*)

Table 4. (*Continued*)

	Study Name/Drug	N/Etiol/ Class	Design	Positive Results
PDE-5 inhibitors	SUPER-1 Oral sildenafil versus placebo[69]	278 PAH I–IV	Double-blind 12-week	• 6MWD • Symptoms • Hemodynamics
	PHIRST-1 Oral tadalafil versus placebo[70]	405 PAH I–IV	Double-blind 16-week	• 6MWD • Delay clinical worsening • Hemodynamics • HRQoL

Epoprostenol was the first FDA-approved therapy used to treat primary PH.[12] It has a short half-life (3–5 min) and is stable at room temperature for only 8 hrs requiring cooling and continuous administration by means of an infusion pump and a permanent tunneled catheter. A thermostable formulation is also now available. Epoprostenol improves symptoms, exercise capacity and hemodynamics and is the only treatment shown to reduce mortality in idiopathic PAH in a randomized study.[57] This landmark study was a 12-week prospective, randomized, multicenter, open-label trial of 81 patients with IPAH/FPAH and New York Heart Association (NYHA) functional class III or IV symptoms treated with epoprostenol versus conventional therapy (anticoagulants, calcium channel blocker, diuretics, digoxin, and oxygen). The primary outcome, median 6 minute walk distance (6MWD), increased by 31 ms (from 315 to 362 ms at 12 weeks in the 41 patients treated with epoprostenol and decreased by 29 ms (from 270 to 204 ms) in the 40 patients treated with conventional therapy alone. Difference in 6MWD between epoprostenol and conventional treatment was 60 ms ($p < 0.002$).[57] Serious adverse events related to the delivery system include pump malfunction, local site infection, catheter obstruction and sepsis.[56]

Iloprost is a chemically stable prostacyclin analogue available for inhaled administration. Inhaled iloprost has been evaluated in a randomized controlled fashion. The Aerosolized Iloprost Randomized study (AIR) in which daily repetitive iloprost inhalations (6 to 9 times,

2.5 to 5 micrograms/inhalation, median 30 micrograms daily) were compared with placebo inhalation in patients with PAH and chronic thromboembolic pulmonary hypertension (CTEPH). The study showed an increase in exercise capacity and improvement in symptoms and PVR in enrolled patients.[58] Inhaled iloprost was well tolerated with flushing and jaw pain being the most frequent side effect.[56]

Treprostinil is a tricyclic benzidine analogue of epoprostenol, with sufficient chemical stability to be administered at ambient temperature. These characteristics allow administration of the compound by the parenteral as well as the subcutaneous route. The effects of treprostinil in PAH were studied in an RCT and showed improvements in exercise capacity, hemodynamics and symptoms.[59] The subcutaneous administration of treprostinil can be accomplished by a microinfusion pump and a small subcutaneous catheter. Infusion site pain was the most common adverse effect of treprostinil.[59] IV treprostinil is approved in the United States in patients with PAH who cannot tolerate the subcutaneous administration (based on bioequivalence).[56] Treprostinil is also available via the inhalation route. In the TRIUMPH trial (inhaled TReprostInil sodium in Patients with severe Pulmonary Parterial Hypertension), PAH subjects treated with inhaled treprostinil in addition to their background therapy with either bosentan or sildenafil showed improvements in 6MWD by 20 ms at peak dose, *N*-terminal pro- B-type natriuretic peptide (NT-proBNP) levels and quality-of-life measures.[60]

Endothelin-1 is a potent vasoconstrictor. It also has mitogenic effects that contribute to pulmonary vascular wall remodeling. Endothelin-1 exerts these properties by binding to 2 distinct receptor isoforms in the pulmonary vascular smooth muscle cells, endothelin A and B receptors. Patients afflicted with PAH have been shown to have elevated levels of endothelin-1 in the pulmonary circulation. Endothelin-1 levels have been shown to be inversely proportional to flow through the pulmonary circuit and correlate with disease severity and prognosis.[61] The list of the pivotal trials among the endothelin receptor antagonists are listed in Table 4.

Bosentan is a dual endothelin A and B receptor antagonist and the first molecule of its class to be synthesized. Bosentan has been evaluated in RCTs in subjects with PAH. These trials have demonstrated improvement in exercise capacity, functional class, hemodynamics, echocardiographic and Doppler variables and time to clinical worsening.[62,63] Increases in hepatic aminotransferases occurred in ~10% of the subjects but were found to be dose-dependent and reversible after dose reduction or discontinuation. Liver function testing should be performed monthly in patients receiving bosentan.[56] Bosentan has been approved for treatment of PAH in patients with NYHA functional class II, III and IV symptoms.

Ambrisentan is a non-sulfonamide, propanoic acid class of endothelin receptor antagonist that is selective for the endothelin A receptor. Ambrisentan has been studied in 2 large RCTs Ambrisentan in PAH, Randomized, double-blind, placebo controlled, multicenter, Efficacy Study 1 and 2 (ARIES) and has demonstrated efficacy on symptoms, exercise capacity, hemodynamics and time to clinical worsening of patients with idiopathic PAH and PAH associated with connective tissue disease and human immunodeficiency virus infection.[56,64] It has been approved for the treatment of NYHA functional class II and III patients. The incidence of abnormal liver function tests range from 0.8–3% but monthly liver function assessment is not mandated in the United States. An increased incidence of peripheral edema has been reported with ambrisentan use.[56]

Macitentan is a dual endothelin antagonist, developed by modifying the structure of bosentan to increase efficacy and safety. Macitentan is characterized by sustained receptor binding and enhanced tissue penetration. In the event driven Study with an Endothelin Receptor Antagonist in PAH to Improve Clinical Outcome (SERAPHIN) study,[65] 742 PAH patients were treated with 3 or 10 mg macitentan as compared with placebo for an average of 100 weeks. The primary endpoint was the time from the initiation of treatment to the first occurrence of a composite endpoint of death, atrial septostomy, lung transplantation, initiation of treatment with intravenous or subcutaneous prostanoids, or worsening of PAH. Macitentan significantly reduced this composite endpoint of morbidity and mortality among patients with PAH and also increased exercise capacity. Benefits were shown both for patients who had not received treatment previously and for those receiving background therapy for PAH. While no liver toxicity was shown, reduction in blood hemoglobin <8 g/dl was observed in 4.3% of patients receiving 10 mg of macitentan.

Nitric Oxide (NO) is a potent vasodilator[61] In PAH, there is a deficiency of NO that contributes to the ultimate development of pulmonary vascular wall remodeling and vasoconstriction. The NO pathway involves two primary enzymes and pathways: Soluble guanylate cyclase (sGC) and phosphodiesterase 5. The sGC stimulators enhance cyclic guanosine monophosphate (cGMP) production.[66] Pre-clinical studies with sGC stimulators have shown antiproliferative and antiremodeling properties in animal models.[56] Phosphodiesterase 5 inhibitors (PDE-5i) result in vasodilation by inhibition of the cGMP degrading enzyme PDE-5. It is known that the pulmonary vasculature contains substantial amounts of PDE-5 hence the interest on the potential clinical benefit in PAH patients. List of the pivotal trials of sGC stimulators and the PDE-5 inhibitors are in Table 4.

Riociguat has a dual mode of action, acting in synergy with endogenous NO and also directly stimulating sGC independent of NO availability. The PAH Soluble Guanylate Cyclase–Stimulator Trial-1 (PATENT-1)is an RCT with 443 PAH patients (44% and 6% on background therapy with ERA or prostanoids, respectively) treated with riociguat up to 2.5 mg 3 times daily. This trial has shown favorable results on exercise capacity, hemodynamics, NYHA functional class and time to clinical worsening.[67] The most common serious adverse event in the placebo group and the 2.5 mg group was syncope (4% and 1%, respectively). Riociguat is approved for PAH and CTEPH patients [56,68] in the US.

Sildenafil is an orally active, potent and selective PDE-5i. The double-blind, placebo-controlled study Sildenafil Use in Pulmonary Arterial Hypertension (SUPER-1) involving 278 patients with symptomatic PAH randomized to placebo or sildenafil (20, 40, or 80 mg) orally three times daily for 12 weeks.[69] Sildenafil dosage of 20 mg three times daily was found to superior to placebo and comparable to the other dosages in improvement in the six minute walk distance.

The approved dose is 20 mg three times daily. Most side effects of sildenafil are mild to moderate and mainly related to vasodilation (headache, flushing, epistaxis).[56]

Tadalafil is a once daily, selective PDE-5i. A RCT Pulmonary arterial Hypertension and ReSponse to Tadalafil trial(PHIRST) in 406 PAH patients (53% on background bosentan therapy) treated with tadalafil 2.5, 10, 20, or 40 mg once daily has shown favorable results on exercise capacity, symptoms, hemodynamics, and time to clinical worsening at the 40 mg once daily dosage.[70]

10. Additional Treatment Considerations

Clinical response is based on attaining reasonable goals of therapy reassessed at 3 to 6 months after initiation of treatment.[56] Goals of therapy include the following: (1) modified NYHA functional class I or II; (2) echocardiography of normal/near-normal RV size and function;(3) hemodynamic parameters showing normalization of RV function (RAP <8 mmHg and CI >2.5 to 3.0 l/min/m2); (4) Six minute walk distance (6MWD) of >380 meters; (5) cardiopulmonary exercise testing, including peak oxygen consumption >15 ml/min/kg; and (6) normal BNP levels.[24]

Combination therapy is an attractive option for the management of PAH, because of the 3 separate signaling pathways known to be involved in the disease. From the REVEAL registry, combination therapy was employed in 41.3% of the patients.[15] The patterns to apply combination therapy may be sequential or initial. Sequential combination therapy is the most widely utilized strategy. From monotherapy there is addition of a second and then third drug in cases of inadequate clinical results or in cases of deterioration. The rationale for initial or upfront combination therapy is based on the known mortality of PAH that is reminiscent of many malignancies and the fact that malignancies and critical medical illnesses are not treated with a stepwise approach to therapy but rather with pre-emptive combination therapy. The experience on RCTs with initial combination therapy is however limited. A multicenter, multi-national, blinded, placebo-controlled trial AMBITION (A Randomized, Multicenter

Study of First-Line Ambrisentan and Tadalafil Combination Therapy in Subjects with Pulmonary Arterial Hypertension) comparing first line monotherapy with tadalafil, monotherapy with ambrisentan and combination therapy with tadalafil and ambrisentan in de novo NYHA functional class II and III PAH patients is underway to address the efficacy to safety ratio of initial combination therapy. Initial combination therapy has been allocated a grade of recommendation II b and level of evidence C in NYHA functional class IV PAH patients in case of non-availability of IV prostanoids.[56]

The long-term outcomes of medically treated patients remain uncertain and lung transplantation should continue to be an important option for those who fail on such therapy and remain in NYHA functional class III or IV. The overall 5-year survival following transplantation for PAH was considered to be 45% to 50%, recently noted to have increased to 52% to 75% at 5 years and to 45% to 66% at 10 years. It is reasonable to consider eligibility for lung transplantation after an inadequate clinical response is confirmed on maximal combination therapy (Fig. 2). However, the option of lung transplantation applicability may be limited in those patients of advanced age.

The creation of an inter-atrial right-to-left shunt through balloon atrial septostomy as a temporizing measure can decompress the right heart chambers and increase left ventricle pre-load and cardiac output. This improves systemic oxygen transport despite arterial oxygen desaturation and decreases sympathetic hyperactivity. The recommended technique is graded balloon dilation atrial septostomy, which produces equivalent improvements in hemodynamics and symptoms but reduced risk compared with the original blade technique.[56] This procedure is viewed as a potential "bridge" to lung transplantation in those patients with advanced PAH who are failing on maximal medical therapy.

11. Prognosis

The prognosis of PAH has improved but remains suboptimal. The natural history of PAH was well described by the NIH Registry with a median survival of 2.8 years; 1-year, 3-year and 5-year survival rates were 68%, 48% and 34% respectively.[3] The French Registry recently characterized survival and important prognostic indicators in patients with PAH, demonstrating improved survival of PAH patients with 1-, 2- and 3-year survival of 85.7%, 69.5% and 54.9% for incident cases.[12] In an elderly cohort of patients, however, estimated 1-, 3 and 5-year survival rates were 76.4%, 50.5% and 37.6% respectively.[6] Predictors of a poor prognosis include: Advanced NYHA functional class, poor exercise capacity as measured by the 6MWT or cardiopulmonary exercise test, high right atrial pressure, significant RV dysfunction, evidence of RV failure, low cardiac index, elevated BNP and underlying diagnosis of scleroderma spectrum of diseases.[1] The diagnosis of PAH in elderly patients is associated with poorer survival likely due to greater vulnerability to the hemodynamic disturbances of PAH.[6]

12. Conclusion

PAH is a chronic and progressive pulmonary vascular disease that leads to right heart failure and ultimately death if left untreated. PAH was previously considered as an illness that affects mostly the young but has been increasingly recognized in the elderly. This may be related to the growing use of echocardiography and right heart catheterization in elderly patients, improved physicians' awareness and rigorous evaluation for PAH as a potential explanation for older patients' symptoms, or the emergence of late onset PAH at advanced age. A high index of suspicion should be maintained to diagnose PAH promptly and a thorough diagnostic work-up should be performed to discriminate between the expected consequences of aging, pulmonary vascular disease and frequent causes of secondary PH such as HFpEF. A right heart catheterization is considered the diagnostic gold standard and is needed prior to initiation of PAH-directed therapy. Currently, several treatment options exist for PAH patients. Utilization of specific PAH therapy has led to improvement of dyspnea, functional status and quality of life in patients with this pulmonary vascular disease.

References

1. McLaughlin VV, Archer SL, Badesch DB. *et al.* (2009) ACCF/AHA 2009 expert consensus document on pulmonary hypertension a report of the American College of Cardiology Foundation Task Force on Expert Consensus Documents and the American Heart Association developed in collaboration with the American College of Chest Physicians; American Thoracic Society, Inc.; and the Pulmonary Hypertension Association. *JACC* **53**: 1573–1619.
2. Montani D, Gunther S, Dorfmuller P *et al.* (2013) Pulmonary arterial hypertension. *Orphanet J Rare Dis* **8**: 97.
3. Rich S, Dantzker DR, Ayres SM *et al.* (1987) Primary pulmonary hypertension. A national prospective study. *Ann Intern Med* **107**: 216–223.
4. Hill NS, Preston I, Roberts K. (2011) Defining the phenotypes for pulmonary hypertension associated with diastolic heart failure. *Circ Heart Fail* **4**: 238–240.
5. Simonneau G, Gatzoulis MA, Adatia I *et al.* (2013) Updated clinical classification of pulmonary hypertension. *JACC* **62**: D34–D41.
6. Shimony A, Fox BD, Afilalo J *et al.* (2012) Pulmonary arterial hypertension in the elderly-clinical characteristics and long-term survival. *Lung* **190**: 645–649.
7. Lador F, Herve P. (2013) A practical approach of pulmonary hypertension in the elderly. *Semin Respir Crit Care Med* **34**: 654–664.
8. Hoeper MM, Huscher D, Ghofrani HA *et al.* (2013) Elderly patients diagnosed with idiopathic pulmonary arterial hypertension: Results from the COMPERA registry. *Int J Cardiol* **168**: 871–880.
9. Appelbaum L, Yigla M, Bendayan D *et al.* (2001) Primary pulmonary hypertension in Israel: A national survey. *Chest* **119**: 1801–1806.
10. Poms AD, Turner M, Farber HW *et al.* (2013) Comorbid conditions and outcomes in patients with pulmonary arterial hypertension: A REVEAL registry analysis. *Chest* **144**: 169–176.
11. Frost AE, Farber HW, Barst RJ *et al.* (2013) Demographics and outcomes of patients diagnosed with pulmonary hypertension with pulmonary capillary wedge pressures 16 to 18 mm Hg: Insights from the REVEAL Registry. *Chest* **143**: 185–195.
12. Humbert M, Sitbon O, Chaouat A *et al.* (2006) Pulmonary arterial hypertension in France: Results from a national registry. *Am J Respir Critic Care Med* **173**: 1023–1030.

13. Ling Y, Johnson MK, Kiely DG *et al.* (2012) Changing demographics, epidemiology, and survival of incident pulmonary arterial hypertension: Results from the pulmonary hypertension registry of the United Kingdom and Ireland. *Am J Respir Critic Care Medicine.* **186**: 790–796.
14. Walker AM, Langleben D, Korelitz JJ *et al.* (2006) Temporal trends and drug exposures in pulmonary hypertension: An American experience. *Am Heart J* **152**: 521–526.
15. Badesch DB, Raskob GE, Elliott CG *et al.* (2010) Pulmonary arterial hypertension: Baseline characteristics from the REVEAL Registry. *Chest* **137**: 376–387.
16. Hyduk A, Croft JB, Ayala C *et al.* (2005) Pulmonary hypertension surveillance — United States, 1980–2002. *Morb Mortal Wkly Rep. Surveill Summ* **54**: 1–28.
17. Foley RJ, Wilcox D, Walsh SJ *et al.* (2011) Survival of geriatric idiopathic pulmonary arterial hypertension patients. *Conn Medicine* **75**: 11–15.
18. Vaupel JW. (2010) Biodemography of human ageing. *Nature* **464**: 536–542.
19. Salive ME. (2013) Multimorbidity in Older Adults. *Epidemiol Rev.*
20. Lam CS, Borlaug BA, Kane GC *et al.* (2009) Age-associated increases in pulmonary artery systolic pressure in the general population. *Circulation* **119**: 2663–2670.
21. Rubenfire M, Lippo G, Bodini BD *et al.* (2009) Evaluating health-related quality of life, work ability, and disability in pulmonary arterial hypertension: An unmet need. *Chest* **136**: 597–603.
22. Murad K, Kitzman DW. (2012) Frailty and multiple comorbidities in the elderly patient with heart failure: Implications for management. *Heart Failure Rev* **17**: 581–588.
23. Gomberg-Maitland M, Bull TM, Saggar R *et al.* (2013) New trial designs and potential therapies for pulmonary artery hypertension. *JACC* **62**: D82–D91.
24. McLaughlin VV, Gaine SP, Howard LS *et al.* (2013) Treatment goals of pulmonary hypertension. *JACC* **62**: D73–D81.
25. Boxer RS, Wang Z, Walsh SJ *et al.* (2008) The utility of the 6-minute walk test as a measure of frailty in older adults with heart failure. *Am J Geriatr Cardiol* **17**: 7–12.
26. Janssens JP, Pache JC, Nicod LP. (1999) Physiological changes in respiratory function associated with ageing. *Euro Respir J* **13**: 197–205.
27. Lalley PM. (2013) The aging respiratory system–pulmonary structure, function and neural control. *Respir Physiol Neurobiol* **187**: 199–210.

28. Vaz Fragoso CA, Gill TM. (2012) Respiratory impairment and the aging lung: A novel paradigm for assessing pulmonary function. *J Gerontol A Biol Sci Med Sci* **67**: 264–275.
29. Knudson RJ, Slatin RC, Lebowitz, MD *et al.* (1976) The maximal expiratory flow-volume curve. Normal standards, variability, and effects of age. *Am Rev Respir Dis* **113**: 587–600.
30. Aguilaniu B, Maitre J, Glenet S *et al.* (2008) European reference equations for CO and NO lung transfer. *Euro Respir J* **31**: 1091–1097.
31. Chen CH, Nakayama M, Nevo E *et al.* (1998) Coupled systolic-ventricular and vascular stiffening with age: Implications for pressure regulation and cardiac reserve in the elderly. *JACC* **32**: 1221–1227.
32. Hosoda Y, Kawano K, Yamasawa F *et al.* (1984) Age-dependent changes of collagen and elastin content in human aorta and pulmonary artery. *Angiology* **35**: 615–621.
33. Farrar JF, Blomfield J, Reye RD. (1965) The structure and composition of the maturing pulmonary circulation. *J Pathol Bacteriol* **90**: 83–96.
34. Mackay EH, Banks J, Sykes B *et al.* (1978) Structural basis for the changing physical properties of human pulmonary vessels with age. *Thorax* **33**: 335–344.
35. Redfield MM, Jacobsen SJ, Burnett JC *et al.* (2003) Burden of systolic and diastolic ventricular dysfunction in the community: Appreciating the scope of the heart failure epidemic. *JAMA* **289**: 194–202.
36. McQuillan BM, Picard MH, Leavitt M *et al.* (2001) Clinical correlates and reference intervals for pulmonary artery systolic pressure among echocardiographically normal subjects. *Circulation* **104**: 2797–2802.
37. Mahjoub H, Levy F, Cassol M *et al.* (2009) Effects of age on pulmonary artery systolic pressure at rest and during exercise in normal adults. *Euro J Echocardiogr* **10**: 635–640.
38. Kovacs G, Berghold A, Scheidl S *et al.* (2009) Pulmonary arterial pressure during rest and exercise in healthy subjects: A systematic review. *Euro Respir J* **34**: 888–894.
39. Kuchel GA. (2010) Aging and Homeostatic Regulation. In: Halter JB, Hazzard WR, Ouslander JG *et al.* eds. *Hazzard's Principles of Geriatric Medicine and Gerontology*. 6th ed. McGraw Hill, New York. 621–630.
40. Burch JB, Augustine AD, Frieden LA *et al.* (2014) Advances in geroscience: Impact on healthspan and chronic disease. *J Gerontol A Biol Sci Med Sci* **69**: S1–S3.

41. Goldman DP, Cutler D, Rowe JW *et al.* (2013) Substantial health and economic returns from delayed aging may warrant a new focus for medical research. *Health affairs* **32**: 1698–1705.
42. Tchkonia T, Zhu Y, van Deursen J *et al.* (2013) Cellular senescence and the senescent secretory phenotype: Therapeutic opportunities. *J Clin Invest* **123**: 966–972.
43. Lourenco AP, Fontoura D, Henriques-Coelho T *et al.* (2012) Current pathophysiological concepts and management of pulmonary hypertension. *Int J Cardiol* **155**: 350–361.
44. Rhodes CJ, Davidson A, Gibbs JS *et al.* (2009) Therapeutic targets in pulmonary arterial hypertension. *Pharmacol Ther* **121**: 69–88.
45. Jeffery TK, Wanstall JC. (2001) Pulmonary vascular remodeling: A target for therapeutic intervention in pulmonary hypertension. *Pharmacol Ther* **92**: 1–20.
46. Jurasz P, Courtman D, Babaie S *et al.* (2010) Role of apoptosis in pulmonary hypertension: From experimental models to clinical trials. *Pharmacol Ther* **126**: 1–8.
47. Shapiro BP, McGoon MD, Redfield MM. (2007) Unexplained pulmonary hypertension in elderly patients. *Chest* **131**: 94–100.
48. de Oliveira RK, Ferreira EV, Ramos RP *et al.* (2014) Usefulness of pulmonary capillary wedge pressure as a correlate of left ventricular filling pressures in pulmonary arterial hypertension. *J Heart Lung Transplant* **33**: 157–162.
49. Thenappan T, Shah SJ, Gomberg-Maitland M *et al.* (2011) Clinical characteristics of pulmonary hypertension in patients with heart failure and preserved ejection fraction. *Circ Heart Fail* **4**: 257–265.
50. Ohara T, Ohte N, Little WC. (2012) Pulmonary hypertension in heart failure with preserved left ventricular ejection fraction: Diagnosis and management. *Curr Opin Cardiol* **27**: 281–287.
51. Afshar M, Collado F, Doukky R. (2012) Pulmonary hypertension in elderly patients with diastolic dysfunction and preserved ejection fraction. *Open Cardiovasc Med J* **6**: 1–8.
52. Rifaie O, El-Damanhory H, Amr M *et al.* (2010) Prevalence and predictors of pulmonary hypertension in elderly patients with isolated diastolic heart failure. *Kardiologia polska* **68**: 655–661.
53. Robbins IM, Newman JH, Johnson RF *et al.* (2009) Association of the metabolic syndrome with pulmonary venous hypertension. *Chest* **136**: 31–36.

54. Shah SJ. (2012) Pulmonary hypertension. *JAMA* **308**: 1366–1374.
55. Halpern SD, Taichman DB. (2009) Misclassification of pulmonary hypertension due to reliance on pulmonary capillary wedge pressure rather than left ventricular end-diastolic pressure. *Chest* **136**: 37–43.
56. Galie N, Corris PA, Frost A *et al.* (2013) Updated treatment algorithm of pulmonary arterial hypertension. *JACC* **62**: D60–72.
57. Barst RJ, Rubin LJ, Long WA *et al.* (1996) A comparison of continuous intravenous epoprostenol (prostacyclin) with conventional therapy for primary pulmonary hypertension. *New Engl J Med* **334**: 296–301.
58. Olschewski H, Simonneau G, Galie N *et al.* (2002) Inhaled iloprost for severe pulmonary hypertension. *New Engl J Med* **347**: 322–329.
59. Simonneau G, Barst RJ, Galie N *et al.* (2002) Continuous subcutaneous infusion of treprostinil, a prostacyclin analogue, in patients with pulmonary arterial hypertension: A double-blind, randomized, placebo-controlled trial. *Am J Respir Critic Care Med* **165**: 800–804.
60. McLaughlin VV, Benza RL, Rubin LJ *et al.* (2010) Addition of inhaled treprostinil to oral therapy for pulmonary arterial hypertension: A randomized controlled clinical trial. *JACC* **55**: 1915–1922.
61. McLaughlin VV, Davis M, Cornwell W. (2011) Pulmonary arterial hypertension. *Curr Prob Cardiol* **36**: 461–517.
62. Rubin LJ, Badesch DB, Barst RJ *et al.* (2002) Bosentan therapy for pulmonary arterial hypertension. *New Engl J Med* **346**: 896–903.
63. Galie N, Rubin L, Hoeper M *et al.* (2008) Treatment of patients with mildly symptomatic pulmonary arterial hypertension with bosentan (EARLY study): A double-blind, randomised controlled trial. *Lancet* **371**: 2093–2100.
64. Galie N, Olschewski H, Oudiz RJ *et al.* (2008) Ambrisentan for the treatment of pulmonary arterial hypertension: Results of the ambrisentan in pulmonary arterial hypertension, randomized, double-blind, placebo-controlled, multicenter, efficacy (ARIES) study 1 and 2. *Circulation* **117**: 3010–3019.
65. Pulido T, Adzerikho I, Channick RN *et al.* (2013) Macitentan and morbidity and mortality in pulmonary arterial hypertension. *New Engl J Med* **369**: 809–818.
66. Humbert M, Sitbon O, Simonneau G. (2004) Treatment of pulmonary arterial hypertension. *New Engl J Med* **351**: 1425–1436.
67. Ghofrani HA, Galie N, Grimminger F *et al.* (2013) Riociguat for the treatment of pulmonary arterial hypertension. *New Engl J Med* **369**: 330–340.

68. Ghofrani HA, D'Armini AM, Grimminger F *et al.* (2013) Riociguat for the treatment of chronic thromboembolic pulmonary hypertension. *New Engl J Med* **369**: 319–329.
69. Galie N, Ghofrani HA, Torbicki A *et al.* (2005) Sildenafil citrate therapy for pulmonary arterial hypertension. *New Engl J Med* **353**: 2148–2157.
70. Galie N, Brundage BH, Ghofrani HA *et al.* (2009) Tadalafil therapy for pulmonary arterial hypertension. *Circulation* **119**: 2894–2903.

Chapter 13

Growth Factors and Aging in Pulmonary Arterial Hypertension

Claudio Bravo*,†, Won-Kyung Cho‡, and Hyung J. Chun*,§

Pulmonary arterial hypertension (PAH) is a rare disease with the hallmark of vascular remodeling of the pulmonary arterioles, associated with formation of plexiform and concentric lesions comprised of proliferating vascular cells. Ultimate clinical outcomes for the majority of PAH patients, despite recent advancements in therapies, are death from right ventricular failure or lung transplant. Recent advances in our understanding of the molecular signaling processes involved in the pathogenesis of disease have identified a number of key growth factors involved in PAH, some of which are targeted by currently available pharmacologic agents, and others that represent potentially attractive therapeutic targets. Here we will provide an overview of the disease process as it relates to aging and expand upon the potential therapeutic targets that can be considered to advance the treatment paradigm.

*Yale Cardiovascular Research Center, Section of Cardiovascular Medicine and
†Bridgeport Hospital, Yale New Haven Health System.
‡Section of Pulmonary, Critical Care, and Sleep Medicine, Department of Internal Medicine, Yale University School of Medicine, New Haven, CT 06511.
§Yale Cardiovascular Research Center, Yale University School of Medicine, 300 George Street, Room 770H, New Haven, CT 06511. Email:hyung.chun@yale.edu

1. Definition and Classification

Pulmonary hypertension (PH) is defined by a resting mean pulmonary artery pressure (mPAP) of ≥25 mmHg.[1] Although initially classified as primary or secondary, depending on whether an identifiable cause was present,[2] newly recognized causes of PH have led to re-classification by the World Health Organization (WHO) into the five groups depending on cause and treatment options (Table 1),[3,4] with group 1 PH being PAH and group 2–5 designated PH. PAH is characterized by PH that is caused by conditions that directly affect small arterial vessels of the lungs and is the only form of PH currently approved for the treatment with pulmonary vasodilator therapy.[1,4]

Table 1.

	Updated Classification of Pulmonary Hypertension 5th WSPH Nice 2013
Group 1	Pulmonary arterial hypertension
	Idiopathic PAH (IPAH)
	Familiar PAH (FPAH)
	Bone morphogenetic protein (BMP) receptor type-2 (BMPR2)
	ALK-1, ENG, SMAD9, CAV1, KCNK3
	Unknown
	Drug and toxin-induced
	Associated with: (APAH)
	Connective tissue disease (CTD)
	HIV infection
	Portal hypertension
	Congenital heart diseases
	Schistosomiasis
	Pulmonary veno-occlusive disease and/or pulmonary capillary hemangiomatosis
	Persistent pulmonary hypertension of the newborn
Group 2	Pulmonary hypertension due to left heart disease
	Left ventricular systolic dysfunction
	Left ventricular diastolic dysfunction
	Valvular disease
	Congenital/acquired left heart inflow/outflow tract obstruction and congenital cardiomyopathies

(*Continued*)

Table 1. (Continued)

	Updated Classification of Pulmonary Hypertension 5th WSPH Nice 2013
Group 3	Pulmonary hypertension due to lung diseases and/or hypoxia Chronic obstructive pulmonary disease Interstitial lung disease Other pulmonary diseases with mixed restrictive and obstructive pattern Sleep-disordered breathing Alveolar hypoventilation disorders Chronic exposure to high altitude Developmental lung diseases
Group 4	Chronic thromboembolic pulmonary hypertension
Group 5	Pulmonary hypertension with unclear multifactorial mechanisms Hematologic disorders: chronic hemolytic anemia, myeloproliferative disorders, splenectomy Systemic disorders: sarcoidosis, pulmonary histiocytosis, lymphangioleiomyomatosis Metabolic disorders: glycogen storage disease, Gaucher disease, thyroid disorders Others: tumoral obstruction, fibrosing mediastinitis, chronic renal failure, segmental PH

We will primarily restrict our discussions on group 1 PH, as the other forms will be discussed elsewhere.

2. Epidemiology

PAH is a relatively uncommon disease with a high mortality and morbidity. The exact prevalence and incidence of PAH are not fully known. In a large USA registry, the incidence and prevalence of group 1 PAH were estimated to be 2.3 and 12.4 per million patients, respectively.[5] European registries have found variable incidence and prevalence, with a French registry demonstrating comparable statistics as the U.S. (2.4 and 15 per million patient respectively) and a U.K. registry demonstrating fewer cases.[6,7] In the Registry to Evaluate Early and Long-term PAH Disease Management (REVEAL) study, 54 sites collected the information of patients with group

1 PAH. In this registry, women predominated over men,[5] and approximately half of the group 1 or PAH was due to APAH and the other half was IPAH. Within APAH, CTD was present in half of these patients with 90% of them being women.[8] Another registry based on three university hospitals in the US, showed that female predominates in all subtype of group 1 PAH, except in the HIV associated group.[9] The mean age of patients with PAH at the time of diagnosis was 36 ± 15 years in a 1987 study, with more recent registries placing the mean age closer to 50.[5–7] Quite surprisingly, another recent European registry even reported 63% of patients being older than 65.[10] It is obvious that the incidence and prevalence of PAH have been increasing in the elderly population, which could be due to greater awareness of disease by physicians or the general population, or increased overall life expectancy. With increased awareness of PH in the older population, a number of factors associated with aging complicate the treatment of these patients, including the vascular changes such as decreased total capillary volume in aged lung[11] and increased pulmonary arterial stiffness,[12,13] which contribute to the demonstrated increase in the right ventricular systolic pressure (RVSP) (estimated to be ~1mmHg per decade).[14] Moreover, the cardiac ventricular and systemic arterial compliances are decreased, which likely lead to ventricular diastolic dysfunction and further complicates the diagnosis of PAH.[15]

3. Pathophysiology

The anatomic changes in the lungs of PAH patients involve vascular remodeling that affects the small pulmonary arteries with subsequent loss of global vascular luminal cross-sectional area. Large pulmonary artery compliance is also decreased in PAH. These changes result in increased pulmonary vascular resistance (PVR) and right heart failure. The mechanisms of lumen-obliterating processes of pulmonary artery are multifactorial, including vasoconstriction associated with endothelial dysfunction, dysregulated cellular growth, inflammation and/or increased extracellular matrix

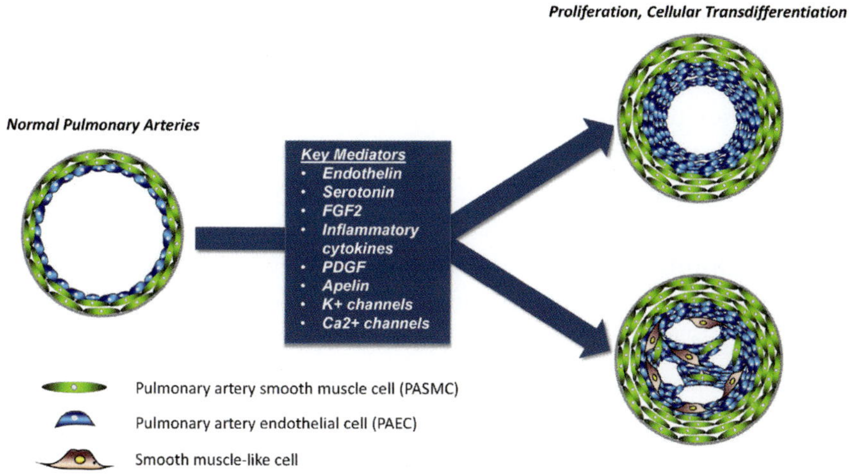

Fig. 1. Mediators of Vascular Remodeling in PAH.

deposition resulting in vascular fibrosis (Fig.1).[16,17] These abnormal vascular remodeling processes involve all vessel layers (intima, media and adventitia).[18–24] Among these, one of the most prominent features of PAH pathology is dysregulated proliferation of vascular cells in the pulmonary arterioles, suggesting the presence of a switch from a quiescent state to a proliferative, apoptosis-resistant state in vascular cells. The proliferating cells encompass multiple cell types, including myofibroblast-like cells[25,26] and mesenchymal progenitor cells,[27] as well as endothelial cells, vascular smooth muscle cells and fibroblasts.[17] These processes altogether contribute to the generation of plexiform arteriopathy (glomeruloid-like vascular structures) and vascular pruning (loss of precapillary vessels).[28,29] Given the proliferative nature of the pulmonary vascular cells in PAH, some have regarded PAH as a quasi-malignant state.[30] Such a hypothesis has been supported by demonstration of endothelial clonality [31,32] and proposed to involve a "second-hit" in a subset of these cells that result in their hyperproliferation, either in conjunction with presence of germline mutations (such as those with bone morphogenic receptor type 2 (BMPR2) mutation) or due to exposure to other toxins.[33–35]

4. Current Therapies and their Targeted Mechanisms in PAH

Four classes of drugs are currently FDA approved for treatment of PAH patients. Thus far, endothelin-1, nitric oxide and prostacyclin pathways are utilized as therapeutic targets in PAH.[36] Despite the small number of patients, these classes of drugs account for over $3 billion in annual sales. Additional agents that are commonly used in this patient population, including calcium channel blockers and diuretics are beyond the scope of this chapter.

4.1. *Prostanoids*

Prostacyclin (PGI2) is a cyclic adenosine monophosphate (cAMP)-pathway-mediated potent pulmonary vasodilator[37] and inhibits platelet aggregation, inflammation and proliferation of the pulmonary artery smooth muscle cell (PASMC).[38] On the counterpart, thromboxane A2 (TXA2) is a vasoconstrictor, proliferation stimulator and platelet activator.[39,40] Patients with PAH have a reduced expression of prostacyclin synthase in the lungs.[41,42] On the other hand, patients with PAH have an increased production of TXA2 that contributes with the physiopathology of this syndrome.[41] This imbalance between prostacyclin and thromboxane levels appears to be important in the generation of PAH.[41] These findings have served in part as the rationale for augmenting prostacyclin signaling as a therapy in PAH.

Epoprostenol is a synthetic prostacyclin that is given via continuous intravenous infusion. Epoprostenol has been found to improve symptoms, exercise capacity and hemodynamics in patients with PAH. In fact, this remains the only treatment with demonstrated survival benefit in patients with IPAH and its survival benefit is further supported by observational studies.[43–49] Continuous infusion of epoprostenol requires a permanently implanted central venous catheter using a portable infusion pump, titration of doses based on therapeutic response and/or toxicities and can lead to significant rebound adverse effects if stopped abruptly.[43–45,50] It is also associated with multiple side effects (including jaw pain, diarrhea and arthralgias) and its cumbersome delivery method is associated with thrombosis, infection or pump malfunction that can be problematic.[51,52] Other forms of prostacyclin analogs include treprostinil, which can be given orally, via inhalation, or infusion (either subcutaneously or intravenously), iloprost, which is given via inhalation[53–55] and beraprost, an orally active prostacyclin analogue.[56,57]

4.2. *Endothelin receptor antagonists*

Another key mediator of PAH targeted by approved therapies is the endothelin signaling pathway. Endothelin-1 (ET-1) is a 21 amino acid vasoactive polypeptide that exerts its effects via two different receptors, namely ET receptor type A (ET_A) and type B (ET_B).[58] ET_A receptors are located predominantly on smooth muscle cells where they mediate vasoconstriction, proliferation and fibrosis,[59] whereas ET_B receptors are found predominantly on vascular endothelial cells where they induce vasodilation. However, in PAH, expression of vasodilatory endothelial ET_B is decreased and expression of both constrictive ET_A and ET_B in the vascular smooth muscle cells is increased.[60–63] Patients with PAH have increased expression of ET-1 in pulmonary vascular cells compared to healthy controls.[64,65] The plasma level of ET-1 has also been found to correlate with the severity and prognosis of PAH.[65,66]

Endothelin-1 receptor antagonists (ERAs) emerged as an initial therapy for group 1 PAH in the late 1990s. Bosentan and macitentan are nonselective ET receptor blockers, while ambrisentan is a selective ET_A blocker. Ambrisentan was found to improve symptoms, as demonstrated by increase in the exercise capacity, improvement in hemodynamics and lengthening of the time to clinical worsening in patients with IPAH and PAH associated with CTD.[67,68] Bosentan also showed improvement of exercise capacity, functional class, hemodynamics and time to clinical worsening.[68–71] Macitentan has a better tissue penetrance and longer sustained receptor binding and showed mortality, morbidity and exercise tolerance benefit; however, this study was not powered to show a benefit in mortality as an independent outcome.[72] The main adverse effects of ERAs are hepatotoxicity and peripheral edema. Thus, caution needs to be taken to treat patients with liver dysfunction.[68,70,72]

4.3. *Phosphodiesterase 5 inhibitors and soluble guanylate cyclase stimulator*

Nitric oxide (NO) is a free radical lipophilic gaseous molecule, which may easily diffuse through pulmonary artery endothelial cell (PAEC) and PASMC membranes and participate in the intracellular molecular signaling. NO is a vasodilator,[73] inhibits platelet activation[74] and inhibits PASMC proliferation.[75] NO is produced by nitric oxide synthase (NOS) from L-arginine.[76] There are at least three isoforms of NOS in mammals: The neuronal NOS (nNOS or NOS1), inducible NOS (iNOS or NOS2) and endothelial NOS (eNOS or NOS3).[77] NO exerts its vasodilatory effect on vascular SMC by increasing cyclic guanosine monophosphate (cGMP) synthesized by the soluble guanylate cyclase (sGC). cGMP is thereafter degraded by phosphodiesterases (PDE), especially the isoform 5.[78] Alternatively, NO signaling pathway involves the oxidation of NO to nitrite[79] or reactions of NO with protein thiols to form S-nitrosothiols (SNOs),[80] which are posttranslational modifications that alter the kinetic of certain proteins. Among NOS isoforms, eNOS is considered to be the main isoform involved in PAH. While the expression level of eNOS has been reported varied in the lungs of patients with PAH and animal models of PH, there is a general consensus that the overall NO bioavailability is decreased.[81–86] The paradox of increased eNOS expression and diminished NO level is potentially explained by a process termed "eNOS uncoupling," a dysfunctional state of the enzyme in which electrons transferring from the NOS reductase domain to the oxygenase domain are diverted to molecular oxygen rather than to L-arginine, forming superoxide rather than NO.[87]

A number of drugs have shown the capability of increasing NO availability. PDE 5 inhibitors such as sildenafil, tadalafil and vardenafil, or sGC stimulator such as riociguat can increase the NO concentration in PAH patients. All of the PDE 5 inhibitors can improve exercise capacity, symptoms, hemodynamics and time to clinical worsening, but have not demonstrated mortality benefits.[88–92] Common side effects include headache, flushing, dyspepsia and epistaxis. The recently approved riociguat, an oral sGC stimulator, has shown to increase the exercise capacity, hemodynamics and time to clinical worsening and has been found to be well tolerated, with syncope as the most frequent side effect.[93]

4.4. *Combination therapy*

Combination therapy, which combines drugs with different mechanisms of action, have shown some additive effect or have been successful to lower dose of each agent. Indication of combination therapy is when patient is refractory to monotherapy. Usually, it consists of, at least, two drugs among prostanoids, ERAs and PDE5 inhibitors.[47,48]

4.5. *Genetics*

Hereditary PAH, or familial PAH, accounts for approximately 6 to 10% of group 1 PAH. An important signaling pathway in the PAH pathogenesis is BMPR2 signaling. In 75% of patients with familial PAH (FPAH), more than 300 independent mutations have been identified in the BMPR2 gene. BMPR2 is a type II receptor member of the transforming growth factor (TGF)-β family. This protein targets the SMAD pathway and the mutations are thought to lead to inactivation of BMPR2 and cause loss of function.[94,95] However, of those who carry the BMPR2 mutation, the disease penetrance is only 20%, suggesting that secondary factors, whether environmental or genetic, may be playing a key role in the disease pathogenesis.[96] BMPR2 mutations have also been identified in 25% of idiopathic or sporadic cases of PAH.[97,98] Moreover, decreased BMPR2 signaling or expression has been reported in diverse forms of PAH regardless of the presence of mutations.[99] These findings suggest that reduction of BMPR2 expression or signaling, perhaps more so than the mutations themselves may be key determinant of developing PAH. Another mutation that involves one of the TGF-β family, the activin receptor-like kinase 1 (ALK-1) gene, has been found but is less frequently seen in patients with PAH. This mutation is common in patients with FPAH secondary to hemorrhagic telangiectasia[100] and induces angiogenesis through an SMAD pathway dependent mechanism as well.[101] Those patients with FPAH due to hemorrhagic telangiectasia may also be carriers of other less frequent mutations, including endoglin[100,102] or SMAD9.[103] More recently, two additional gene mutations have been described in PAH: Caveolin-1 (CAV1) which encodes a membrane protein of caveolae, abundant in the endothelial cells of the lung[104] and KCNK3, a gene encoding for potassium channel superfamily *K* member-3.[93]

5. Emerging Therapeutic Targets and Strategies: Focus on the Growth Factors

Despite the existing approved PAH therapies and the demonstrated mutations that contribute to disease pathogenesis, PAH subjects continue to succumb to right heart failure and high rates of mortality.[105,106] These limitations in our treatment armament highlight the need to identify and test additional therapeutic targets that can potentially provide greater mechanistic insights into the disease pathogenesis. Some of these factors are discussed below.

5.1. *Serotonin*

Serotonin (5-hydroxy-tryptamine: 5-HT) is a neurotransmitter with vasoconstrictive properties in the pulmonary vascular system[107,108] and stimulates proliferation of PAECs, PASMCs and fibroblasts.[109,110] The role of serotonin in PAH development became important after patients receiving anorexic drugs that interfere with serotonin (5-HT) handling, specifically derivatives from fenfluramine,[111,112] developed PAH and fond to have increased plasmat levels of serotonin.[113] Elevated 5-HT levels in plasma of patients with IPAH also have been reported.[113] Further, a recent study reported that the L-allelic variant of the serotonin transporter (5-HTT) gene promoter, which is associated with 5-HTT overexpression and increased PASMC growth, was present in homozygous form in 65% of patients with PAH compared to 27% of controls.[114] Studies in mice overexpressing 5-HTT showed worse hypoxia induced PH compared to the wild type littermates.[115,116] Conversely, mice either lacking 5-HTT or treated with the 5-HTT inhibitor fluoxetine had attenuated progression of PH.[117,118] Taken together, the serotonin pathway appears to be an important mediator in PAH, but clinical trials to modulate the serotonin pathway have been disappointing likely due to its complex signaling pathways.[114,119,120]

5.2. *Fibroblast growth factor*

Normal angiogenesis is known to involve multiple angiogenic growth factors and cytokines. Fibroblast growth factor 2 (FGF2 or bFGF) has been documented to have a key role in endothelial and vascular smooth muscle cell migration, proliferation, and synthesis of extracellular matrix proteins.[121] Based on previous animal data suggesting elevated FGF2 levels in PH,[122,123] serum and urine FGF2 levels were assessed in a cohort of patients with PAH. Interestingly, FGF2 was found to be significantly increased in PAH subjects.[124] A more recent study demonstrated that the PAECs express significantly greater levels of FGF2 and that it can be targeted by either short interfering RNA against FGF2 or using a pharmacologic FGFR1 inhibitor (SU-5402) to ameliorate PH in experimental rodent models.[122] Our recent study further demonstrated that pulmonary artery endothelial expression of FGF2 and FGFR1 are regulated by two microRNAs, namely miR-424 and miR-503, whose expression is regulated by apelin/APJ signaling and decreased in PAECs of PAH subjects.[125]

Overall, these studies identify a potential key role for overproduction of FGF2 and heightened FGF-mediated proliferative response as a key mediator of pathogenesis of PAH. It is likely that such a mechanism is a key contributor to promotion of both PASMC[122] and PAEC[126] proliferation. Recent literature in the oncology field has identified a number of FGF signaling inhibitors that have demonstrated efficacy in both pre-clinical and clinical models, which could potentially be used in experimental models of PH and have the potential to progress to clinical trials based on results.[127]

5.3. *Platelet derived growth factor*

Compelling evidence from animal models of PH[128,129] and patients with PAH[130,131] supports that the platelet derived growth factor (PDGF) pathway plays an important role in the pathophysiology of PAH. The PDGF ligand binds to the PDGF receptor (PDGFR).[132] There are at least two isoforms of this receptor, PDGF-α and PDGF-β. The binding of the endogenous ligand to this receptor activates its tyrosine kinase activity,[132,133] inducing hyperplasia of PASMC[134] and protecting against apoptosis.[133] In normal blood vessels the expression of PDGF ligand and PDGFR is low, but is markedly upregulated in lungs of monocrotaline[135] or hypoxia[136,137] induced animal models of PH, similarly to what is described in lungs from patients with PAH.[130,138] The importance of PDGF has been confirmed in genetically modified mice. Overexpression of the constitutively active PDGF-β worsen the PH course in chronically hypoxic mice, compared to their wild type littermate.[139] Furthermore, the pharmacological inhibition of PDGFR with imatinib, an FDA approved drug for the treatment of several hematologic neoplastic diseases, reversed the vascular remodeling in animal models of PH.[140] Case reports of patients with PAH experimentally treated with imatinib showed dramatic functional capacity and hemodynamic improvement.[141,142] Unfortunately, in a larger, phase III clinical trial (Imatinib in PAH, a Randomized, Efficacy Study (IMPRES)), the adverse effects associated to the drug led to frequent discontinuation of the medication and failure of approval, although improvements in hemodynamic and functional outcomes had been reached.[143]

5.4. *Inflammatory mediators*

A role for inflammation in PAH has been initially suggested based on the finding of both innate and adaptive inflammatory cells, including macrophages, mast cells, lymphocytes and dendritic cells, in lungs from patients with PAH.[144] In addition, PAH often accompanies chronic inflammatory diseases such as autoimmune (systemic sclerosis) or infectious diseases (HIV, human gamma herpes virus or hepatitis C).[145] Recently, a positive correlation between the average perivascular inflammation score, the severity of vascular remodeling and mean pulmonary arterial pressure has been reported.[146] Beyond increased perivascular and intravascular immune cell infiltration, increased expression of chemokines including RANTES (regulated upon activation normal *T* cell expressed and secreted), fractalkine and monocyte chemotactic protein-1 has also been reported in the lungs of patients with IPAH.[147–149] Furthermore, patients with PAH exhibit higher circulating as well pulmonary expression of interleukin-1 IL-1β, IL-6 and TNF-α.[150] TNF-α has been implicated to play a key role in proliferation of PASMCs in many PH experimental models.[151] Recently, lung specific overexpression of IL-6 in mice replicated the pathological lesions observed in advanced PAH including distal arteriolar muscularization, plexogenic arteriopathy and increased PVR.[152] In addition, serum level of IL-6 is inversely correlated with adverse outcome, including survival.[153] Further, the roles of another inflammatory cytokine, namely IL-13, in PH have been suggested by using lung-specific IL-13-overexpressing transgenic mice or an animal model of Schistosomiasis.[154,155]

Maladaptation of the immune response has been implicated as a contributor to chronic inflammatory response in PAH. For instance, several types of autoantibodies directed against antinuclear antigens, endothelial cells and fibroblasts are often found in PAH and these autoantibodies have been suggested in endothelial cell apoptosis.[156–158] Moreover, idiopathic PAH patients are reported to have increased circulating regulatory *T* cells, which control the balance between Th1 and Th2 responses as well as self-tolerance, as compared to controls, suggesting altered immune control by CD4+ *T* lymphocytes in PAH.[159–161]

Collectively, these data indicate that a number of different inflammatory pathways are involved in the pathogenesis of PAH. Therefore, some novel therapeutic approaches to slow down the progression of disease by controlling the immune/inflammatory component have been tried. Recently, low-dose FK506, an immunosuppressant, was tried in animal model of PH with a good outcome, through a mechanism that appears to involve BMPR2 signaling pathway.[162] Although TNF-α appears to be one of key inflammatory mediators of pulmonary hypertension,[163] the results of antagonizing this cytokine have been mixed in experimental PH models.[164,165] Therefore, further studies will be needed in terms of clinical application of anti-inflammatory approach in PAH.

5.5. *Apelin*

The GPCR ligand apelin has recently emerged as a potential regulator of pulmonary vascular homeostasis, with roles in PAH.[125,166,167] Apelin has been found to augment cardiac contractility and induce vasorelaxation, at least in part via an NO dependent manner. Its only known receptor thus far is APJ, which is highly expressed in the pulmonary endothelium. Apelin expression has been found to be decreased in the serum of patients with PAH, as well as in the PAECs.[167,168] Apelin administration to experimental models of PH led to amelioration of disease and apelin null mice were found to have worsening PH compared to controls in the chronic hypoxia model. More recent studies have identified a key role for apelin as a suppressor of FGF2 expression from PAECs, and also found to inhibit PASMC proliferation.[168] Moreover, microRNAs that are downstream of apelin, namely miR-424 and miR-503, were found to be decreased in PAH PAECs, and restoration of these microRNAs in experimental PH model inhibited the aberrant proliferation of PAH

PAECs and also reverse experimental PH models.[125] These studies have led to beginning of clinical trials in the U.K. to test the efficacy of intravenous apelin peptide administration in improving the pulmonary vascular resistance in patients with PAH. Overall, these studies identify apelin as an intriguing potential therapeutic target, although further work is required to validate the role of this pathway in clinical PAH.

5.6. *K^+ channels/Ca^{2+} channels*

Altered function of K^+ channels and Ca^{2+} channels has been reported in PAH. Down-regulated or dysfunctional voltage-gated *K*+ channels (most notably Kv1.5 and Kv1.2) results in depolarization of membrane potentials of PASMC allowing calcium influx via the voltage gated calcium channels and induction of muscle contraction as well as SMC proliferation. All these processes contribute to PAH.[169–171] It has been shown that iptakalim, an ATP sensitive potassium channel activator, prevents PASMC proliferation and induces vasodilation.[172] In addition, Ca2+ signalling through transient receptor potential (TRP) ion channels has been reported to play a role in IPAH, where TRPC3 and TRPC6 expression are upregulated in PASMCs.[173]

6. Special Considerations of the PAH Pathogenesis in Elderly Population

The vasculature undergoes functional and structural changes with aging. The vascular wall undergoes structural remodeling including intimal and medial thickening leading to vascular stiffness. Further, alterations in the function of endothelial cells are well known. For instance impaired PGI_2-mediated vasodilation, increased ET-1-mediated vasoconstriction and decreased eNOS activity have been reported with aging.[174–176] Furthermore, antithrombotic and vasodilatory properties of the endothelium are reduced with aging, whereas inflammatory activity and oxidative stress increase.[177] In addition, the activity and expression of many molecules that are known to play the key roles in the development of PAH seem to change with aging, including PDGF and serotonin.[178,179] Also a recent study showed arterial stiffness in middle-aged and older adults is associated with decreased plasma level of apelin.[180] Taken together, aging seems to impose a burden on pulmonary circulation system, which might explain increased prevalence and incidence of PAH in the elderly population.

7. Conclusions

Undoubtedly the incidence and prevalence of PAH in the elderly population is increasing. However the diagnosis of PAH in the elderly population is complicated by the aging effects on the cardiovascular system. In particular, heart failure with preserved ejection fraction such as diastolic dysfunction of left heart, which can lead to pulmonary venous hypertension, is more common in the elderly population. Therefore, a more careful hemodynamic assessment through procedures such as right heart catheterization will be needed in this population to obtain definitive classification of PH. Recent advances in treatment have given us more flexibilities in our management of patients with PAH, although it remains a fatal disease. Given the importance of early diagnosis of PAH, increased awareness of disease by physicians will be important to improve clinical outcome, especially in the elderly population.

References

1. Hoeper MM *et al.* (2013) Definitions and diagnosis of pulmonary hypertension. *JACC* **62**(25 Suppl): D42–D50.
2. Anonymous (1973) Primary pulmonary hypertension and SLE. *New Engl J Med* **288**(20): 1078–1079.
3. Rich Se. (1998) Executive summary from the World Symposium on Primary Pulmonary Hypertension, Evian, France, September 6–10. *co-sponsored by The World Health Organization.*
4. Simonneau G *et al.* (2013) Updated clinical classification of pulmonary hypertension. *JACC* **62**(25 Suppl): D34–D41.

5. Frost AE *et al.* (2011) The changing picture of patients with pulmonary arterial hypertension in the United States: How REVEAL differs from historic and non-US Contemporary Registries. *Chest* **139**(1): 128–137.
6. Humbert M *et al.* (2006) Pulmonary arterial hypertension in France: Results from a national registry. *Am J Respir Critic Care Med* **173**(9): 1023–1030.
7. Ling Y *et al.* (2012) Changing demographics, epidemiology, and survival of incident pulmonary arterial hypertension: Results from the pulmonary hypertension registry of the United Kingdom and Ireland. *Am J Respir Critic Care Med* **186**(8): 790–796.
8. Badesch DB *et al.* (2010) Pulmonary arterial hypertension: Baseline characteristics from the REVEAL Registry. *Chest* **137**(2): 376–387.
9. Thenappan T, Shah SJ, Rich S *et al.* (2007) A USA-based registry for pulmonary arterial hypertension: 1982–2006. *Euro Respir J* **30**(6): 1103–1110.
10. Hoeper MM *et al.* (2013) Elderly patients diagnosed with idiopathic pulmonary arterial hypertension: Results from the COMPERA registry. *Int J Cardiol* **168**(2): 871–880.
11. Aguilaniu B, Maitre J, Glenet S *et al* (2008) European reference equations for CO and NO lung transfer. *Euro Respir J* **31**(5): 1091–1097.
12. Hosoda Y *et al.* (1984) Age-dependent changes of collagen and elastin content in human aorta and pulmonary artery. *Angiology* **35**(10): 615–621.
13. Mitchell GF *et al.* (2004) Changes in arterial stiffness and wave reflection with advancing age in healthy men and women: The Framingham Heart Study. *Hypertension* **43**(6): 1239–1245.
14. Lam CS *et al.* (2009) Age-associated increases in pulmonary artery systolic pressure in the general population. *Circulation* **119**(20): 2663–2670.
15. Redfield MM *et al.* (2003) Burden of systolic and diastolic ventricular dysfunction in the community: Appreciating the scope of the heart failure epidemic. *JAMA* **289**(2): 194–202.
16. Tuder RM *et al.* (2013) Relevant issues in the pathology and pathobiology of pulmonary hypertension. *JACC* **62**(25 Suppl): D4–D12.
17. Chan SY, Loscalzo J. (2008) Pathogenic mechanisms of pulmonary arterial hypertension. *J Mol Cell Cardiol* **44**(1): 14–30.
18. Hassell KL. (1998) Altered hemostasis in pulmonary hypertension. *Blood Coagul Fibrinolysis* **9**(2): 107–117.

19. Price LC *et al.* (2012) Inflammation in pulmonary arterial hypertension. *Chest* **141**(1): 210–221.
20. Schermuly RT, Ghofrani HA, Wilkins MR *et al.* (2011) Mechanisms of disease: Pulmonary arterial hypertension. *Nat Rev. Cardiol* **8**(8): 443–455.
21. Rabinovitch M. (2007) Pathobiology of pulmonary hypertension. *Ann Rev Pathol* **2**: 369–399.
22. Tuder RM *et al.* (2009) Development and pathology of pulmonary hypertension. *JACC* **54**(1 Suppl): S3–S9.
23. Voelkel NF *et al.* (2006) Right ventricular function and failure: Report of a National Heart, Lung, and Blood Institute working group on cellular and molecular mechanisms of right heart failure. *Circulation* **114**(17): 1883–1891.
24. Bristow MR *et al.* (1998) The pressure-overloaded right ventricle in pulmonary hypertension. *Chest* **114**(1 Suppl): 101S–106S.
25. Yi ES *et al.* (2000) Distribution of obstructive intimal lesions and their cellular phenotypes in chronic pulmonary hypertension. A morphometric and immunohistochemical study. *Am J Respir Critic Care Med* **162**(4): 1577–1586.
26. Maruoka M *et al.* (2012) Characterization of myofibroblasts in chronic thromboembolic pulmonary hypertension. *Int J Cardiol* **159**(2): 119–127.
27. Firth AL *et al.* (2010) Multipotent mesenchymal progenitor cells are present in endarterectomized tissues from patients with chronic thromboembolic pulmonary hypertension. *Am J Physiol Cell Physiol* **298**(5): C1217–C1225.
28. Rubin LJ. (1997) Primary pulmonary hypertension. *New Engl J Med* **336**(2): 111–117.
29. Frid MG *et al.* (2006) Hypoxia-induced pulmonary vascular remodeling requires recruitment of circulating mesenchymal precursors of a monocyte/macrophage lineage. *Am J Pathol* **168**(2): 659–669.
30. Rai PR *et al.* (2008) The cancer paradigm of severe pulmonary arterial hypertension. *Am J Respir Critic Care Med* **178**(6): 558–564.
31. Lee SD *et al.* (1998) Monoclonal endothelial cell proliferation is present in primary but not secondary pulmonary hypertension. *J Clin Invest* **101**(5): 927–934.
32. Voelkel NF *et al.* (1998) Primary pulmonary hypertension between inflammation and cancer. *Chest* **114**(3 Suppl): 225S–230S.

33. Yuan JX, Rubin LJ. (2005) Pathogenesis of pulmonary arterial hypertension: The need for multiple hits. *Circulation* **111**(5): 534–538.
34. Austin ED , Loyd JE. (2007) Genetics and mediators in pulmonary arterial hypertension. *Clin Chest Med* **28**(1): 43–57.
35. Tuder RM, Radisavljevic Z, Shroyer KR *et al.* (1998) Monoclonal endothelial cells in appetite suppressant-associated pulmonary hypertension. *Am J Respir Critic Care Med* **158**(6): 1999–2001.
36. Farber HW, Loscalzo J. (2004) Pulmonary arterial hypertension. *New Engl J Med* **351**(16): 1655–1665.
37. Gerber JG, Voelkel N, Nies AS *et al.* (1980) Moderation of hypoxic vasoconstriction by infused arachidonic acid: Role of PGI2. *J Appl Physiol* **49**(1): 107–112.
38. Hara S *et al.* (1995) Overexpression of prostacyclin synthase inhibits growth of vascular smooth muscle cells. *Biochem Biophys Res Commun* **216**(3): 862–867.
39. Golino P *et al.* (1989) Local platelet activation causes vasoconstriction of large epicardial canine coronary arteries *in vivo.* Thromboxane A2 and serotonin are possible mediators. *Circulation* **79**(1): 154–166.
40. Huang RY *et al.* (2014) Thromboxane A2 exerts promoting effects on cell proliferation through mediating cyclooxygenase-2 signal in lung adenocarcinoma cells. *J Cancer Res Clin Oncol* **140**(3): 375–386.
41. Christman BW *et al.* (1992) An imbalance between the excretion of thromboxane and prostacyclin metabolites in pulmonary hypertension. *New Engl J Med* **327**(2): 70–75.
42. Tuder RM *et al.* (1999) Prostacyclin synthase expression is decreased in lungs from patients with severe pulmonary hypertension. *Am J Respir Critic Care Med* **159**(6): 1925–1932.
43. McLaughlin VV, Shillington A, Rich S. (2002) Survival in primary pulmonary hypertension: The impact of epoprostenol therapy. *Circulation* **106**(12): 1477–1482.
44. Sitbon O *et al.* (2002) Long-term intravenous epoprostenol infusion in primary pulmonary hypertension: Prognostic factors and survival. *JACC* **40**(4): 780–788.
45. Barst RJ *et al.* (1996) A comparison of continuous intravenous epoprostenol (prostacyclin) with conventional therapy for primary pulmonary hypertension. *New EnglJ Med* **334**(5): 296–301.
46. Galie N *et al.* (2013) Updated treatment algorithm of pulmonary arterial hypertension. *JACC* **62**(25 Suppl): D60–D72.

47. Galie N *et al.* (2009) Guidelines for the diagnosis and treatment of pulmonary hypertension: the Task Force for the Diagnosis and Treatment of Pulmonary Hypertension of the European Society of Cardiology (ESC) and the European Respiratory Society (ERS), endorsed by the International Society of Heart and Lung Transplantation (ISHLT). *Euro Heart J* **30**(20): 2493–2537.
48. Barst RJ *et al.* (2009) Updated evidence-based treatment algorithm in pulmonary arterial hypertension. *JACC* **54**(1 Suppl): S78–S84.
49. McLaughlin VV *et al.* (2009) ACCF/AHA 2009 expert consensus document on pulmonary hypertension: A report of the American College of Cardiology Foundation Task Force on Expert Consensus Documents and the American Heart Association: Developed in collaboration with the American College of Chest Physicians, American Thoracic Society, Inc., and the Pulmonary Hypertension Association. *Circulation* **119**(16): 2250–2294.
50. Rubin LJ *et al.* (1990) Treatment of primary pulmonary hypertension with continuous intravenous prostacyclin (epoprostenol). Results of a randomized trial. *Ann Intern Med* **112**(7): 485–491.
51. Oudiz RJ *et al.* (2004) Micrococcus-associated central venous catheter infection in patients with pulmonary arterial hypertension. *Chest* **126**(1): 90–94.
52. Kitterman N *et al.* (2012) Bloodstream infections in patients with pulmonary arterial hypertension treated with intravenous prostanoids: Insights from the REVEAL REGISTRY(R). *Mayo Clin Proc* **87**(9): 825–834.
53. McLaughlin VV *et al.* (2006) Randomized study of adding inhaled iloprost to existing bosentan in pulmonary arterial hypertension. *Am J Respir Critic Care Med* **174**(11): 1257–1263.
54. Hoeper MM *et al.* (2006) Combining inhaled iloprost with bosentan in patients with idiopathic pulmonary arterial hypertension. *Euro Respir J* **28**(4): 691–694.
55. Higenbottam T, Butt AY, McMahon A *et al.*(1998) Long-term intravenous prostaglandin (epoprostenol or iloprost) for treatment of severe pulmonary hypertension. *Heart* **80**(2): 151–155.
56. Simonneau G *et al.* (2002) Continuous subcutaneous infusion of treprostinil, a prostacyclin analogue, in patients with pulmonary arterial hypertension: A double-blind, randomized, placebo-controlled trial. *Am J Respir Critic Care Med* **165**(6): 800–804.

57. Barst RJ *et al.* (2003) Beraprost therapy for pulmonary arterial hypertension. *JACC* **41**(12): 2119–2125.
58. Sakurai T *et al.* (1990) Cloning of a cDNA encoding a non-isopeptide-selective subtype of the endothelin receptor. *Nature* **348**(6303): 732–735.
59. Zamora MA, Dempsey EC, Walchak SJ *et al.* (1993) BQ123, an ETA receptor antagonist, inhibits endothelin-1-mediated proliferation of human pulmonary artery smooth muscle cells. *Am J Respir cell Mol Biol* **9**(4): 429–433.
60. Maron BA *et al.* (2012) Aldosterone inactivates the endothelin-B receptor via a cysteinyl thiol redox switch to decrease pulmonary endothelial nitric oxide levels and modulate pulmonary arterial hypertension. *Circulation* **126**(8): 963–974.
61. Dupuis J. (2001) Endothelin-receptor antagonists in pulmonary hypertension. *Lancet* **358**(9288): 1113–1114.
62. Sato K *et al.* (1995) Effects of separate and combined ETA and ETB blockade on ET-1-induced constriction in perfused rat lungs. *Am J Physiol* **269**(5): L668–L672.
63. Shichiri M, Kato H, Marumo F *et al.* (1997) Endothelin-1 as an autocrine/paracrine apoptosis survival factor for endothelial cells. *Hypertension* **30**(5): 1198–1203.
64. Giaid A *et al.* (1993) Expression of endothelin-1 in the lungs of patients with pulmonary hypertension. *New Engl J Med* **328**(24): 1732–1739.
65. Stewart DJ, Levy RD, Cernacek P *et al.* (1991) Increased plasma endothelin-1 in pulmonary hypertension: Marker or mediator of disease? *Ann Intern Med* **114**(6): 464–469.
66. Rubens C *et al.* (2001) Big endothelin-1 and endothelin-1 plasma levels are correlated with the severity of primary pulmonary hypertension. *Chest* **120**(5): 1562–1569.
67. Galie N *et al.* (2005) Ambrisentan therapy for pulmonary arterial hypertension. *JACC* **46**(3): 529–535.
68. Galie N *et al.* (2008) Ambrisentan for the treatment of pulmonary arterial hypertension: Results of the ambrisentan in pulmonary arterial hypertension, randomized, double-blind, placebo-controlled, multicenter, efficacy (ARIES) study 1 and 2. *Circulation* **117**(23): 3010–3019.
69. Channick RN *et al.* (2001) Effects of the dual endothelin-receptor antagonist bosentan in patients with pulmonary hypertension: A randomised placebo-controlled study. *Lancet* **358**(9288): 1119–1123.

70. Rubin LJ *et al.* (2002) Bosentan therapy for pulmonary arterial hypertension. *New Engl J Med* **346**(12): 896–903.
71. Humbert M *et al.* (2004) Combination of bosentan with epoprostenol in pulmonary arterial hypertension: BREATHE-2. *Euro Respir J* **24**(3): 353–359.
72. Pulido T *et al.* (2013) Macitentan and morbidity and mortality in pulmonary arterial hypertension. *New Engl J Med* **369**(9): 809–818.
73. Palmer RM, Ferrige AG, Moncada S. (1987) Nitric oxide release accounts for the biological activity of endothelium-derived relaxing factor. *Nature* **327**(6122): 524–526.
74. Loscalzo J. (2001) Nitric oxide insufficiency, platelet activation, and arterial thrombosis. *Circulation research* **88**(8): 756–762.
75. Sato J *et al.* (2000) eNOS gene transfer to vascular smooth muscle cells inhibits cell proliferation via upregulation of p27 and p21 and not apoptosis. *Cardiovascular Res* **47**(4): 697–706.
76. Moncada S, Higgs A. (1993) The L-arginine-nitric oxide pathway. *New Engl J Med* **329**(27): 2002–2012.
77. RG K, SM. (1995) Nitric oxide synthases in mammals. *Biochem J* **1**(298): 249–258.
78. Coggins MP, Bloch KD. (2007) Nitric oxide in the pulmonary vasculature. *Arterioscler Thromb Vasc Biol* **27**(9): 1877–1885.
79. Kim-Shapiro DB, Schechter AN, Gladwin MT. (2006) Unraveling the reactions of nitric oxide, nitrite, and hemoglobin in physiology and therapeutics. *Arterioscler Thromb Vasc Biol* **26**(4): 697–705.
80. Hess DT, Matsumoto A, Kim SO *et al.* (2005) Protein S-nitrosylation: Purview and parameters. *Nat Rev. Mol Cell Biol* **6**(2): 150–166.
81. Sharma S *et al.* (2008) Altered carnitine homeostasis is associated with decreased mitochondrial function and altered nitric oxide signaling in lambs with pulmonary hypertension. *Am J Physiol Lung Cell Mol Physiol* **294**(1): L46–L56.
82. Xue C, Johns RA (1995) Endothelial nitric oxide synthase in the lungs of patients with pulmonary hypertension. *New Engl J Med* **333**(24): 1642–1644.
83. Giaid A, Saleh D (1995) Reduced expression of endothelial nitric oxide synthase in the lungs of patients with pulmonary hypertension. *New Engl J Med* **333**(4): 214–221.
84. Kaneko FT *et al.* (1998) Biochemical reaction products of nitric oxide as quantitative markers of primary pulmonary hypertension. *Am J Respir Critic Care Med* **158**(3): 917–923.

85. Demoncheaux EA *et al.* (2005) Decreased whole body endogenous nitric oxide production in patients with primary pulmonary hypertension. *J Vascul Res* **42**(2): 133–136.
86. Kovacs G *et al.* (2009) Borderline pulmonary arterial pressure is associated with decreased exercise capacity in scleroderma. *Am J Respir Critic Care Med* **180**(9): 881–886.
87. Beckman JS , Koppenol WH (1996) Nitric oxide, superoxide, and peroxynitrite: The good, the bad, and ugly. *Am J Physiol* **271**(5): C1424–C1437.
88. Rubin LJ *et al.* (2011) Long-term treatment with sildenafil citrate in pulmonary arterial hypertension: The SUPER-2 study. *Chest* **140**(5): 1274–1283.
89. Galie N *et al.* (2005) Sildenafil citrate therapy for pulmonary arterial hypertension. *New Engl J Med* **353**(20): 2148–2157.
90. Jing ZC*et al.* (2011) Vardenafil in pulmonary arterial hypertension: A randomized, double-blind, placebo-controlled study. *Am J Respir Critic cCare Med* **183**(12): 1723–1729.
91. Oudiz RJ *et al.* (2012) Tadalafil for the treatment of pulmonary arterial hypertension: A double-blind 52-week uncontrolled extension study. *JACC* **60**(8): 768–774.
92. Galie N *et al.* (2009) Tadalafil therapy for pulmonary arterial hypertension. *Circulation* **119**(22): 2894–2903.
93. Ghofrani HA *et al.* (2013) Riociguat for the treatment of pulmonary arterial hypertension. *New Engl J Med* **369**(4): 330–340.
94. International PPHC *et al.* (2000) Heterozygous germline mutations in BMPR2, encoding a TGF-beta receptor, cause familial primary pulmonary hypertension. *Nat Genet* **26**(1): 81–84.
95. Deng Z *et al.* (2000) Familial primary pulmonary hypertension (gene PPH1) is caused by mutations in the bone morphogenetic protein receptor-II gene. *Am J Hum Genet* **67**(3): 737–744.
96. Cogan J *et al.* (2012) Role of BMPR2 alternative splicing in heritable pulmonary arterial hypertension penetrance. *Circulation* **126**(15): 1907–1916.
97. Machado RD *et al.* (2009) Genetics and genomics of pulmonary arterial hypertension. *JACC* **54**(1 Suppl): S32–S42.
98. Soubrier F *et al.* (2013) Genetics and genomics of pulmonary arterial hypertension. *JACC* **62**(25 Suppl): D13–D21.
99. Davies RJ, Morrell NW. (2008) Molecular mechanisms of pulmonary arterial hypertension: Role of mutations in the bone morphogenetic protein type II receptor. *Chest* **134**(6): 1271–1277.

100. Harrison RE *et al.* (2003) Molecular and functional analysis identifies ALK-1 as the predominant cause of pulmonary hypertension related to hereditary haemorrhagic telangiectasia. *J Med Genet* **40**(12): 865–871.
101. McLaughlin VV *et al.* (2009) ACCF/AHA 2009 expert consensus document on pulmonary hypertension a report of the American College of Cardiology Foundation Task Force on Expert Consensus Documents and the American Heart Association developed in collaboration with the American College of Chest Physicians; American Thoracic Society, Inc.; and the Pulmonary Hypertension Association. *JACC* **53**(17): 1573–1619.
102. Chaouat A *et al.* (2004) Endoglin germline mutation in a patient with hereditary haemorrhagic telangiectasia and dexfenfluramine associated pulmonary arterial hypertension. *Thorax* **59**(5): 446–448.
103. Nasim MT *et al.* (2011) Molecular genetic characterization of SMAD signaling molecules in pulmonary arterial hypertension. *Human mutation* **32**(12): 1385–1389.
104. Austin ED *et al.* (2012) Whole exome sequencing to identify a novel gene (caveolin-1) associated with human pulmonary arterial hypertension. *Circulation. Cardiovasc Genet* **5**(3): 336–343.
105. Benza RL *et al.* (2012) An evaluation of long-term survival from time of diagnosis in pulmonary arterial hypertension from the REVEAL Registry. *Chest* **142**(2): 448–456.
106. Vonk-Noordegraaf A *et al.* (2013) Right heart adaptation to pulmonary arterial hypertension: Physiology and pathobiology. *JACC* **62**(25 Suppl): D22–D33.
107. Jain S, Ventura H, deBoisblanc B. (2007) Pathophysiology of pulmonary arterial hypertension. *Semin Cardiothorac Vascu Anesth* **11**(2): 104–109.
108. Weir EK, Hong Z, Varghese A. (2004) The serotonin transporter: A vehicle to elucidate pulmonary hypertension? *Circulation Res* **94**(9): 1152–1154.
109. Marcos E *et al.* (2004) Serotonin-induced smooth muscle hyperplasia in various forms of human pulmonary hypertension. *Circulation Res* **94**(9): 1263–1270.
110. Lee SL, Wang WW, Lanzillo JJ *et al.* (1994) Serotonin produces both hyperplasia and hypertrophy of bovine pulmonary artery smooth muscle cells in culture. *Am J Physiol* **266**(1): L46–L52.

111. Douglas JG, Munro JF, Kitchin AH *et al.* (1981) Pulmonary hypertension and fenfluramine. *Br Med J* **283**(6296): 881–883.
112. Abenhaim L *et al.* (1996) Appetite-suppressant drugs and the risk of primary pulmonary hypertension. International Primary Pulmonary Hypertension Study Group. *New Engl J Med* **335**(9): 609–616.
113. Herve P *et al.* (1995) Increased plasma serotonin in primary pulmonary hypertension. *Am J Med* **99**(3): 249–254.
114. Eddahibi S *et al.* (2001) Serotonin transporter overexpression is responsible for pulmonary artery smooth muscle hyperplasia in primary pulmonary hypertension. *J Clin Invest* **108**(8): 1141–1150.
115. MacLean MR *et al.* (2004) Overexpression of the 5-hydroxytryptamine transporter gene: Effect on pulmonary hemodynamics and hypoxia-induced pulmonary hypertension. *Circulation* **109**(17): 2150–2155.
116. Guignabert C *et al.* (2006) Transgenic mice overexpressing the 5-hydroxytryptamine transporter gene in smooth muscle develop pulmonary hypertension. *Circulation Res* **98**(10): 1323–1330.
117. Guignabert C *et al.* (2005) Serotonin transporter inhibition prevents and reverses monocrotaline-induced pulmonary hypertension in rats. *Circulation* **111**(21): 2812–2819.
118. Eddahibi S *et al.* (2000) Attenuated hypoxic pulmonary hypertension in mice lacking the 5-hydroxytryptamine transporter gene. *J Clin Invest* **105**(11): 1555–1562.
119. Eddahibi S *et al.* (2006) Cross talk between endothelial and smooth muscle cells in pulmonary hypertension: Critical role for serotonin-induced smooth muscle hyperplasia. *Circulation* **113**(15): 1857–1864.
120. Thomas M, Ciuclan L, Hussey MJ *et al.* (2013) Targeting the serotonin pathway for the treatment of pulmonary arterial hypertension. *Pharmacol Ther* **138**(3): 409–417.
121. Vlodavsky I *et al.* (1987) Endothelial cell-derived basic fibroblast growth factor: Synthesis and deposition into subendothelial extracellular matrix. *Proc Natl Acad Sci USA* **84**(8): 2292–2296.
122. Izikki M *et al.* (2009) Endothelial-derived FGF2 contributes to the progression of pulmonary hypertension in humans and rodents. *J Clin Invest* **119**(3): 512–523.
123. Wedgwood S *et al.* (2007) Fibroblast growth factor-2 expression is altered in lambs with increased pulmonary blood flow and pulmonary hypertension. *Pediatr Res* **61**(1): 32–36.

124. Benisty JI *et al.* (2004) Elevated basic fibroblast growth factor levels in patients with pulmonary arterial hypertension. *Chest* **126**(4): 1255–1261.
125. Kim J *et al.* (2013) An endothelial apelin-FGF link mediated by miR-424 and miR-503 is disrupted in pulmonary arterial hypertension. *Nat Med* **19**(1): 74–82.
126. Tu L *et al.* (2011) Autocrine fibroblast growth factor-2 signaling contributes to altered endothelial phenotype in pulmonary hypertension. *Am J Respir Cell Mol Biol* **45**(2): 311–322.
127. Harding TC *et al.* (2013) Blockade of nonhormonal fibroblast growth factors by FP-1039 inhibits growth of multiple types of cancer. *Sci Transl Med* **5**(178): 178ra139.
128. Balasubramaniam V *et al.* (2003) Role of platelet-derived growth factor in vascular remodeling during pulmonary hypertension in the ovine fetus. *Am J Physiol. Lung Cell Mol Physiol* **284**(5): L826–L833.
129. Jankov RP *et al.* (2005) A role for platelet-derived growth factor beta-receptor in a newborn rat model of endothelin-mediated pulmonary vascular remodeling. *Am J Physiol. Lung Cell Mol Physiol* **288**(6): L1162–L1170.
130. Humbert M *et al.* (1998) Platelet-derived growth factor expression in primary pulmonary hypertension: Comparison of HIV seropositive and HIV seronegative patients. *Euro Respir J* **11**(3): 554–559.
131. Perros F *et al.* (2008) Platelet-derived growth factor expression and function in idiopathic pulmonary arterial hypertension. *Am J Respir Critic Care Med* **178**(1): 81–88.
132. Heldin CH, Westermark B. (1999) Mechanism of action and in vivo role of platelet-derived growth factor. *Physiol Rev* **79**(4): 1283–1316.
133. Rosenkranz S, Kazlauskas A. (1999) Evidence for distinct signaling properties and biological responses induced by the PDGF receptor alpha and beta subtypes. *Growth factors* **16**(3): 201–216.
134. Yu Y *et al.* (2003) PDGF stimulates pulmonary vascular smooth muscle cell proliferation by upregulating TRPC6 expression. *Am J Physiol. Cell Physiol* **284**(2): C316–C330.
135. Arcot SS, Lipke DW, Gillespie MN *et al.* (1993) Alterations of growth factor transcripts in rat lungs during development of monocrotaline-induced pulmonary hypertension. *Biochem Pharmacol* **46**(6): 1086–1091.
136. Katayose D *et al.* (1993) Increased expression of PDGF A- and B-chain genes in rat lungs with hypoxic pulmonary hypertension. *Am J Physiol* **264**(2): L100–L106.

137. Kwapiszewska G *et al.* (2005) Expression profiling of laser-microdissected intrapulmonary arteries in hypoxia-induced pulmonary hypertension. *Respir Res* **6**: 109.
138. Lanner MC, Raper M, Pratt WM *et al.* (2005) Heterotrimeric G proteins and the platelet-derived growth factor receptor-beta contribute to hypoxic proliferation of smooth muscle cells. *Am J Respir Cell Mol Biol* **33**(4): 412–419.
139. Dahal BK *et al.* (2011) Hypoxic pulmonary hypertension in mice with constitutively active platelet-derived growth factor receptor-beta. *Pulmonary Circulation* **1**(2): 259–268.
140. Schermuly RT *et al.* (2005) Reversal of experimental pulmonary hypertension by PDGF inhibition. *J Clin Invest* **115**(10): 2811–2821.
141. Souza R, Sitbon O, Parent F *et al.* (2006) Long term imatinib treatment in pulmonary arterial hypertension. *Thorax* **61**(8): 736.
142. Ghofrani HA, Seeger W, Grimminger F. (2005) Imatinib for the treatment of pulmonary arterial hypertension. *New Engl J Med* **353**(13): 1412–1413.
143. Hoeper MM *et al.* (2013) Imatinib mesylate as add-on therapy for pulmonary arterial hypertension: Results of the randomized IMPRES study. *Circulation* **127**(10): 1128–1138.
144. Pullamsetti SS *et al.* (2011) Inflammation, immunological reaction and role of infection in pulmonary hypertension. *Clin Microbiol Infect* **17**(1): 7–14.
145. Hassoun PM *et al.* (2009) Inflammation, growth factors, and pulmonary vascular remodeling. *JACC* **54**(1 Suppl): S10–S19.
146. Stacher E *et al.* (2012) Modern age pathology of pulmonary arterial hypertension. *Am J Respir Critic Care Med* **186**(3): 261–272.
147. Dorfmuller P *et al.* (2002) Chemokine RANTES in severe pulmonary arterial hypertension. *Am J Respir Critic Care Med* **165**(4): 534–539.
148. Balabanian K *et al.* (2002) CX(3)C chemokine fractalkine in pulmonary arterial hypertension. *Am J Respir Critic Care Medicine* **165**(10): 1419–1425.
149. Itoh T *et al.* (2006) Increased plasma monocyte chemoattractant protein-1 level in idiopathic pulmonary arterial hypertension. *Respirol* **11**(2): 158–163.
150. Humbert M *et al.* (1995) Increased interleukin-1 and interleukin-6 serum concentrations in severe primary pulmonary hypertension. *Am J Respir Critic Care Med* **151**(5): 1628–1631.

151. Cracowski JL *et al.* (2014) Proinflammatory cytokine levels are linked to death in pulmonary arterial hypertension. *Euro Respir J* **43**(3): 915–917.
152. Steiner MK *et al.* (2009) Interleukin-6 overexpression induces pulmonary hypertension. *Circulation Res* **104**(2): 236–244.
153. Soon E *et al.* (2010) Elevated levels of inflammatory cytokines predict survival in idiopathic and familial pulmonary arterial hypertension. *Circulation* **122**(9): 920–927.
154. Graham BB *et al.* (2010) Schistosomiasis-induced experimental pulmonary hypertension: Role of interleukin-13 signaling. *Am J Pathol* **177**(3): 1549–1561.
155. Cho WK *et al.* (2013) IL-13 receptor alpha2-arginase 2 pathway mediates IL-13-induced pulmonary hypertension. *Am J Physiol Lung Cell Mol Physiol* **304**(2): L112–L124.
156. Tamby MC *et al.* (2005) Anti-endothelial cell antibodies in idiopathic and systemic sclerosis associated pulmonary arterial hypertension. *Thorax* **60**(9): 765–772.
157. Tamby MC *et al.* (2006) Antibodies to fibroblasts in idiopathic and scleroderma-associated pulmonary hypertension. *Euro Respir J* **28**(4): 799–807.
158. Bordron A *et al.* (1998) The binding of some human antiendothelial cell antibodies induces endothelial cell apoptosis. *J Clin Invest* **101**(10): 2029–2035.
159. Ulrich S, Nicolls MR, Taraseviciene L *et al.* (2008) Increased regulatory and decreased CD8+ cytotoxic T cells in the blood of patients with idiopathic pulmonary arterial hypertension. *Respir Int Rev Thorac Dis* **75**(3): 272–280.
160. Tamosiuniene R *et al.* (2011) Regulatory T cells limit vascular endothelial injury and prevent pulmonary hypertension. *Circulation Res* **109**(8): 867–879.
161. Huertas A *et al.* (2012) Leptin and regulatory T-lymphocytes in idiopathic pulmonary arterial hypertension. *Euro Respir J* **40**(4): 895–904.
162. Spiekerkoetter E *et al.* (2013) FK506 activates BMPR2, rescues endothelial dysfunction, and reverses pulmonary hypertension. *J Clin Invest*1 **23**(8): 3600–3613.
163. Fujita M *et al.* (2002) Pulmonary hypertension in TNF-alpha-overexpressing mice is associated with decreased VEGF gene expression. *J Appl Physiol* **93**(6): 2162–2170.

164. Wang Q *et al.* (2013) Monocrotaline-induced pulmonary arterial hypertension is attenuated by TNF-alpha antagonists via the suppression of TNF-alpha expression and NF-kappaB pathway in rats. *Vascul Pharmacol* **58**(1–2): 71–77.
165. Henriques-Coelho T, Brandao-Nogueira A, Moreira-Goncalves D *et al.* (2008) Effects of TNF-alpha blockade in monocrotaline-induced pulmonary hypertension. *Portuguese J Cardiol* **27**(3): 341–348.
166. Falcao-Pires I *et al.* (2009) Apelin decreases myocardial injury and improves right ventricular function in monocrotaline-induced pulmonary hypertension. *Am J Physiol Heart Circ Physiol* **296**(6): H2007–H2014.
167. Chandra SM *et al.* (2011) Disruption of the apelin-APJ system worsens hypoxia-induced pulmonary hypertension. *Arterioscler Thromb Vasc Biol* **31**(4): 814–820.
168. Alastalo TP *et al.* (2011) Disruption of PPARgamma/beta-catenin-mediated regulation of apelin impairs BMP-induced mouse and human pulmonary arterial EC survival. *J Clin Invest* **121**(9): 3735–3746.
169. Yuan JX *et al.* (1998) Dysfunctional voltage-gated K+ channels in pulmonary artery smooth muscle cells of patients with primary pulmonary hypertension. *Circulation* **98**(14): 1400–1406.
170. Moudgil R, Michelakis ED, Archer SL. (2006) The role of K+ channels in determining pulmonary vascular tone, oxygen sensing, cell proliferation, and apoptosis: Implications in hypoxic pulmonary vasoconstriction and pulmonary arterial hypertension. *Microcirculation* **13**(8): 615–632.
171. Pozeg ZI *et al.* (2003) In vivo gene transfer of the O2-sensitive potassium channel Kv1.5 reduces pulmonary hypertension and restores hypoxic pulmonary vasoconstriction in chronically hypoxic rats. *Circulation* **107**(15): 2037–2044.
172. Xie W, Wang H, Wang H *et al.* (2004) Effects of iptakalim hydrochloride, a novel KATP channel opener, on pulmonary vascular remodeling in hypoxic rats. *Life sciences* **75**(17): 2065–2076.
173. Yu Y *et al.* (2004) Enhanced expression of transient receptor potential channels in idiopathic pulmonary arterial hypertension. *Proc Natl Acad Sci USA* **101**(38): 13861–13866.
174. Nicholson WT, Vaa B, Hesse C *et al.* (2009) Aging is associated with reduced prostacyclin-mediated dilation in the human forearm. *Hypertension* **53**(6): 973–978.

175. Van Guilder GP, Westby CM, Greiner JJ *et al.* (2007) Endothelin-1 vasoconstrictor tone increases with age in healthy men but can be reduced by regular aerobic exercise. *Hypertension* **50**(2): 403–409.
176. Cau SB, Carneiro FS, Tostes RC. (2012) Differential modulation of nitric oxide synthases in aging: Therapeutic opportunities. *Front Physiol* **3**:218.
177. Minamino T, Komuro I. (2007) Vascular cell senescence: Contribution to atherosclerosis. *Circulation Res* **100**(1): 15–26.
178. Yang XP, Pei ZH, Ren J. (2009) Making up or breaking up: The tortuous role of platelet-derived growth factor in vascular ageing. *Clin Exp Pharmacol Physiol* **36**(8): 739–747.
179. Meltzer CC *et al.* (1998) Serotonin in aging, late-life depression, and Alzheimer's disease: The emerging role of functional imaging. *Neuropsychopharmacol* **18**(6): 407–430.
180. Fujie S *et al.* (2014) Reduction of arterial stiffness by exercise training is associated with increasing plasma apelin level in middle-aged and older adults. *PloS one* **9**(4): e93545.

Chapter 14

Chronic Obstructive Lung Disease in the Elderly

Jessica F. Most* and Carolyn L. Rochester†

1. Epidemiology

The burden of chronic obstructive pulmonary disease (COPD) has increased over the last several decades, with COPD presently affecting 210 million people worldwide[1]. COPD is now the 3rd leading cause of death in the United States,[2] and 15 million Americans report they are currently living with COPD.[3] This may be a considerable underestimate of the burden of COPD as the disease remains underdiagnosed, with up to 50% of patients with airway obstruction unaware they have COPD.[4] Older age (>65 yrs) is associated with a higher prevalence of COPD,[5] and age confers a 2-fold risk of developing COPD per decade.[6] One in 4 men and 1 in 6 women over the age of 55 will develop COPD in their lifetime,[7] although the overall risk for developing COPD varies with gender, smoking status, and country of origin.[6] COPD is also a leading cause of hospitalizations among American adults, especially those over the age of 55.[8] Age is also a predictor of longer length of hospital stay,[8] and patients over

*College of Medicine, Drexel University, Division of Pulmonary, Critical Care and Sleep Medicine E-mail: Jessica.Most@drexelmed.edu
†Yale University School of Medicine, Department of Internal Medicine, Section of Pulmonary, Critical Care and Sleep; E-mail: carolyn.rochester@yale.edu

age 85 are 3 times more likely to die in the hospital and in the 90 days post-discharge as compared to those under age 65.[9]

2. Pathophysiology

COPD is "characterized by persistent airflow limitation that is usually progressive and associated with an enhanced chronic inflammatory response in the airways and lung to noxious particles or gases. Exacerbations and comorbidities contribute to the overall severity in individual patients".[10] The structural and functional changes in the respiratory system in COPD develop as a result of a complex set of interactions between susceptible hosts and the environment. Exposure to tobacco smoke is the principal cause of COPD; other risk factors include exposures to pollutants, dusts, chemicals, fumes, frequent childhood respiratory infections, history of low birth weight or infant bronco pulmonary dysplasia, low socioeconomic status and history of asthma.[10]

Although incompletely reversible airflow obstruction is a key defining feature of COPD, COPD is a heterogeneous disease, and the structural changes in the airways and lung parenchyma vary among individuals. Airflow obstruction may result from inflammation, increased mucus production and bronchoconstriction in the large airways, or more predominantly from structural remodeling of the distal bronchioles <2 mm in diameter and/or from the presence of emphysema.[11,12] Emphysema may be present in varying distribution in the lungs, but is associated with loss of intact alveolar–capillary units, loss of elastic recoil, reduced gas transfer capacity and dynamic airways compression during exhalation. Airflow obstruction resulting from the above noted structural changes in the airways and/or lung parenchyma leads to increased resistive work of breathing and often leads to lung hyperinflation, either at rest and/or during exercise. Hyperinflation in turn leads to impaired respiratory muscle mechanics, increased elastic work of breathing, and increased dead space/tidal volume ratio (by posing constraint on tidal volume). It can also cause or contribute to cardiovascular impairment by increasing pulmonary artery pressure, reducing right ventricular preload and increasing left ventricular afterload. Airflow obstruction also leads to gas exchange disturbances by causing ventilation-perfusion (V/Q) mismatch. The severity of gas exchange disturbances depends on the severity of the underlying structural derangements. While hypoxemia is the principal consequence of V/Q mismatch in COPD, hypercarbia can also ensue, particularly when the structural derangements in the lung are severe, such that despite high minute ventilation the carbon dioxide is no longer cleared effectively from the body, or when the work of breathing is so high that ventilatory failure occurs. Pulmonary hypertension may also be present at rest among persons with advanced disease. Each of the above noted physiologic disturbances present at rest among patients with COPD worsen during acute exacerbations of the disease.

For any degree of lung function impairment, patients vary widely with regard to symptoms and level of physical functional impairment. This likely relates, at least in part, to the presence of varying body composition and the presence of comorbidities (discussed below). Importantly, a multidimensional disease assessment measure — the BODE index — which incorporates body mass index (BMI), severity of airflow obstruction (FEV1%), dyspnea severity (MRC dyspnea score) and exercise capacity (6 minute walk test) is a better discriminator of mortality risk[13] and other clinical outcomes than FEV1 alone. Other multidimensional disease assessment tools — DOSE,[14] COTE,[15] ADO,[16] CODEX[17] are also useful to characterize patients more fully than measures of lung function alone. Published guidelines recommend routine assessment not only of presence and severity of pulmonary function impairment and gas exchange disturbances, but also of the severity of symptoms, frequency of exacerbations, and degree of exercise impairment for patients with COPD.[10]

Also importantly, it is now clear that there exist varying clinical subsets of patients with COPD, including persons with asthma/COPD overlap,[18,19] COPD/OSA overlap,[20] persons with concurrent bronchiectasis,[21] and those with combined pulmonary fibrosis and emphysema syndrome (CPFES).[22] Health care practitioners must be aware of these subgroups, as patients with these conditions may require additional selected therapies, and some of these conditions, especially COPD/OSA overlap and CPFES are associated with worse clinical outcomes than either condition alone.[22,23]

3. Diagnosis of Copd in the Elderly

The Global Initiative for Chrnoic Obstructive Lung Disease (GOLD) advocates that the diagnosis of COPD be based on spirometry demonstrating the presence of a reduced post-bronchodilator FEV1/FVC ratio less than 0.7, together with a history of exposure to relevant risk factors and the presence of respiratory symptoms.[10] Indeed the FEV1/FVC ratio is used in most prevalence studies to define the presence of COPD, since a single cut-off value is practical for routine use. However, the use of the fixed FEV1/FVC ratio <0.7 as the best means to define COPD is controversial, because the normal values for FEV1/FVC ratio vary with age.[24–26] Normal aging, wherein elasticity of the lung decreases over time, is associated with reductions in FVC, FEV1 and FEV1/FVC %; normal age-related decline in lung function is particularly substantial after the age of 70.[27,28]

An alternate way used commonly to define the presence of "abnormal" airflow obstruction is the "lower limit of normal" (LLN) for age, based on spirometry values below the lower 5th percentile of normal age-related reference values from medical screening populations of healthy, never-smoker adults.[25,29] The American Thoracic Society recommends the use of equations based on the Third National Health and Nutrition Examination Survey (NHANES III) to calculate predicted and LLN reference values for adults in the United States.[25] Based on this, an FEV1/FVC ratio of <0.7 is considered abnormal for persons under age 70, whereas an FEV1/FVC ratio of <0.65 is considered abnormal for persons over age 70. It must be noted that the NHANES III-derived values were based on persons ranging in age from 8–80 years[30] and little data is available regarding normal values for persons over the age of 80. Moreover, the use of LLN spirometry values to define COPD is likely also imperfect since the choice of a 5% cutoff for healthy never smokers may not account for other factors that may result in COPD.[31]

Overall, however, the estimated prevalence of COPD tends to be higher when the fixed ratio is used in epidemiologic studies for diagnosing COPD than when the LLN criteria are used.[31–37] For both the fixed FEV1/FVC and LLN methods, the estimated prevalence of

COPD is less when post-bronchodilator testing results are used as compared with pre-bronchodilator tests.[38] Both the fixed ratio method and the LLN method of diagnosis have been associated with several clinically relevant outcomes[34] including hospitalization rates and mortality.[35,39]

Importantly, because of the normal age-related decline in spirometry values, the use of the fixed FEV1/FVC ratio <0.7 to define COPD often leads to over-diagnosis of COPD (i.e. obstructive lung disease) in the elderly as compared to the LLN method,[31,40] particularly among persons with milder degrees of airflow obstruction.[34] Over-diagnosis of COPD in the elderly may lead to adverse clinical outcomes by virtue of initiation of potentially unnecessary medications such as inhaled bronchodilators (long-acting beta-agonists (LABA) or long-acting anticholinergics (LAMA)) and/or inhaled corticosteroids (ICS) which may lead to untoward side effects (discussed below). Over-diagnosis of COPD also has potential to cause the patient to experience concern, anxiety, and/or depression related to having a disease condition. Although it is not currently possible to draw firm conclusions regarding which spirometric diagnostic method is preferable in general to define the presence of airflow obstruction, clinicians should exercise caution in making a diagnosis of COPD based on the fixed FEV1/FVC ratio <0.7 alone among persons over the age of 70, particularly if the only spirometric abnormality is a mildly reduced FEV1/FVC ratio in the absence of concomitant reduction in FEV1, a scooped appearance of the expiratory limb of the flow volume loop, or symptoms suggestive of the disease. Where the diagnosis may be in question, the clinician should consider evaluating whether the FEV1/FVC ratio falls below the LLN for age as confirmatory evidence for the diagnosis. A recent systematic review found that where there are discordant findings between fixed FEV1/FVC ratio and LLN methods, a diagnosis other than COPD should be considered as the basis for the patients" symptoms, especially among elderly persons with mild degrees of airflow obstruction.[34]

The LLN method may also be a better predictor of mortality in this patient group.[34] In one longitudinal study, persons age 65–80 with FEV1/FVC ratios <0.7 and less than the LLN for age had higher mortality risk than persons with fixed FEV1/FVC ratio <0.7 alone.[41] However, Mannino and colleagues demonstrated that elderly persons with FEV1/FVC ratio <0.7 but greater than the LLN also had higher hospitalization and mortality rates than persons with FEV1/FVC ratio >0.7 (normal).[39] This increased mortality risk among persons with FEV1/FVC <0.7 but greater than the LLN was recently corroborated in another population based sample of middle-aged men.[42] However, this patient group had lower mortality rates compared with those with FEV1/FVC ratios <0.7 and less than the LLN. This suggests that some airways disease may be present in persons with FEV1/FVC <0.7 but greater than the LLN, and that the requirement for the FEV1/FVC ratio to also fall below the LLN for age to establish the diagnosis may under-diagnose COPD in some elderly persons.[32,42] Longitudinal follow-up of a patient's symptoms and lung function is necessary to identify the presence of COPD, and distinguish disease based on the abnormal FEV1/FVC ratio from age-related lung function decline in this patient group.

The forced expiratory volume in 1 second/forced expiratory volume in 6 seconds (FEV1/FEV6s) ratio less than predicted normal is an alternate available method to establish a diagnosis of COPD in the elderly.[43,44] The FEV 6s maneuver may be easier to perform than the full FVC maneuver for elderly persons, and may reduce the risk of syncope.[43] A reduced FEV1/FEV6 sec ratio <LLN Is also associated with increased risk of mortality in persons over the age of 65.[43]

4. Lung Aging and Disease Pathogenesis

The pathogenesis of COPD has been reviewed in detail elsewhere.[12,45–47] Different combinations of pathogenetic processes occur in individuals; this likely accounts, at least in part, for the heterogeneity of structural changes in the airways and lung parenchyma as well as varying systemic manifestations and comorbidities found among COPD patients. Inflammation, protease-antiprotease imbalance, and oxidant-antioxidant imbalance are three key components that contribute to development of COPD. Additional mechanisms that may amplify and/or perpetuate tissue damage include acute and/or latent viral infection, recurrent bacterial infections, alterations in mechanical forces, activation of proinflammatory transcription factors, impaired activity of macrophage histone deacetylase (an enzyme important for turning off proinflammatory genes), autoimmunity, alterations in extracellular matrix, and dysregulated tissue repair.[12,45] Premature aging, with cellular senescence and immunoscenescence is another suspected mechanism in the pathogenesis of COPD.[12,45,46,48–51]

Normal lung aging is characterized by degeneration of collagen and elastin, with resultant airspace enlargement,[49] decline in lung function,[52] and reduced function of the mucociliary escalator[48] as well as by reduced strength and endurance of the respiratory muscles (as a consequence of type IIa muscle fiber atrophy)[52] and reduced cough strength.[48] In addition, older persons have elevated systemic levels of pro-inflammatory cytokines,[53] yet have a reduced functional immune response.[48,49,54] Collectively, decline in the adaptive immune response and upregulation of the innate immune response leads to a pro-inflammatory state[49,55] and an increased propensity to tissue damage that likely contributes to the pathogenesis of COPD[48,49] in susceptible individuals. Molecular processes related to aging that are particularly relevant to COPD pathogenesis are increased oxidative stress,[50,52] activation of the transcription factor *nF-kB*, impaired ability to repair damaged DNA, telomere shortening in lung cells and peripheral leukocytes,[46,50,51,56–58] altered *T* cell mediated immune responses,[49,55] decreased epithelial barrier function,[59] altered host defense properties of monocytes, macrophages, and neutrophils;[55] apoptosis;[46] and dysregulated extracellular matrix production, maintenance and/or repair.[51] This topic is considered in further detail in Chapter **14** of this book.

As noted previously, COPD is a heterogeneous disease, and several phenotypes can be recognized.[60–63] The extent to which accelerated aging and/or immunosenescence per se (relative to other concurrent pathogenic processes) may contribute to the development of particular disease phenotypes is as yet unclear. However, some evidence suggests that aging mechanisms such as telomere shortening[56] alveolar cell senescence,[64] mesenchymal cell senescence[65] and failure of extracellular matrix proteins[51] may predispose patients particularly to the development of emphysema. Other aging-related processes such as epithelial cell senescence, impaired secretion clearance, mesenchymal stem cell senescence, immunosenescence, and autoimmunity may predispose patients to development of small airways inflammation and remodeling.[51,66] Premature aging mechanisms may also account in part for some of the systemic comorbidities associated with COPD.[51] Further research is needed to elucidate the molecular mechanisms underlying the varying phenotypes of COPD.

5. Comorbidities and COPD

Comorbidities are frequently recognized among persons with COPD as important contributors to the disease state, and this is especially true in the elderly COPD patient. Some important comorbidities that are prevalent in the advanced age COPD population and have a significant impact on morbidity and mortality include: cardiovascular disease, cognitive impairment, depression, and ambulatory dysfunction. It is also recognized that the care of a multimorbid patient requires a team approach, and various disease management strategies are under investigation for the COPD patient with comorbidities.

Cardiovascular disease is the leading cause of mortality in those with mild to moderate COPD,[67,68] and 1 in 3 patients with COPD will die from cardiovascular related causes.[69] This correlation seems to go beyond shared risk factors, as FEV1 has been shown to be an independent predictor of cardiovascular related deaths.[70] The reason for this synergy is unclear; it is known that increased COPD severity is associated with increased risk of cardiovascular disease and cardiac events,[71] and that there is particular vulnerability for acute myocardial infarction during or following acute exacerbations of COPD (AECOPD).[72] The presence of COPD also imparts an increased risk of hospitalization due to cardiovascular causes as compared to healthy age-matched controls.[73,74] As is true for COPD, the risk of heart failure increases with age. The combination of COPD and heart failure is frequently unrecognized; up to 20% of COPD patients have previously undiagnosed left ventricular failure.[75,76] Elderly patients are also less likely to have non-invasive cardiac testing for complaints of dyspnea and are less likely to be referred to a cardiologist,[77] thus are more likely to remain underdiagnosed. Plasma BNP levels can be a useful diagnostic marker to identify heart failure in these patients.[78,79] Given the high prevalence of this comorbid condition, all elderly patients with protracted dyspnea or activity limitation should be screened for evidence of systolic and/or diastolic heart failure,[80] especially if the dyspnea severity is out of proportion to the severity of pulmonary function impairment. Occult cardiac ischemia should also be considered.

Reduced FEV1 is an independent risk factor for the development of atrial fibrillation and increases the risk of hospitalization for this condition.[77] The presence of atrial fibrillation also doubles the overall mortality risk in COPD patients.[78] Recent use of oral corticosteroids(OCS) increases risk for developing new onset atrial fibrillation,[79] suggesting COPD patients are at highest risk during an AECOPD. COPD also adversely affects the success of cardioversion for atrial fibrillation.[80] Unfortunately, the optimal treatment for atrial fibrillation in COPD patients is not known, as this patient population is frequently excluded from studies of atrial fibrillation.

Beta blockers have been shown to decrease hospital admissions and mortality in those with heart failure. Unfortunately, older age and presence of COPD are associated with lower rates of beta blocker prescription.[81] Beta blockers do not adversely affect FEV1 or induce bronchospasm, nor reduce the response to inhaled bronchodilators in the vast majority of patients with COPD.[82,83] Treatment with selective beta-blockers is not only considered safe, but has been associated with a reduced risk of COPD exacerbations in addition to their mortality benefit.[82–84] Beta blockers should not be withheld from COPD patients with concomitant heart failure or ischemic heart disease.

Cognitive impairment among COPD patients may be associated with increased mortality and is associated with functional impairment including difficulty with medication management.[85] Age and hypoxemia both predispose patients to cognitive impairment, with up to 77% of hypoxemic COPD patients exhibiting impairment,[85] however even non-hypoxemic COPD patients exhibit impaired cognitive performance, mainly in verbal memory and constructive ability[86] when compared to healthy age matched controls.[87] Approximately 20% of nursing home patients in the US have COPD, and up to two-thirds of these patients suffer from short term memory problems; 40% have moderate or severe cognitive impairments.[88] Cognitive impairment may make it difficult to perform spirometry (thus impeding the diagnosis of COPD[89]), may contribute to loss of functional independence,[90] and may substantially impact the patient's ability to use inhaled therapies effectively.[91] It is not yet clear whether the pattern of cognitive impairment is specific to the disease.[85] Further work is required to address the mechanisms underlying cognitive impairment in COPD, identify appropriate screening measures, and address impact of cognitive impairment on morbidity and mortality in COPD.

Depression is the most common psychiatric disorder in the elderly, and it is thought to be both underdiagnosed and undertreated in this population[92]. Depression frequently coexists with COPD, and may lead to cognitive impairment and contribute to poor disease control.[90,93] Among patients with stable COPD, 10 to 42% of patients are clinically depressed, and these percentages are increased following acute exacerbations.[94] Rates of depression exceed 60% among oxygen-dependent COPD patients.[95] Those with depression and COPD have decreased quality of life,[96] with increased levels of disability,[97] and are more likely to experience exacerbations and to be hospitalized.[98] Depression incidence increases with age, and the elderly are less likely to report depressive symptoms, less likely to be diagnosed by their physicians with depression,[99] and are less likely to receive treatment for depression.[100] Depression is unlikely to remit spontaneously in the elderly,[100] and both screening for and treatment of depression are warranted in the elderly COPD patient since such persons are at risk not only for increased symptom burden but also for an increase in 3-year mortality.[92,101]

Adults with COPD have a 10-fold increased risk of disability compared to adults without chronic conditions,[102] and the development of impairment in non-pulmonary systems such as abnormal body composition, decreased muscle strength, and poor balance is a stronger predictor of disability than respiratory impairment.[103] Sarcopenia, osteoporosis, and reduced activity levels lead to high rates of deconditioning, disability, and frailty in the elderly COPD population. The basis of skeletal muscle dysfunction in COPD patients is likely multifactorial[104] and contributing factors vary in individual patients. Deconditioning is one prominent cause of skeletal muscle dysfunction. Patients with COPD are inactive compared with healthy persons,[105] and activity levels decrease further during and after exacerbations.[106] Many patients have not returned to their prior activity level one year post-exacerbation.[106] Age-related sarcopenia, tissue hypoxia, electrolyte disturbances, low anabolic hormone levels and systemic corticosteroids can also contribute to skeletal muscle dysfunction in COPD.[104] Importantly, the presence of skeletal muscle dysfunction is associated with reduced strength, endurance, and maximal exercise capacity.[107]

Weight loss is an independent predictor of mortality in frail elderly patients,[108] and disease-related malnutrition is a common problem in COPD, affecting 10–45% of COPD patients. Age and severity of COPD both independently predict nutritional status.[107] Both the severity of COPD (based on GOLD stage)[10] and age negatively correlate with body functionality, and GOLD stage also correlates with body composition.[107] Malnutrition in the elderly is a complex disorder including both psychosocial and physical factors including dependency, disability, depression, and comorbidity.[109] Moreover, muscle dysfunction associated with COPD relates not only to nutritional impairment, but also to dysregulation of protein synthesis versus degradation, dysregulation of myonuclear turnover, and other skeletal muscle alterations including mitochondrial dysfunction, decreased oxidative enzyme capacity and a shift from type I to type II muscle fibers which are less resistant to fatigue.[110] Nutritional support has been shown to improve respiratory muscle strength and endurance,[111] however given the multitude of factors that contribute to malnutrition and skeletal muscle loss in the elderly COPD patient a more complex intervention is likely required to affect outcomes.

Frailty is a complex concept loosely defined as difficulty responding appropriately to a disruption in homeostasis due to loss of functionality and physiologic reserve, and it is independently associated with the risk of falls, disability, and mortality in the elderly population.[111] Nearly 25–50% of those over the age of 85 are considered to be frail.[112] All of the previously mentioned comorbidities including malnutrition, skeletal muscle dysfunction, and loss of fat free body mass contribute to frailty. The clinical syndrome of frailty is defined as three or more of the following conditions: Unintentional weight loss (>10 lbs/yr), self-reported fatigue, weakness, slow walking speed, low physical activity, and balance/gait abnormalities.[113] Frailty can substantially impact the disease course of COPD with one study finding that frailty increased the risk of long-term mortality of the elderly COPD patient by 80%.[114] There is a bidirectional relationship between disability and an increased likelihood of falls in the frail adult. COPD is also associated with a high incidence of falls in the elderly, second only to osteoarthritis.[115] Balance is an important predictor of falls, and many manifestations of COPD including: Dyspnea, hypoxemia,[116] lower limb muscle weakness, nutritional depletion, depression, and cognitive impairment have been implicated in the increased risk of falls in the COPD patient.[117] Interventions such as pulmonary rehabilitation(PR), to be discussed more below, may have a positive impact on the frail COPD patient.

Lastly, approximately half of patients with COPD have osteoporosis,[118] and this comorbidity also remains underdiagnosed. The prevalence of osteoporosis increases with increased disease severity and age. Those patients with lower BMI and reduced fat-free mass, as well as women are at higher risk,[119] and while the use of OCS is associated with the development of osteoporosis, COPD remains an independent risk factor in the absence of corticosteroid treatment. Hip fractures resulting from osteoporosis and osteoarthritis can further impair patients functional status. Vertebral compression fractures are common;[120] severe back pain and increased kyphosis resulting from vertebral compression fracture can worsen mechanics of breathing, gas exchange, functional limitations, and may precipitate overt respiratory failure. Screening and treatment for osteoporosis in the older adult is essential.

Currently in the United States, COPD patients with milder disease tend to be cared for by primary care providers (or may not seek medical care) and they are only referred to pulmonary specialists and/or PR programs once their disease in more advanced or difficult to manage. The multimorbid patient is also referred commonly to a variety of other health care specialists, which may lead to fragmentation of patient care, as well as recommendation of complex and often conflicting pharmacologic and non-pharmacologic treatment regimens that are difficult, if not impossible, for patients to follow. The concept of "patient centered medical homes" has received significant attention in recent years. This approach may be beneficial for the elderly COPD patient. A recent VA study among patients with an average age of 70 found that a COPD disease management program reduced hospitalizations and emergency room visits by 41%.[121] There has been a general finding that these types of interventions are associated with improved health care quality and patient experiences.[122] However, not all studies of disease management programs have demonstrated clinical benefit, and one randomized controlled trial raised concerns about such programs by demonstrating increased mortality in the disease management patient group.[123] More research is needed in this area to determine if an integrated care approach has the potential to improve patient satisfaction and medical compliance, as well as lead to health-preserving behavior change, earlier recognition and prevention of severe exacerbations, reduced hospitalizations, and ultimately favorably alter the course of the disease.

6. Therapeutic Interventions for Elderly Persons with COPD

6.1. *Pharmacologic therapies*

The pharmacotherapy available to treat persons with COPD has been reviewed in detail elsewhere.[10,124–127] Inhaled medications available for treatment of COPD include short- and long-acting beta agonists (LABA) and anticholinergics (LAMA). Both of these classes of agents improve lung function, reduce symptoms, improve exercise tolerance, improve quality of life, and reduce the risk of exacerbations.[10,124,125] Dual class bronchodilator therapy improves lung function more than either class of agent alone.[128] Combination therapy with long-acting bronchodilators plus inhaled corticosteroid (ICS) also improves lung function and reduces symptoms and exacerbations for persons with COPD. Combination therapy is indicated for persons with severe lung function impairment whose symptoms remain incompletely controlled or who have frequent exacerbations despite bronchodilator therapy.[10,129,130] "Triple therapy" with LABA, LAMA, and ICS may be required for symptom control among persons with severe airflow obstruction, severe symptoms, and a history of frequent exacerbations.[131] None of these agents has been proven definitively to alter the course of the disease, although the TORCH study demonstrated a near significant decrease in mortality among persons using combination therapy,[130] and *posthoc* analysis of the TORCH data demonstrated that LABA/ICS treatment was associated with slower decline in FEV1 over time.[129]

Since COPD is most common among persons of advancing age, therapeutic recommendations for COPD have been largely derived from trials involving subjects with an average age of 65 years.[124,129] Current treatment recommendations may only partially apply to the advanced elderly population. To date, there have been no studies evaluating the effect of age on the pharmacokinetics of tiotropium, β-2 agonists, or inhaled corticosteroids.[132] It is known that β-adrenergic response decreases with increasing age, and a higher concentration of β-agonists may be needed for adequate bronchodilator response in older subjects. One study found that older patients had smaller degrees of bronchodilation with salbutamol than younger patients, an effect that was not seen for ipratropium.[133] However, a large population-based retrospective cohort study including 46,403 patients found a higher mortality rate and higher rates of hospitalization and emergency room visits over a 5.5 year follow-up period among elderly COPD patients (mean age 77) who were initially prescribed long-acting anticholinergic medication as compared to persons initially prescribed a long-acting beta-agonist.[134] In contrast, another study found tiotropium led to an increased time to first exacerbation when compared to salmeterol.[135] Thus, at present, it remains unclear which class of agent is the preferred primary bronchodilator in the elderly in regard to improving patient outcomes.

Polypharmacy is common in the older patient due to the predisposition of elderly persons to have multiple medical problems. There are five key considerations in prescribing medication to the elderly patient: (1) determine the evidence of efficacy in older patients, (2) assess the likelihood of adverse drug events, (3) discuss the harm/benefit analysis with the patient, (4) choose appropriate dose, formulation, and delivery of the drugs, and (5) careful patient monitoring.[136] As noted, inhaled therapy is the preferred mode of delivery for most COPD medications. Unfortunately, older age is associated with reduced ability to used inhaled devices due to both physical and cognitive limitations.

Difficulties with use of metered dose inhalers (MDIs) include poor breath-actuation timing, inability to dispense medication due to hand weakness or incoordination, and issues with retaining knowledge in regards to proper technique for use. Multiple studies have demonstrated that the majority of patients over the age of 65 cannot use MDIs effectively, with only 14% over the age of 75 able to use an MDI competently.[137,138] Dry powdered inhalers (DPIs) are advantageous, as they do not require timing of actuation or increased hand strength for drug administration. However, many patients are unable to generate a strong enough peak inspiratory flow for adequate drug delivery. A recent study found that 1 in 5 patients were unable to generate sufficient inspiratory flow for drug delivery, and age, gender, height, and FVC percent predicted were independent predictors of suboptimal peak inspiratory flow rate.[139] Nebulized medication may be the optimal delivery mechanism for the elderly patient, and most preferred COPD medications with the exception of long acting anticholinergics are available in nebulized form.

Overdosage of drugs that are cleared renally is another potential concern in the elderly and sarcopenia can blunt the rise in serum creatinine (Cr) associated with a reduced glomerular filtration rate (GFR). Chronic renal failure has been described as "the neglected comorbidity" in COPD: One group of investigators found a prevalence of overt renal failure in 22% and concealed renal failure (normal Cr with low GFR) in 21% of their cohort of COPD patients.[140] This is an important consideration in patients receiving renally cleared medication such as antibiotics for an acute exacerbation.

Potential side effects of β-agonists include tremor, tachycardia and palpitations, and cardiac dysrhythmias.[141] Adverse effects for anticholinergic agents include dry mouth, constipation, headache, pharyngitis, urinary tract infection, urinary retention, and worsening of narrow angle glaucoma.[132] Controversy exists regarding the cardiovascular risks of both β-agonists and long-acting anticholinergic agents, with some trials suggesting an increase in cardiovascular events with both classes of medications,[142,143] but other large, prospective randomized controlled trials involving tiotropium (UPLIFT),[144] salmeterol (TORCH),[130] formoterol,[145] and indacaterol[146] failing to show excess cardiovascular events with these medications. Lastly, inhaled corticosteroid use is associated with oropharyngeal candidiasis, skin bruising, decreased bone density, cataracts, and most importantly an increased risk of pneumonia.[141,147–150]

The choice of inhaled therapy should be based on a combination of the severity of lung function impairment, symptoms and exacerbation frequency, as well as a patient's ability to use the delivery device, risk of side effects, comorbidities, and use of other medications. In general, inhaled therapies should not be withheld from the elderly as long as the risks and benefits of each treatment option are weighed and the patient is monitored closely.

Selected additional therapies may be considered for persons whose COPD is inadequately controlled despite bronchodilators and/or inhaled corticosteroids. Phosphodiesterase-4 inhibitors can improve symptoms, lung function, and reduce exacerbation risk among persons with severe airflow obstruction (FEV1 <50% predicted), clinical features of chronic bronchitis, and history of frequent exacerbations.[10,151,152] Theophylline can also be considered as a third line treatment. Recent clinical trials have shown that daily macrolide therapy can reduce the frequency of exacerbations particularly for those 65 or older.[153,154] However those with cardiovascular disease and prolonged QT intervals were excluded from these trials, and macrolide therapy has been associated with increased risk of cardiac arrest. Moreover, azithromycin was associated with hearing loss in some patients.[153,154] The long term risk of selection for antibiotic-resistant respiratory pathogens is also unclear. The potential for these adverse effects should be considered carefully before addition of regular macrolide therapy to the medical regimen for elderly persons with COPD.

6.2. *Non-pharmacologic therapies*

6.2.1. *Immunizations*

Immunization against influenza and pneumococcus is recommended for elderly COPD patients.[155] Influenza vaccination has been shown to reduce hospitalizations and death among elderly persons.[156] Unfortunately, there has not been a dramatic decrease in morbidity and mortality due to influenza in this population in the last two decades.[157] High dose inactivated influenza vaccination can be considered; it has been associated with improved antibody response,[158] although it has yet to be determined if this leads to meaningful clinical outcomes.[159] The 23-valent pneumococcal polysaccharide vaccine (PPV) may not be effective in those over the age of 65[160] and studies have failed to show a decrease in all-cause mortality in COPD patients.[161] Much of the decreased mortality in the elderly from pneumococcal vaccination is attributed to a decrease in pneumococcal infection in the young leading to herd immunity.[162] It is recommended that those over 65 receive one PPV, and while it is known that immunity wanes over time, it is not clear if a repeat immunization is warranted. It is also unclear what the role of protein conjugated vaccines in the elderly is at this time, but this may prove to be an effective adjunct or alternative.[162]

6.2.2. *Supplemental oxygen therapy*

The use and benefits of long-term supplemental oxygen therapy (LTOT) has been the subject of a recent comprehensive review.[163] Patients with resting PaO_2 <55 mmHg or arterial oxygen saturation

<88% at rest, with exertion and/or during sleep while breathing room air generally qualify for initiation of supplemental oxygen therapy. Oxygen may also be prescribed if patients' PaO_2 is 55–59 mmHg and SaO_2 88–89% if they have known pulmonary hypertension, or clinical findings suggestive of cor pulmonale or polycythemia (with Hct >55%).[127,164] The requirement for supplemental oxygen is a poor prognostic feature for elderly persons with COPD.[165–168] Persons on LTOT who require hospitalization and mechanical ventilation for COPD exacerbation have especially high mortality rates, hospital readmission risk and often ultimately require institution-based skilled nursing care.[169] The Medical Research Council[170] and Nocturnal Oxygen Therapy [171] trials demonstrated that use of supplemental O2 more than 15 hours per day improves survival for severely hypoxemic patients with COPD as compared with no O_2 treatment. However, O_2 therapy does not as clearly provide survival benefit among persons with less severe hypoxemia or persons who only have nocturnal O_2 desaturations.[172] Additional benefits of supplemental oxygen therapy for severely hypoxemic patients with COPD include improvements in pulmonary artery pressure, exercise tolerance, quality of life, sleep quality, and possibly improved cognitive function.[163,170,171]

There are some practical considerations regarding prescription of O_2 for elderly COPD patients. Although choice of an O_2 delivery system that adequately corrects the hypoxemia is of principal concern, the system chosen must also be manageable for the patient. The placement of long cords for use with stationary concentrators enables patients to walk freely in their homes without carrying portable equipment, but also poses a potential fall risk. When possible, use of lightweight portable systems is desirable (where relevant), as elderly persons may have difficulty carrying tanks weighing more than a few pounds. This in turn can impact patient compliance with prescribed therapy. Rollator walkers with brakes, seat, and basket can be helpful to enable elderly patients requiring LTOT to remain mobile in and outside of their homes; O2 tanks can be placed in the basket and the patient can sit to rest as needed. Patient cognition and home safety should also be considered in prescribing LTOT to elderly COPD patients; caution must be undertaken to ensure the patient (and family members) avoids smoking, cooking flames, or other heating systems to reduce the risk of fire.[173]

6.2.3. *Pulmonary rehabilitation*

Pulmonary rehabilitation (PR) is "a comprehensive intervention based on a thorough patient assessment followed by patient-tailored therapies that include, but are not limited to, exercise training, education, and behavior change, designed to improve the physical and psychological condition of people with chronic respiratory disease and to promote the long-term adherence to health-enhancing behaviors".[174] Core components of PR include patient assessment, exercise training, pulmonary education including self-management techniques, and outcomes assessment. PR has been demonstrated convincingly to improve exercise capacity, reduce symptoms such as dyspnea and leg fatigue, improve quality of life, and reduce urgent healthcare utilization and hospitalizations[174–177] for patients with COPD. It is effective and beneficial both for persons in the chronic stable state of disease as well as for persons recovering from COPD exacerbations.[174,178,179] Indeed PR is one of the most effective therapeutic interventions available for COPD patients. PR undertaken early (within ~1 month) of hospitalization for acute COPD exacerbation substantially reduces the risk of 30 day hospital readmission.[178,179] Persons who remain symptomatic despite optimized medical therapy should be referred for PR.

Given that multiple medical comorbidities are common among elderly persons with COPD, and that general frailty may be present, the question could be raised as to whether elderly persons achieve gains in PR comparable to those gained by younger persons. Studies published to date indeed demonstrate that elderly patients with COPD do benefit from PR.[174,175,180–183] Notably, since COPD is principally diagnosed in persons over the age of 65, many of the clinical studies documenting benefits of PR have been comprised of an elderly patient population. Two recent studies compared outcomes of PR in persons of varying age. In one study ($n = 200$), persons over the age of 70 achieved significant gains in the shuttle walk test, Borg dyspnea scores, and quality of life (based on the Chronic Respiratory Disease Questionnaire) following 6 weeks of outpatient PR that were comparable to the gains made by persons under age 70.[184] In another, comparable gains were made following inpatient PR among elderly persons > age 75 as compared with persons age 65–75.[181] Even persons with severe airflow obstruction can benefit,[174,175,185] and severity of lung function impairment is not a useful criteria by which to exclude patients from PR. Housebound persons unable to attend outpatient hospital-based programs can benefit from a carefully structured supervised home-based program.[180]

Evidence to date also suggests that the presence of multiple comorbidities also does not preclude or limit gains made in PR.[186,187] However, as for all patients participating in PR, patient assessment, including careful medical history, physical examination, review of prior medical records, symptom and exercise capacity assessments prior to PR are crucial to gain understanding of the factors leading to patients' symptoms, functional impairments and activity limitation. Assessment and awareness of baseline exercise capacity and medical comorbidities (particularly cardiovascular disease, arthritis, osteoporosis, and anemia) are essential for formulating a safe exercise training prescription as well as for patient monitoring during PR and for individualizing and optimizing the education program. Some comorbidities may be identified for the first time by PR staff; close partnering between PR program staff and referring clinicians is desirable, especially for the multimorbid elderly patient.

The exercise training component of most PR programs includes multimodality aerobic and strength exercise training of the lower and upper extremities. Aerobic exercise typically includes cycle ergometry and/or treadmill walking. Safety concerns may arise in regards to use of these types of exercise equipment for some elderly patients. Free hallway walking and Nordic walking[188] are effective alternate methods of exercise training for elderly persons unable to perform cycle or treadmill exercise. Walking aids such as rollator walkers are effective in improving walking exercise tolerance for severely debilitated persons.[189–191] Impaired balance and fall risk is an important safety consideration for some elderly patients with COPD participating in PR.[192]

Balance training incorporated into PR can improve balance performance, muscle strength, and functional ability for such persons.[193] Tai Chi is another exercise training method that can be used successfully for elderly patients with COPD.[194]

Anxiety, depression and fatigue typically improve following patient participation in PR.[195–197] Cognitive impairment, a consideration for some persons, has potential to limit gains made by participants in PR, by virtue of reducing the patient's ability to learn health-enhancing behaviors and incorporate new knowledge and routines into daily life, although some data suggests improved cognitive function post-PR.[85] Cognitive impairment may also be newly identified while patients are participating in PR, and this can prompt referral of patients for formal neurocognitive evaluation where needed.

Overall, PR is a highly effective therapeutic intervention for elderly persons with COPD; patients should not be excluded by virtue of advanced age. As is routine in PR practice, safety precautions should be undertaken based on each individual's medical conditions.

6.2.4. *Lung transplantation*

COPD is one of the most common conditions for which patients are referred for lung transplantation.[198,199] Lung transplantation can improve exercise tolerance, quality of life, and survival for selected persons with COPD who have failed medical therapies.[198,200] Median survival following lung transplantation is 5 to 6 years.[198] The survival benefit from double lung transplant (DLT) may exceed that gained from single lung transplant (SLT)[201] for COPD patients, however limited donor organ availability may preclude DLT.

Historically, the age of 60 was considered the cutoff limit for bilateral lung transplant candidacy and 65 was considered the age limit for SLT.[202] Several considerations factor into the assignment of a limitation of patient candidacy for lung transplantation based on age. These include: (a) a limited number of available organs for transplant, (b) the risk of worse outcomes related to dysfunction of other organs with more advanced age, and (c) the desire to perform transplantation when the reduction in life expectancy based on the disease is greater than that related to age, other comorbidities, or the expected wait time for a suitable organ donor.

In 2006, updated International Guidelines for selection of lung transplantation candidates were published.[203] Age over 65 is now considered to be a relative, rather than absolute contraindication to lung transplantation. The choice of timing for referral of patients with COPD for lung transplantation can be difficult, and identifying elderly persons with low life expectancy particularly related to their COPD as compared with other factors can be especially tricky. In general, poor prognostic features with increased risk of mortality in COPD include hypoxemia, hypercarbia, elevated pulmonary artery pressures, FEV1 and diffusing capacity less than 20% predicted, low exercise capacity, low BMI, and history of hospitalization for acute COPD exacerbation associated with hypercarbia.[204–208] As noted previously, The BODE Index[13] is a better predictor of mortality than FEV1 alone. However, the rate of deterioration of lung function is variable,[209,210] and even some persons with severe airflow limitation can remain clinically stable for extended periods of time. Patients should not be considered for transplant referral until and unless they are worsening clinically despite optimal pharmacologic and non-pharmacologic (O2, smoking cessation, pulmonary rehabilitation ± lung volume reduction surgery (LVRS)) therapy.[203] Persons with a BODE index score greater than 5 can also be considered for lung transplantation referral.[203] The indications for transplantation according to the 2006 Guidelines[203] are shown in Table 1.

Persons over the age of 65 should not be referred if they have any of the absolute contraindications to lung transplantation or several of the relative contraindications to transplantation as detailed in the 2006 Guidelines.[203]

In 2005, a Lung Allocation Score (LAS) was implemented in the United States that prioritizes patients on the transplant wait list based on their risk of death while on the wait list relative to their expected post-transplant survival.[211,212] Since clinical deterioration in COPD may occur more slowly than for some other conditions such as pulmonary fibrosis, patients with COPD tend to have lower

Table 1. Guidelines for referral and transplantation for COPD patients.[203]

Clinical Features	**Recommendation**
BODE index score >5	Consider Referral
BODE index score 7–9	Refer for Transplant
Pulmonary HTN AND/OR Cor pulmonale	Refer for Transplant
FEV1 <20% predicted AND Diffusing capacity <20% OR Homogeneous distribution of emphysema	Refer for Transplant

LAS scores than patients with other conditions who are waiting for transplantation.[198,213,214] Among patients with COPD awaiting transplant, lower LAS scores have also been associated with improved survival to transplant.[215]

Lung transplantation improves physical and social functioning, and improves patient quality of life.[216–219] Three month post-transplant survival rates for patients with COPD are approximately 91%, higher than other patient groups.[220] The median survival rate for lung transplant recipients with COPD who survive at least one year is 6.8 years, less than that seen for other conditions.[220] This likely at least in part reflects the older age and greater number of comorbid medical conditions as compared to other patients, such as those with cystic fibrosis. Debate exists as to whether in general, lung transplantation affords a long-term survival benefit for patients with COPD as compared to the natural history of the disease, and studies relating to performance of single (SLT) versus bilateral lung transplantation (BLT) have yielded varied clinical outcomes, including survival.[198]

Lung transplantation can be undertaken successfully among carefully selected persons with COPD over the age of 60 but under the age of 70.[221] One large retrospective analysis of outcomes of

8363 adult lung transplant recipients from the United Network for Organ Sharing data, in which 40% of those who had undergone lung transplantation had COPD, showed that 30 and 90 day mortality were not greater for persons over age 60 than for the younger age groups.[222] Overall, however, age >60 years was associated with a 37% increased risk of death (hazard ratio 1.37; 95% C.I. 1.16–1.62; $p < 0.001$). Persons over age 70 had significantly increased risk of both 30 day (HR 2.9; $p = 0.02$) and 1 year (HR 2.2; $p = 0.08$) mortality; the 1 year mortality rate was 42%. In this study, older patients were also less likely to return to prior baseline functional status as compared with younger patients. Interestingly, the older patients had lower likelihood of organ rejection; this was postulated to be related to the aging immune system. Overall, the investigators concluded that persons over the age of 70 should not undergo lung transplantation.

Carefully selected patients with low exercise capacity, upper lung zone predominant heterogeneous distribution of emphysema may gain a survival advantage from LVRS.[223] LVRS can serve as a bridge to transplantation for some patients.[224] Lung transplantation can be undertaken successfully following prior LVRS,[225,226] although in one recent retrospective study patients who had lung transplantation following LVRS were found to have longer transplantation operative scores, longer hospital length of stay, and reduced long-term post-transplant survival (median 49 months) versus transplant alone (median 96 months, $p = 0.0008$).[227]

Low baseline performance status is associated with worse 1-year post-transplant mortality.[228] Functional performance status and exercise capacity are expected to improve in PR, and as such patients are typically required to undertake PR prior to lung transplantation.[229] PR is also an opportunity wherein the patient can learn how to prepare optimally for surgery, can learn more about what the surgery, what the post-op recovery period will entail, as well as benefits and risks of immunosuppressive medications. Engaging the patient fully in the process of preparation for and recovery from transplantation has potential to improve post-operative outcomes. PR is also beneficial to improve exercise tolerance, reduce symptoms, and improve QOL in the post-transplantation period.[230–232] Pre-transplantation PR may also be a time when patients who are not optimally suited to undergo transplantation may be identified; also, persons who are unable or unwilling to participate may potentially have worse post-transplant outcomes.

7. Palliative Care for Elderly Persons with End-Stage COPD

Palliative care teams can provide great assistance to patients and their caregivers in regard to managing refractory symptoms such as dyspnea, coping with frequent hospitalizations, serving as a liaison between patients and multiple primary and specialty care providers, and helping with end-of-life decision making. Although short-term outcomes for COPD patients can be difficult to predict, mortality is particularly high among elderly persons with COPD and multiple comorbidities who require hospitalization and assisted ventilation for exacerbations of COPD.[169,233] Providers should consider seeking input from palliative care teams (where available) for such persons, as well as for those with severe refractory disabling symptoms despite routine medical therapy (including O2 and PR), persons having difficulty discussing or making end of life decisions, or persons who experience prolonged hospitalization or who require prolonged skilled nursing care.[234–238]

References

1. Organization WH. (2007). Chronic Respiratory Diseases. In *Global surveillance, prevention and control of chronic respiratory diseases: A comprehensive approach* pp. 21–31. Switzerland: WHO Press
2. Hoyert DL, Xu J. (2012) Deaths: Preliminary data for 2011. *Natl Vital Stat Rep* **61**: 1–51.
3. Prevention CfDCa. (2012) Chronic obstructive pulmonary disease among adults — United States, 2011. *MMWR* **61**: 938–943.
4. Mannino DM, Gagnon RC, Petty TL *et al.* (2000) Obstructive lung disease and low lung function in adults in the United States: Data from the National Health and Nutrition Examination Survey, 1988–1994. *Arch Intern Med* **160**: 1683–1689.

5. Halbert RJ, Natoli JL, Gano A i. (2006) Global burden of COPD: systematic review and meta-analysis. *Euro Respir J* **28**: 523–532.
6. Buist AS, McBurnie MA, Vollmer WM *et al.* (2007) International variation in the prevalence of COPD (The BOLD Study): A population-based prevalence study. *The Lancet* **370**: 741–750.
7. van Durme YMTA, Verhamme KMC, Stijnen T *et al.* (2009) Prevalence, incidence, and lifetime risk for the development of copd in the elderly: The rotterdam study. *Chest* **135**: 368–377.
8. Mannino DM. (2002) COPD*: Epidemiology, prevalence, morbidity and mortality, and disease heterogeneity. *chest* **121**: 121S–126S.
9. Connolly MJ, Lowe D, Anstey K *et al.* (2006) Admissions to hospital with exacerbations of chronic obstructive pulmonary disease: Effect of age related factors and service organisation. *Thorax* **61**: 843–848.
10. Disease GIfCOL. (2013) Global Strategy For The Diagnosis, Management, And Prevention Of Chronic Obstructive Pulmonary Disease www.goldcopd.com
11. Hogg JC, Chu F, Utokaparch S *et al.* (2004) The nature of small-airway obstruction in chronic obstructive pulmonary disease. *New Engl J Med* **350**: 2645–2653.
12. Macnee W. (2007) Pathogenesis of chronic obstructive pulmonary disease. *Clin Chest Med* **28**: 479–513.
13. Celli BR, Cote CG, Marin JM *et al.* (2004) The body-mass index, airflow obstruction, dyspnea, and exercise capacity index in chronic obstructive pulmonary disease. *New Engl J Med* **350**: 1005–1012.
14. Jones RC, Donaldson GC, Chavannes NH *et al.* (2009) Derivation and validation of a composite index of severity in chronic obstructive pulmonary disease: The DOSE Index. *Am J Respir Crit Care Med* **180**: 1189–1195.
15. Divo M, Cote C, de Torres JP *et al.* (2012) Comorbidities and risk of mortality in patients with chronic obstructive pulmonary disease. *Am J Respir Critical Care Med* **186**: 155–161.
16. Puhan MA, Garcia-Aymerich J, Frey M *et al.* (2009) Expansion of the prognostic assessment of patients with chronic obstructive pulmonary disease: The updated BODE index and the ADO index. *Lancet* **374**: 704–711.
17. Almagro P, Soriano JB, Cabrera FJ *et al.* (2014) Short- and medium-term prognosis in patients hospitalized for COPD exacerbation: The CODEX index. *Chest* **145**: 972–980.
18. de Marco R, Pesce G, Marcon A *et al.* (2013) The coexistence of asthma and chronic obstructive pulmonary disease (COPD):

Prevalence and risk factors in young, middle-aged and elderly people from the general population. *PLoS ONE* **8**: e62985.

19. Menezes AM, Montes de Oca M, Perez-Padilla R *et al.* (2014) Increased risk of exacerbation and hospitalization in subjects with an overlap phenotype: COPD-asthma. *Chest* **145**: 297–304.
20. Rizzi M, Palma P, Andreoli A *et al.* (1997) Prevalence and clinical feature of the "overlap syndrome", obstructive sleep apnea (OSA) and chronic obstructive pulmonary disease (COPD), in OSA population. *Sleep Breathing* **2**: 68–72.
21. Martinez-Garcia MA, Soler-Cataluna JJ, Donat Sanz Y *et al.* (2011) Factors associated with bronchiectasis in patients with COPD. *Chest* **140**: 1130–1137.
22. Jankowich MD, Rounds SI. (2012) Combined pulmonary fibrosis and emphysema syndrome: A review. *Chest* **141**: 222–231.
23. Marin JM, Soriano JB, Carrizo SJ *et al.* (2010) Outcomes in patients with chronic obstructive pulmonary disease and obstructive sleep apnea: The overlap syndrome. *Am J Respir Crit Care Med* **182**: 325–331.
24. Swanney MP, Ruppel G, Enright PL *et al.* (2008) Using the lower limit of normal for the FEV1/FVC ratio reduces the misclassification of airway obstruction. *Thorax* **63**: 1046–1051.
25. Pellegrino R, Viegi G, Brusasco V *et al.* (2005) Interpretative strategies for lung function tests. *Eur Respir J* **26**: 948–968.
26. Mikulski MA, Gerke AK, Lourens S *et al.* (2013) Agreement between fixed-ratio and lower limit of normal spirometry interpretation protocols decreases with age: is there a need for a new GOLD standard? *J Occup Environ Med* **55**: 802–808.
27. Ware JH, Dockery DW, Louis TA *et al.* (1990) Longitudinal and cross-sectional estimates of pulmonary function decline in never-smoking adults. *Am J Epidemiol* **132**: 685–700.
28. Janssens JP, Pache JC, Nicod LP. (1999) Physiological changes in respiratory function associated with ageing. *Eur Respir J* **13**: 197–205.
29. Garcia-Rio F, Pino JM, Dorgham A *et al.* (2004) Spirometric reference equations for European females and males aged 65–85 yrs. *Eur Respir J* **24**: 397–405.
30. Hankinson JL, Odencrantz JR, Fedan KB. (1999) Spirometric reference values from a sample of the general U.S. population. *Am J Respir Crit Care Medicine* **159**: 179–187.
31. Colak Y, Lokke A, Marott JL *et al.* (2013) Impact of diagnostic criteria on the prevalence of COPD. *Clin Respir J* **7**: 297–303.

32. Guder G, Brenner S, Angermann CE *et al.* (2012) "GOLD or lower limit of normal definition? A comparison with expert-based diagnosis of chronic obstructive pulmonary disease in a prospective cohort-study". *Respir Res* **13**: 13.
33. Schirnhofer L, Lamprecht B, Vollmer WM *et al.* (2007) COPD prevalence in Salzburg, Austria: Results from the Burden of Obstructive Lung Disease (BOLD) Study. *Chest* **131**: 29–36.
34. van Dijk WD, Gupta N, Tan WC *et al.* (2014) Clinical relevance of diagnosing COPD by fixed ratio or lower limit of normal: A systematic review. *COPD* **11**: 113–120.
35. Mohamed Hoesein FA, Zanen P, Lammers JW. (2011) Lower limit of normal or FEV1/FVC <0.70 in diagnosing COPD: An evidence-based review. *Respir Med* **105**: 907–915.
36. Aggarwal AN, Gupta D, Agarwal R *et al.* (2011) Comparison of the lower confidence limit to the fixed-percentage method for assessing airway obstruction in routine clinical practice. *Respir Care* **56**: 1778–1784.
37. Szanto O, Montnemery P, Elmstahl S. (2010) Prevalence of airway obstruction in the elderly: results from a cross-sectional spirometric study of nine age cohorts between the ages of 60 and 93 years. *Prim Care Respir J* **19**: 231–236.
38. Tilert T, Dillon C, Paulose-Ram R *et al.* (2013) Estimating the U.S. prevalence of chronic obstructive pulmonary disease using pre- and post-bronchodilator spirometry: The National Health and Nutrition Examination Survey (NHANES) 2007–2010. *Respir Res* **14**: 103.
39. Mannino DM, Sonia Buist A, Vollmer WM. (2007) Chronic obstructive pulmonary disease in the older adult: What defines abnormal lung function? *Thorax* **62**: 237–241.
40. Brazzale DJ, Upward AL, Pretto JJ. (2010) Effects of changing reference values and definition of the normal range on interpretation of spirometry. *Respirology* **15**: 1098–1103.
41. Vaz Fragoso CA, Concato J, McAvay G *et al.* (2010) Chronic obstructive pulmonary disease in older persons: A comparison of two spirometric definitions. *Respir Med* **104**: 1189–1196.
42. Wollmer P, Engstrom G. (2013) Fixed ratio or lower limit of normal as cut-off value for FEV1/VC: An outcome study. *Respir Med* **107**: 1460–1462.
43. Sorino C, Sherrill D, Guerra S *et al.* (2011) Prognostic value of FEV1/FEV6 in elderly people. *Clin Physiol Func Imag* **31**: 101–107.

44. Ferguson GT, Enright PL, Buist AS *et al.* (2000) Office spirometry for lung health assessment in adults: A consensus statement from the National Lung Health Education Program. *Chest* **117**: 1146–1161.
45. MacNee W, Tuder RM. (2009) New paradigms in the pathogenesis of chronic obstructive pulmonary disease I. *Proc Am Thorac Soc* **6**: 527–531.
46. Tuder RM, Petrache I. (2012) Pathogenesis of chronic obstructive pulmonary disease. *J Clin Invest* **122**: 2749–2755.
47. Cosio MG, Saetta M, Agusti A. (2009) Immunologic aspects of chronic obstructive pulmonary disease. *New Engl J Med* **360**: 2445–2454.
48. Lowery EM, Brubaker AL, Kuhlmann E *et al.* (2013) The aging lung. *Clin Interv Aging* **8**: 1489–1496.
49. Sharma G, Hanania NA, Shim YM. (2009) The aging immune system and its relationship to the development of chronic obstructive pulmonary disease. *Proc Am Thorac Soc* **6**: 573–580.
50. Ito K, Barnes PJ. (2009) COPD as a disease of accelerated lung aging. *Chest* **135**: 173–180.
51. Chilosi M, Carloni A, Rossi A *et al.* (2013) Premature lung aging and cellular senescence in the pathogenesis of idiopathic pulmonary fibrosis and COPD/emphysema. *Transl Res* **162**: 156–173.
52. Boron WF BE. (2012) The physiology of aging. In Boron WF (ed.), *Medical Physiology*, pp.1281–1292. Philadelphia, PA: Elsevier Health Sciences.
53. Ershler WB, Keller ET. (2000) Age-associated increased interleukin-6 gene expression, late-life diseases, and frailty. *Ann Rev Med* **51**: 245–270.
54. Panda A, Arjona A, Sapey E *et al.* (2009) Human innate immunosenescence: causes and consequences for immunity in old age. *Trends Immunol* **30**: 325–333.
55. Shaykhiev R, Crystal RG. (2013) Innate immunity and chronic obstructive pulmonary disease: A mini-review. *Gerontol* **59**: 481–489.
56. Alder JK, Guo N, Kembou F *et al.* (2011) Telomere length is a determinant of emphysema susceptibility. *Am J Respir Crit Care Med* **184**: 904–912.
57. Lee J, Sandford AJ, Connett JE *et al.* (2012) The relationship between telomere length and mortality in chronic obstructive pulmonary disease (COPD). *PLoS ONE* **7**: e35567.
58. Calado RT, Dumitriu B. (2013) Telomere dynamics in mice and humans. *Semin Hematol* **50**: 165–174.

59. Ghadially R, Brown BE, Sequeira-Martin SM *et al.* (1995) The aged epidermal permeability barrier. Structural, functional, and lipid biochemical abnormalities in humans and a senescent murine model. *J Clin Invest* **95**: 2281–2290.
60. Han MK, Agusti A, Calverley PM *et al.* (2010) Chronic obstructive pulmonary disease phenotypes: The future of COPD. *Am J Respir Crit Care Med* **182**: 598–604.
61. Burgel PR, Paillasseur JL, Caillaud D *et al.* (2010) Clinical COPD phenotypes: A novel approach using principal component and cluster analyses. *Eur Respir J* **36**: 531–539.
62. Garcia-Aymerich J, Gomez FP, Benet M *et al.* (2011) Identification and prospective validation of clinically relevant chronic obstructive pulmonary disease (COPD) subtypes. *Thorax* **66**: 430–437.
63. Castaldi PJ, Dy J, Ross J *et al.* (2014) Cluster analysis in the COPD Gene study identifies subtypes of smokers with distinct patterns of airway disease and emphysema. *Thorax* **69**: 415–422.
64. Tsuji T, Aoshiba K, Nagai A. (2006) Alveolar cell senescence in patients with pulmonary emphysema. *Am J Respir Crit Care Med* **174**: 886–893.
65. Muller KC, Welker L, Paasch K *et al.* (2006). Lung fibroblasts from patients with emphysema show markers of senescence *in vitro*. *Respir Res* 7: 32
66. Amsellem V, Gary-Bobo G, Marcos E *et al.* (2011) Telomere dysfunction causes sustained inflammation in chronic obstructive pulmonary disease. *Am J Respir Crit Care Med* **184**: 1358–1366.
67. Sin DD. (2009) Is COPD really a cardiovascular disease? *Chest* **136**: 329–330.
68. Finkelstein J, Cha E, Scharf SM. (2009) Chronic obstructive pulmonary disease as an independent risk factor for cardiovascular morbidity. *Int J Chron Obstruct Pulmon Dis* **4**: 337–349.
69. Chatila WM, Thomashow BM, Minai OA *et al.* (2008) Comorbidities in chronic obstructive pulmonary disease. *Proc Am Thorac Soc* **5**: 549–555.
70. Anthonisen NR, Skeans MA, Wise RA *et al.* (2005) The Effects of a Smoking Cessation Intervention on 14.5-Year Mortality A Randomized Clinical Trial. *Ann Intern Med* **142**: 233–239.
71. Curkendall SM, Lanes S, de Luise C *et al.* (2006) Chronic obstructive pulmonary disease severity and cardiovascular outcomes. *Eur J Epidemiol* **21**: 803–813.

72. Donaldson GC, Hurst JR, Smith CJ *et al.* (2010) Increased risk of myocardial infarction and stroke following exacerbation of COPD. *Chest* **137**: 1091–1097.
73. Curkendall SM, deLuise C, Jones JK *et al.* (2006) Cardiovascular disease in patients with chronic obstructive pulmonary disease, Saskatchewan Canada: Cardiovascular disease in COPD patients. *Ann Epidemiol* **16**: 63–70.
74. Huiart L, Ernst P, Suissa S. (2005) Cardiovascular morbidity and mortality in COPD*. *Chest* **128**: 2640–2646.
75. Rutten FH, Moons KG, Cramer MJ *et al.* (2005) Recognising heart failure in elderly patients with stable chronic obstructive pulmonary disease in primary care: Cross sectional diagnostic study. *BMJ* **331**: 1379.
76. Rutten FH, Vonken EJ, Cramer MJ *et al.* (2008) Cardiovascular magnetic resonance imaging to identify left-sided chronic heart failure in stable patients with chronic obstructive pulmonary disease. *Am Heart J* **156**: 506–512.
77. Buch P, Friberg J, Scharling H *et al.* (2003) Reduced lung function and risk of atrial fibrillation in The Copenhagen City Heart Study. *Eur Respir J* **21**: 1012–1016.
78. Fuso L, Antonelli Incalzi R, Pistelli R *et al.* (1995) Predicting mortality of patients hospitalized for acutely exacerbated chronic obstructive pulmonary disease. *Am J Med* **98**: 272–277.
79. van der Hooft CS, Heeringa J, Brusselle GG *et al.* (2006) COrticosteroids and the risk of atrial fibrillation. *Arch Intern Med* **166**: 1016–1020.
80. Pisters R, Nieuwlaat R, Prins MH *et al.* (2012) Clinical correlates of immediate success and outcome at 1-year follow-up of real-world cardioversion of atrial fibrillation: The Euro Heart Survey. *Europace* **14**: 666–674.
81. Maggioni AP, Sinagra G, Opasich C *et al.* (2003) Treatment of chronic heart failure with β adrenergic blockade beyond controlled clinical trials: The BRING-UP experience. *Heart* **89**: 299–305.
82. Salpeter S, Ormiston T, Salpeter E. (2005) Cardioselective beta-blockers for chronic obstructive pulmonary disease. *Cochrane Database Syst Rev* **4**: CD003566
83. Rutten FH, Zuithoff N, Hak E *et al.* (2010) {beta}-Blockers May reduce mortality and risk of exacerbations in patients with chronic obstructive pulmonary disease. *Arch Intern Med.* **170**: 880.

84. Etminan M, Jafari S, Carleton B *et al.* (2012) Beta-blocker use and COPD mortality: a systematic review and meta-analysis. *BMC Pulm Med* **12**: 48.
85. Dodd JW, Getov SV, Jones PW. (2010) Cognitive function in COPD. *Eur Respir J* **35**: 913–922.
86. Incalzi RA, Gemma A, Marra C *et al.* (1993) Chronic obstructive pulmonary disease. An original model of cognitive decline. *Am Rev Respir Dis* **148**: 418–424.
87. Liesker JJW, Postma DS, Beukema RJ *et al.* (2004) Cognitive performance in patients with COPD. *Respir Med* **98**: 351–356.
88. Zarowitz BJ, O'Shea T. (2012) Chronic obstructive pulmonary disease: Prevalence, characteristics, and pharmacologic treatment in nursing home residents with cognitive impairment. *J Managed Care Pharm* **18**: 598–606.
89. Bellia V, Pistelli R, Catalano F *et al.* (2000) Quality Control of Spirometry in the Elderly. *Am J Respir Crit Care Med* **161**: 1094–1100.
90. Antonelli-Incalzi R, Corsonello A, Trojano L *et al.* (2008) Correlation between cognitive impairment and dependence in hypoxemic COPD. *J Clin Exp Neuropsychol* **30**: 141–150.
91. Board M, Allen SC. (2006) A simple drawing test to identify patients who are unlikely to be able to learn to use an inhaler. *Int J Clin Practice* **60**: 510–513.
92. Adamson JA, Price GM, Breeze E *et al.* (2005) Are older people dying of depression? Findings from the medical research council trial of the assessment and management of older people in the community. *J Am Geriatr Soc* **53**: 1128–1132.
93. Incalzi RA, Scarlata S, Pennazza G *et al.* (2014) Chronic obstructive pulmonary disease in the elderly. *Euro J Intern Med* **25**: 320–328.
94. Maurer J, Rebbapragada V, Borson S *et al.* (2008) Anxiety and depression in COPD: Current understanding, unanswered questions, and research needs. *Chest* **134**: 43S–56S.
95. Lacasse Y, Rousseau L, Maltais F. (2001) Prevalence of depressive symptoms and depression in patients with severe oxygen-dependent chronic obstructive pulmonary disease. *J Cardiopulm Rehabil Prev.* **21**: 80–86.
96. Cully JA, Graham DP, Stanley MA *et al.* (2006) Quality of life in patients with chronic obstructive pulmonary disease and comorbid anxiety or depression. *Psychosomatics* **47**: 312–319.

97. Yohannes AM, Baldwin RC, Connolly MJ. (2003) Prevalence of sub-threshold depression in elderly patients with chronic obstructive pulmonary disease. *Int J Geriatr Psychiatry* **18**: 412–416.
98. Xu W, Collet J-P, Shapiro S, Lin Y *et al.* (2008) Independent effect of depression and anxiety on chronic obstructive pulmonary disease exacerbations and hospitalizations. *Am J Respir Crit Care Med* **178**: 913–920.
99. Maurer J, Rebbapragada V, Borson S *et al.* (2008) Anxiety and depression in copd: Current understanding, unanswered questions, and research needs. *Chest* **134**: 43S–56S.
100. Livingston G, Watkin V, Milne B *et al.* (1997) The natural history of depression and the anxiety disorders in older people: The Islington community study. *J Affect Disorders* **46**: 255–262.
101. Fan VS, Ramsey SD, Giardino ND *et al.* (2007) Sex, depression, and risk of hospitalization and mortality in chronic obstructive pulmonary disease. *Arch Intern Med* **167**: 2345.
102. Eisner MD, Yelin EH, Trupin L *et al.* (2002) The influence of chronic respiratory conditions on health status and work disability. *Am J Public Health* **92**: 1506–1513.
103. Maltais F, Decramer M, Casaburi R *et al.* (2014) An official american thoracic society/european respiratory society statement: Update on limb muscle dysfunction in chronic obstructive pulmonary disease. *Am J Respir Crit Care Med* **189**: e15–e62.
104. (1999) Skeletal muscle dysfunction in chronic obstructive pulmonary disease. *Am J Respir Crit Care Med.* **159**: S2–S40.
105. Pitta F, Troosters T, Spruit MA *et al.* (2005) Characteristics of physical activities in daily life in chronic obstructive pulmonary disease. *Am J Respir Crit Care Med* **171**: 972–977.
106. Pitta F, Troosters T, Probst VS *et al.* (2006) Physical activity and hospitalization for exacerbation of COPD*. *Chest* **129**: 536–544.
107. Battaglia S, Spatafora M, Paglino G *et al.* (2011) Ageing and COPD affect different domains of nutritional status: The ECCE study. *Eur Respir J* **37**: 1340–1345.
108. Payette H, Coulombe C, Boutier V *et al.* (1999) Weight loss and mortality among free-living frail elders: a prospective study. *J Gerontol A Biol Sci Med Sci* **54**: M440–M445.
109. Chen CC-H, Schilling LS, Lyder CH. (2001) A concept analysis of malnutrition in the elderly. *J Adv Nursing* **36**: 131–142.

110. Remels AH, Gosker HR, van der Velden J *et al.* (2007) Systemic inflammation and skeletal muscle dysfunction in chronic obstructive pulmonary disease: State of the art and novel insights in regulation of muscle plasticity. *Clin Chest Med* **28**: 537–552.
111. Collins PF, Elia M, Stratton RJ. (2013) Nutritional support and functional capacity in chronic obstructive pulmonary disease: A systematic review and meta-analysis. *Respirology* **18**: 616–629.
112. Crisafulli E, Morandi A, Olivini A *et al.* (2014) Rehabilitation and supportive therapy in elderly patients with Chronic Obstructive Pulmonary Disease. *Euro J Intern Med* **25**: 329–335.
113. Crisafulli E, Venturelli E, Iattoni A *et al.* (2011) Co-morbidities in chronic respiratory patients: limitations or opportunities for caring? *J Med Pers* **9**: 99–103.
114. Galizia G, Cacciatore F, Testa G *et al.* (2011) Role of clinical frailty on long-term mortality of elderly subjects with and without chronic obstructive pulmonary disease. *Aging Clin Exp Res* **23**: 118–125.
115. Lawlor DA, Patel, Rita, Ebrahim S. (2003) Association between falls in elderly women and chronic diseases and drug use: cross sectional study. BMJ 327: 712–7
116. Ozalevli S, Ilgin D, Narin S *et al.* (2011) Association between disease-related factors and balance and falls among the elderly with COPD: A cross-sectional study. *Aging Clin Exp Res* **23**: 372–377.
117. Hodges PW. (2013) Equilibrium, balance and increased risk of falls related to COPD. *COPD and Comorbidity* **14**: 45.
118. Jorgensen NR, Schwarz P, Holme I *et al.* (2007) The prevalence of osteoporosis in patients with chronic obstructive pulmonary disease — A cross sectional study. *Respir. Med.* **101**: 177–185.
119. Bolton CE, Ionescu AA, Shiels KM *et al.* (2004) Associated loss of fat-free mass and bone mineral density in chronic obstructive pulmonary disease. *Am J Respir Crit Care Med.* **170**: 1286–1293.
120. Nuti R, Siviero P, Maggi S *et al.* (2009) Vertebral fractures in patients with chronic obstructive pulmonary disease: The EOLO Study. *Osteoporos Int* **20**: 989–998.
121. Rice KL, Dewan N, Bloomfield HE *et al.* (2010) Disease management program for chronic obstructive pulmonary disease. *Am J Respir Crit Care Med* **182**: 890–896.
122. Grumbach K, Grundy P. (2010). Outcomes of implementing patient centered medical home interventions. In *Patient-Centered Primary Care Collaborative*

123. Fan VS, Gaziano JM, Lew R *et al.* (2012) A comprehensive care management program to prevent chronic obstructive pulmonary disease hospitalizations: A randomized, controlled trial. *Ann Intern Med* **156**: 673–683.
124. Albertson TE, Schivo M, Zeki AA *et al.* (2013) The pharmacological approach to the elderly COPD patient. *Drugs Aging* **30**: 479–502.
125. Possick JD, Most J, Rochester CL. (2013) Advances in the Outpatient Management of Chronic Obstructive Pulmonary Disease. *Clin Pulm Med* **20**: 259–270.
126. Nazir SA, Erbland ML. (2009) Chronic obstructive pulmonary disease: An update on diagnosis and management issues in older adults. *Drugs Aging* **26**: 813–831.
127. Celli BR. (2008) Update on the management of COPD. *Chest* **133**: 1451–1462.
128. van Noord JA, Aumann JL, Janssens E *et al.* (2006) Effects of tiotropium with and without formoterol on airflow obstruction and resting hyperinflation in patients with COPD. *Chest* **129**: 509–517.
129. Celli BR, Thomas NE, Anderson JA *et al.* (2008) Effect of pharmacotherapy on rate of decline of lung function in chronic obstructive pulmonary disease: Results from the TORCH study. *Am J Respir Crit Care Med* **178**: 332–338.
130. Calverley PMA, Anderson JA, Celli B *et al.* (2007) Salmeterol and fluticasone propionate and survival in chronic obstructive pulmonary disease. *New Engl J Med* **356**: 775–789.
131. Aaron SD, Vandemheen KL, Fergusson D *et al.* (2007) Tiotropium in combination with placebo, salmeterol, or fluticasone-salmeterol for treatment of chronic obstructive pulmonary disease: A randomized trial. *Ann Intern Med* **146**: 545–555.
132. Valente S, Pasciuto G, Bernabei R. (2010) Do we need different treatments for very elderly COPD patients? *Respiration* **80**: 357–368.
133. Ullah MI, Newman GB, Saunders KB. (1981) Influence of age on response to ipratropium and salbutamol in asthma. *Thorax* **36**: 523–529.
134. Gershon A, Croxford R, To T *et al.* (2011) Comparison of inhaled long-acting beta-agonist and anticholinergic effectiveness in older patients with chronic obstructive pulmonary disease: A cohort study. *Ann Intern Med* **154**: 583–592.
135. Vogelmeier C, Hederer B, Glaab T *et al.* (2011) Tiotropium versus Salmeterol for the Prevention of Exacerbations of COPD. *New Engl J Med* **364**: 1093–1103.

136. Hilmer SN, McLachlan AJ, Le Couteur DG. (2007) Clinical pharmacology in the geriatric patient. *Fundam Clin Pharmacol* **21**: 217–230.
137. Giraud V, Roche N. (2002) Misuse of corticosteroid metered-dose inhaler is associated with decreased asthma stability. *Eur Respir J* **19**: 246–251.
138. Brennan VK, Osman LM, Graham H *et al.* (2005) True device compliance: The need to consider both competence and contrivance. *Respir Med* **99**: 97–102.
139. Mahler DA, Waterman LA, Gifford AH. (2013) Prevalence and COPD phenotype for a suboptimal peak inspiratory flow rate against the simulated resistance of the Diskus® dry powder inhaler. *J Aerosol Med Pulm Drug Deliv* **26**: 174–179.
140. Antonelli Incalzi R, Fuso L, De Rosa M *et al.* (1997) Co-morbidity contributes to predict mortality of patients with chronic obstructive pulmonary disease. *Eur Respir J* **10**: 2794–2800.
141. Dzierba AL, Jelic S. (2009) Chronicobstructive pulmonary disease in the elderly. *Drugs Aging* **26**: 447–456.
142. Singh S, Loke YK, Furberg CD. (2008) Inhaled anticholinergics and risk of major adverse cardiovascular events in patients with chronic obstructive pulmonary disease: A systematic review and meta-analysis. *JAMA* **300**: 1439–1450.
143. Gershon A, Croxford R, Calzavara A *et al.* (2013) Cardiovascular safety of inhaled long-acting bronchodilators in individuals with chronic obstructive pulmonary disease. *JAMA Intern Med* **173**: 1175–1185.
144. Tashkin DP, Celli B, Senn S *et al.* (2008) A 4-Year trial of tiotropium in chronic obstructive pulmonary disease. *New Engl J Med* **359**: 1543–1554.
145. Campbell SC, Criner GJ, Levine BE *et al.* (2007) Cardiac safety of formoterol 12μg twice daily in patients with chronic obstructive pulmonary disease. *Pulm Pharmacol Ther* **20**: 571–579.
146. Worth H, Chung KF, Felser JM *et al.* (2011) Cardio- and cerebrovascular safety of indacaterol vs formoterol, salmeterol, tiotropium and placebo in COPD. *Respir Med* **105**: 571–579.
147. Jenkins CR, Jones PW, Calverley PM *et al.* (2009) Efficacy of salmeterol/fluticasone propionate by GOLD stage of chronic obstructive pulmonary disease: Analysis from the randomised, placebo-controlled TORCH study. *Respir Res* **10**: 59.

148. Ernst P, Gonzalez AV, Brassard P *et al.* (2007) Inhaled corticosteroid use in chronic obstructive pulmonary disease and the risk of hospitalization for Pneumonia. *Am J Respir Crit Care Med* **176**: 162–166.
149. Burge PS, Calverley PMA, Jones PW *et al.* (2000) Randomised, double blind, placebo controlled study of fluticasone propionate in patients with moderate to severe chronic obstructive pulmonary disease: the ISOLDE trial. *BMJ* 320: 1297–303.
150. Pauwels RA, Löfdahl C-G, Laitinen LA *et al.* (1999) Long-term treatment with inhaled budesonide in persons with mild chronic obstructive pulmonary disease who continue smoking. *New Engl J Med* **340**: 1948–1953.
151. Rennard SI, Calverley PM, Goehring UM *et al.* (2011) Reduction of exacerbations by the PDE4 inhibitor roflumilast — the importance of defining different subsets of patients with COPD. *Respir Res* **12**: 18.
152. Chong J, Poole P, Leung B *et al.* (2011) Phosphodiesterase 4 inhibitors for chronic obstructive pulmonary disease. *Cochrane Database Syst Rev*: CD002309.
153. Albert RK, Connett J, Bailey WC *et al.* (2011) Azithromycin for prevention of exacerbations of COPD. *New Engl J Med* **365**: 689–698.
154. Han MK, Tayob N, Murray S *et al.* (2014) Predictors of chronic obstructive pulmonary disease exacerbation reduction in response to daily Azithromycin Therapy. *Am J Respir Crit Care Med* **189**: 1503–1508.
155. Control CfD. (2014) Advisory committee on immunization practices recommended immunization schedule for adults aged 19 years or older — United States, 2014. *Morbid Mortal Wkly Rep* **63**:
156. Nichol KL, Nordin J, Mullooly J *et al.* (2003) Influenza vaccination and reduction in hospitalizations for cardiac disease and stroke among the elderly. *New Engl J Med* **348**: 1322–1332.
157. Simonsen L, Reichert TA, Viboud C *et al.* (2005) Impact of influenza vaccination on seasonal mortality in the us elderly population. *Arch Intern Med* **165**: 265–272.
158. Falsey AR, Treanor JJ, Tornieporth N *et al.* (2009) Randomized, double-blind controlled phase 3 trial comparing the immunogenicity of high-dose and standard-dose influenza vaccine in adults 65 years of age and older. *J Infect Dis* **200**: 172–180.
159. DiazGranados CA, Dunning AJ, Jordanov E *et al.* (2013) High-dose trivalent influenza vaccine compared to standard dose vaccine in

elderly adults: Safety, immunogenicity and relative efficacy during the 2009–2010 season. *Vaccine* **31**: 861–866.

160. Alfageme I, Vazquez R, Reyes N *et al.* (2006) Clinical efficacy of anti-pneumococcal vaccination in patients with COPD. *Thorax* **61**: 189–195.
161. Schembri S, Morant S, Winter JH *et al.* (2009) Influenza but not pneumococcal vaccination protects against all-cause mortality in patients with COPD. *Thorax* **64**: 567–572.
162. Plotkin S, Jackson LA, Janoff EN. (2008) Pneumococcal vaccination of elderly adults: New paradigms for protection. *Clin Infect Dis* **47**: 1328–1338.
163. Criner GJ. (2013) Ambulatory home oxygen: What is the evidence for benefit, and who does it help? *Respir Care* **58**: 48–64.
164. Rabe KF, Hurd S, Anzueto A *et al.* (2007) Global strategy for the diagnosis, management, and prevention of chronic obstructive pulmonary disease: GOLD executive summary. *Am J Respir Crit Care Med* **176**: 532–555.
165. Katsura H, Ogata M, Kida K. (2001) Factors determining outcome in elderly patients with severe COPD on long-term domiciliary oxygen therapy. *Monaldi Arch Chest Dis = Archivio Monaldi per le malattie del torace / Fondazione clinica del lavoro, IRCCS [and] Istituto di clinica tisiologica e malattie apparato respiratorio, Universita di Napoli, Secondo ateneo* **56**: 195–201.
166. Crockett AJ, Cranston JM, Moss JR *et al.* (2001) Survival on long-term oxygen therapy in chronic airflow limitation: From evidence to outcomes in the routine clinical setting. *Intern Med J* **31**: 448–454.
167. Dubois P, Jamart J, Machiels J *et al.* (1994) Prognosis of severely hypoxemic patients receiving long-term oxygen therapy. *Chest* **105**: 469–474.
168. Law S, Boyd S, Macdonald J *et al.* (2014) Predictors of survival in patients with chronic obstructive pulmonary disease receiving long-term oxygen therapy. *BMJ Support Palliat Care* **4**: 140–145.
169. Hajizadeh N, Goldfeld K, Crothers K. (2014) What happens to patients with COPD with long-term oxygen treatment who receive mechanical ventilation for COPD exacerbation? A 1-year retrospective follow-up study. *Thorax* **205–248**:
170. (1981) Long term domiciliary oxygen therapy in chronic hypoxic cor pulmonale complicating chronic bronchitis and emphysema. Report of the Medical Research Council Working Party. *Lancet* **1**: 681–686.

171. (1980) Continuous or nocturnal oxygen therapy in hypoxemic chronic obstructive lung disease: A clinical trial. Nocturnal oxygen therapy trial group. *Ann Intern Med* **93**: 391–398.
172. Cranston JM, Crockett AJ, Moss JR *et al.* (2005) Domiciliary oxygen for chronic obstructive pulmonary disease. *Cochrane Database Syst Rev*: CD001744.
173. (2008) Fatal fires associated with smoking during long-term oxygen therapy –Maine, Massachusetts, New Hampshire, and Oklahoma, 2000–2007. *MMWR. Morbid Mortal Wkly Rep* **57**: 852–854.
174. Spruit MA, Singh SJ, Garvey C *et al.* (2013) An official american thoracic society/european respiratory society statement: Key concepts and advances in pulmonary rehabilitation. *Am J Respir Crit Care Med* **188**: e13–e64.
175. Ries AL, Bauldoff GS, Carlin BW *et al.* (2007) Pulmonary Rehabilitation: Joint ACCP/AACVPR Evidence-Based Clinical Practice Guidelines. *Chest* **131**: 4S–42S.
176. Bolton CE, Bevan-Smith EF, Blakey JD *et al.* (2013) British Thoracic Society guideline on pulmonary rehabilitation in adults. *Thorax* **68** (Suppl 2):ii1–ii30.
177. Marciniuk DD, Brooks D, Butcher S *et al.* (2010) Optimizing pulmonary rehabilitation in chronic obstructive pulmonary disease-practical issues: A Canadian thoracic society clinical practice guideline. *Can Respir J* **17**: 159–168.
178. Seymour JM, Moore L, Jolley CJ *et al.* (2010) Outpatient pulmonary rehabilitation following acute exacerbations of COPD. *Thorax* **65**: 423–428.
179. Puhan MA, Gimeno-Santos E, Scharplatz M *et al.* (2011) Pulmonary rehabilitation following exacerbations of chronic obstructive pulmonary disease. *Cochrane Database Syst Rev*: CD005305.
180. Boxall AM, Barclay L, Sayers A *et al.* (2005) Managing chronic obstructive pulmonary disease in the community. A randomized controlled trial of home-based pulmonary rehabilitation for elderly housebound patients. *J Cardiopulm Rehabil* **25**: 378–385.
181. Katsura H, Kanemaru A, Yamada K *et al.* (2004) Long-term effectiveness of an inpatient pulmonary rehabilitation program for elderly COPD patients: Comparison between young-elderly and old-elderly groups. *Respirol* **9**: 230–236.

182. Baltzan MA, Kamel H, Alter A *et al.* (2004) Pulmonary rehabilitation improves functional capacity in patients 80 years of age or older. *Can Respir J* **11**: 407–413.
183. Couser JI, Jr., Guthmann R, Hamadeh MA *et al.* (1995) Pulmonary rehabilitation improves exercise capacity in older elderly patients with COPD. *Chest* **107**: 730–734.
184. Sundararajan L, Balami J, Packham S. (2010) Effectiveness of outpatient pulmonary rehabilitation in elderly patients with chronic obstructive pulmonary disease. *J Cardiopulm Rehabil Prev* **30**: 121–125.
185. Di Meo F, Pedone C, Lubich S *et al.* (2008) Age does not hamper the response to pulmonary rehabilitation of COPD patients. *Age Ageing* **37**: 530–535.
186. Hornikx M, Van Remoortel H, Demeyer H *et al.* (2013) The influence of comorbidities on outcomes of pulmonary rehabilitation programs in patients with COPD: a systematic review. *Bio Med Res Int* **2013**: 146–148.
187. Crisafulli E, Gorgone P, Vagaggini B *et al.* (2010) Efficacy of standard rehabilitation in COPD outpatients with comorbidities. *Eur Respir J* **36**: 1042–1048.
188. Breyer MK, Breyer-Kohansal R, Funk GC *et al.* (2010) Nordic walking improves daily physical activities in COPD: A randomised controlled trial. *Respir Res* **11**: 112.
189. Solway S, Brooks D, Lau L *et al.* (2002) The short-term effect of a rollator on functional exercise capacity among individuals with severe COPD. *Chest* **122**: 56–65.
190. Honeyman P, Barr P, Stubbing DG. (1996) Effect of a walking aid on disability, oxygenation, and breathlessness in patients with chronic airflow limitation. *J Cardiopulm Rehabil* **16**: 63–67.
191. Vaes AW, Annegarn J, Meijer K *et al.* (2012) The effects of a "new" walking aid on exercise performance in patients with COPD: A randomized crossover trial. *Chest* **141**: 1224–1232.
192. Janssens L, Brumagne S, McConnell AK *et al.* (2013) Proprioceptive changes impair balance control in individuals with chronic obstructive pulmonary disease. *PLoS ONE* **8**: e57949.
193. Beauchamp MK, Janaudis-Ferreira T, Parreira V *et al.* (2013) A randomized controlled trial of balance training during pulmonary rehabilitation for individuals with COPD. *Chest* **144**: 1803–1810.
194. Leung RWM, McKeough ZJ, Peters MJ *et al.* (2013) Short-form Sun-style t'ai chi as an exercise training modality in people with COPD. *Eur Respir J* **41**: 1051–1057.

195. Coventry PA, Hind D. (2007) Comprehensive pulmonary rehabilitation for anxiety and depression in adults with chronic obstructive pulmonary disease: Systematic review and meta-analysis. *J Psychosom Res* **63**: 551–565.
196. Coventry PA. (2009) Does pulmonary rehabilitation reduce anxiety and depression in chronic obstructive pulmonary disease? *Curr Opin Pulm Med* **15**: 143–149.
197. Harrison SL, Greening NJ, Williams JE *et al.* (2012) Have we underestimated the efficacy of pulmonary rehabilitation in improving mood? *Respir Med* **106**: 838–844.
198. Shah RJ, Kotloff RM. (2013) Lung transplantation for obstructive lung diseases. *Semin Respir Crit Care Med* **34**: 288–296.
199. Christie JD, Edwards LB, Kucheryavaya AY *et al.* (2011) The Registry of the international society for heart and lung transplantation: Twenty-eighth adult lung and heart-lung transplant report–2011. *J Heart Lung Transplant* **30**: 1104–1122.
200. Merlo CA, Orens JB. (2010) Candidate selection, overall results, and choosing the right operation. *Semin Respir Crit Care Med* **31**: 99–107.
201. Thabut G, Christie JD, Ravaud P *et al.* (2008) Survival after bilateral versus single lung transplantation for patients with chronic obstructive pulmonary disease: A retrospective analysis of registry data. *Lancet* **371**: 744–751.
202. Maurer JR, Frost AE, Estenne M *et al.* (1998) International guidelines for the selection of lung transplant candidates. The International Society for Heart and Lung Transplantation, the American Thoracic Society, the American Society of Transplant Physicians, the European Respiratory Society. *J Heart Lung Transplant* **17**: 703–709.
203. Orens JB, Estenne M, Arcasoy S *et al.* (2006) International guidelines for the selection of lung transplant candidates: 2006 update–a consensus report from the Pulmonary Scientific Council of the International Society for Heart and Lung Transplantation. *J Heart Lung Transplant* **25**: 745–755.
204. Connors Jr. AF, Dawson NV, Thomas C *et al.* (1996) Outcomes following acute exacerbation of severe chronic obstructive lung disease. The SUPPORT investigators (Study to Understand Prognoses and Preferences for Outcomes and Risks of Treatments). *Am J Respir Crit Care Med* **154**: 959–967.
205. Oga T, Nishimura K, Tsukino M *et al.* (2003) Analysis of the factors related to mortality in chronic obstructive pulmonary disease: Role of

exercise capacity and health status. *Am J Respir Crit Care Med* **167**: 544–549.

206. Swallow EB, Reyes D, Hopkinson NS *et al.* (2007) Quadriceps strength predicts mortality in patients with moderate to severe chronic obstructive pulmonary disease. *Thorax* **62**: 115–120.
207. Spruit MA, Polkey MI, Celli B *et al.* (2012) Predicting outcomes from 6-minute walk distance in chronic obstructive pulmonary disease. *Journal of the American Medical Directors Association* **13**: 291–297.
208. (2001) Patients at high risk of death after lung-volume-reduction surgery. *New Engl J Med* **345**: 1075–1083.
209. Vestbo J, Edwards LD, Scanlon PD *et al.* (2011) Changes in forced expiratory volume in 1 second over time in COPD. *New Engl J Med* **365**: 1184–1192.
210. Nishimura M, Makita H, Nagai K *et al.* (2012) Annual change in pulmonary function and clinical phenotype in chronic obstructive pulmonary disease. *Am J Respir Crit Care Med* **185**: 44–52.
211. Egan TM, Murray S, Bustami RT *et al.* (2006) Development of the new lung allocation system in the United States. *Am J Transplant* **6**: 1212–1227.
212. Egan TM, Kotloff RM. (2005) Pro/Con debate: Lung allocation should be based on medical urgency and transplant survival and not on waiting time. *Chest* **128**: 407–415.
213. Yusen RD, Shearon TH, Qian Y *et al.* (2010) Lung transplantation in the United States, 1999–2008. *Am J Transplant* **10**: 1047–1068.
214. McCurry KR, Shearon TH, Edwards LB *et al.* (2009) Lung transplantation in the United States, 1998–2007. *Am J Transplant* **9**: 942–958.
215. Nunley DR, Bauldoff GS, Holloman CH *et al.* (2009) The lung allocation score and survival in lung transplant candidates with chronic obstructive pulmonary disease. *Lung* **187**: 383–387.
216. TenVergert EM, Vermeulen KM, Geertsma A *et al.* (2001) Quality of life before and after lung transplantation in patients with emphysema versus other indications. *Psychological Rep* **89**: 707–717.
217. Gross CR, Savik K, Bolman RM *et al.* (1995) Long-term health status and quality of life outcomes of lung transplant recipients. *Chest* **108**: 1587–1593.
218. Limbos MM, Joyce DP, Chan CK *et al.* (2000) Psychological functioning and quality of life in lung transplant candidates and recipients. *Chest* **118**: 408–416.

219. Vermeulen KM, Groen H, van der Bij W *et al.* (2004) The effect of bronchiolitis obliterans syndrome on health related quality of life. *Clin Transplant* **18**: 377–383.
220. Christie JD, Edwards LB, Kucheryavaya AY *et al.* (2012) The registry of the international society for heart and lung transplantation: 29th adult lung and heart-lung transplant report-2012. *J Heart Lung Transplant* **31**: 1073–1086.
221. Smith PW, Wang H, Parini V *et al.* (2006) Lung transplantation in patients 60 years and older: Results, complications, and outcomes. *Ann Thorac Surg* **82**: 1835–1841.
222. Weiss ES, Merlo CA *et al.* (2009) Impact of advanced age in lung transplantation: An analysis of United Network for Organ Sharing data. *J Am Coll Surg* **208**: 400–409.
223. Fishman A, Martinez F, Naunheim K *et al.* (2003) A randomized trial comparing lung-volume-reduction surgery with medical therapy for severe emphysema. *New Engl J Med* **348**: 2059–2073.
224. Tutic M, Lardinois D, Imfeld S *et al.* (2006) Lung-volume reduction surgery as an alternative or bridging procedure to lung transplantation. *Annals Thorac Surg* **82**: 208–213.
225. Burns KE, Keenan RJ, Grgurich WF. (2002) Outcomes of lung volume reduction surgery followed by lung transplantation: A matched cohort study. *Ann Thorac Surg* **73**: 1587–1593.
226. Nathan SD, Edwards LB, Barnett SD *et al.* (2004) Outcomes of COPD lung transplant recipients after lung volume reduction surgery. *Chest* **126**: 1569–1574.
227. Backhus L, Sargent J, Cheng A *et al.* (2014) Outcomes in lung transplantation after previous lung volume reduction surgery in a contemporary cohort. *J Thorac Cardiovasc Surg* **147**: 1678–1683.
228. Grimm J, Valero V, Kilic A *et al.* (2014) Performance status impacts mortality following lung transplantation. *J Heart Lung Transplant* **33**: S80–S80.
229. Li M, Mathur S, Chowdhury NA *et al.* (2013) Pulmonary rehabilitation in lung transplant candidates. *J Heart Lung Transplant* **32**: 626–632.
230. Langer D, Burtin C, Schepers L *et al.* (2012) Exercise training after lung transplantation improves participation in daily activity: A randomized controlled trial. *Am J Transplant* **12**: 1584–1592.
231. Wickerson L, Mathur S, Brooks D. (2010) Exercise training after lung transplantation: a systematic review. *J Heart Lung Transplant* **29**: 497–503.

232. Munro PE, Holland AE, Bailey M *et al.* (2009) Pulmonary rehabilitation following lung transplantation. *Transplant Proc* **41**: 292–295.
233. Seneff MG, Wagner DP, Wagner RP *et al.* (1995) Hospital and 1-year survival of patients admitted to intensive care units with acute exacerbation of chronic obstructive pulmonary disease. *JAMA* **274**: 1852–1857.
234. Carlucci A, Guerrieri A, Nava S. (2012) Palliative care in COPD patients: Is it only an end-of-life issue? *Eur Respir Rev* **21**: 347–354.
235. Janssen DJ, McCormick JR. (2014) Palliative care and pulmonary rehabilitation. *Clin Chest Med* **35**: 411–421.
236. Lanken PN, Terry PB, Delisser HM *et al.* (2008) An official American Thoracic Society clinical policy statement: Palliative care for patients with respiratory diseases and critical illnesses. *Am J Respir Crit Care Med* **177**: 912–927.
237. Gelberg J, McIvor RA. (2010) Overcoming gaps in the management of chronic obstructive pulmonary disease in older patients: New insights. *Drugs Aging* **27**: 367–375.
238. Curtis JR. (2008) Palliative and end-of-life care for patients with severe COPD. *Eur Respir J* **32**: 796–803.

Chapter 15

Genomics of Lung Aging and Idiopathic Pulmonary Fibrosis

Brenda Juan-Guardela* and Naftali Kaminski*,†

1. Introduction

Idiopathic pulmonary fibrosis (IPF) is a chronic interstitial lung disease of unknown etiology that affects elderly adults. IPF is thought to result from repeated cycles of alveolar epithelial cell injury causing fibroblast proliferation and exaggerated accumulation of extracellular matrix in the lung parenchyma.[1] The incidence and prevalence of IPF increases significantly with age, being higher among patients older than 75 years,[2] therefore IPF has been generally considered a disease of aging.

Aging or senescence is determined by molecular and phenotypic changes in an organism that ultimately lead to functional decline and death. Even though aging is considered a physiologic process in humans, it is unclear why IPF is more prevalent in elderly adults. Genome-Scale Transcript Profiling technologies such as microarrays and RNA sequencing have facilitated the study of the pathogenesis IPF by providing an unbiased catalog of the genomic and

* Section of Pulmonary, Critical Care and Sleep Medicine; Yale University School of Medicine, 300 Cedar Street, TAC-S44ID, New Haven, CT 06510, USA.
† Corresponding author.

transcriptional changes that characterize the IPF lung. While the relationship between IPF and aging has not been directly studied at the genome-scale level, the results from genomic studies in IPF have provided several clues to this relationship, as did genomic studies in human cell lines.

To better comprehend the relationship between IPF and aging, we will focus in this chapter on the contribution of genomic studies in understanding the hallmarks of aging in IPF. These hallmarks were defined by López-Otín as genomic instability, epigenetic alterations, telomere attrition, loss of proteostasis, deregulated nutrient sensing, mitochondrial dysfunction, stem cell exhaustion, altered intercellular communication and cellular senescence.[3]

2. Hallmarks of Aging in IPF

2.1. *Genomic instability*

Genomic stability is maintained by powerful repair mechanisms to ensure DNA integrity. The misbalance between DNA damage and repair leads to accumulation of mutations resulting in cell death.[4] There is evidence that supports that DNA damage and mutations may contribute to senescence.[5] Examples of this, are several progeroid syndromes, such as Werner syndrome and Bloom syndrome that have been associated with DNA helicase defects and others such as Cockayne syndrome, Xeroderma pigmantosum and Trichothiodystrophy that have been linked to nucleotide excision repair mutations, implying a possible connection that resembles the process of natural aging.[6,7] Generally speaking, pulmonary fibrosis is not commonly described in these syndromes.

Strong evidence supports that genomic instability occurs in the IPF lung. For example, microsatellite instability (MSI) and loss of heterozygocity (LOH) are frequently found in sputum obtained from patients with IPF.[8] Vassilakis *et al.*, assessed the incidence of MSI and LOH in sputum of IPF patients compared to healthy controls. They found that 50% of the IPF patients had at least one of these genetic variations. However, there was no difference in the subgroup analysis of IPF patients with any genetic variation (MSI and/or LOH positive) and the ones without (MSI/LOH negative) in relation to age. Smoking per se, did not appear to be related to MSI and LOH in this study, since IPF smokers did not have increased frequency of these genetic abnormalities when compared to IPF non-smokers. Comparative proteome analysis of lung tissue from patients with IPF and controls showed an increased expression of DNA damage stress, specifically DNA damage-binding protein 1, indicating a potential role in disease pathogenesis.[9] Likewise, increased expression levels of p21 and p53 related to DNA damage have been described in IPF lung epithelial cells possibly as a compensatory mechanism to repair DNA.[10] A recent large genome-wide association study (GWAS) revealed that genetic variations in TERC and TERT, (discussed below), were associated with fibrotic interstitial pneumonias.[11]

2.2. *Epigenetic changes*

Changes in the epigenome are strongly associated with aging.[12] Epigenome refers to modifications of the chromatin without changes in the DNA sequence. The epigenetic mechanisms that regulate gene expression include DNA methylation, histone modifications and non-coding RNA expression. The first mechanism is related to gene silencing through enzymes (DNA methyltransferases) that add a methyl group to the 5′ position of the cytosine. Hypermethylation of CpG islands in gene promoters represses transcription, in contrast to hypomethylation that promotes gene expression. The second mechanism involves histone acetylation, methylation, phosphorylation and ubiquitination. These changes are considered histone marks, which may represent a key step between signaling pathways that extend lifespan and the expression profiles of genes related to longevity.[13] Lastly, non-coding RNA expression is critical for gene regulation at the transcriptional and post-transcriptional level. Among the most widely studied non-coding RNAs are microRNAs, which negatively regulate the expression of a targeted mRNA and long non-coding RNAs (lncRNAs), which have been associated with chromatin modifying complexes to regulate gene expression.

DNA methylation has been linked to aging and longevity in different organisms[14] and both DNA hypomethylation and hypermethylation have been reported with age.[15] Christensen *et al.*, evaluated methylation changes associated with age in normal human tissues from 10 different anatomical sites and found that *ESR1, GSTP1, IGF2*, *MGMT, MYOD1, RARB*, and *RASSF1* had significant alterations in age-associated hypermethylation.[16] Another study in elderly individuals evaluated DNA methylation in the Alu and LINE-1 sequences and aging.[17] This study showed that while DNA methylation in the Alu sequences declined over time as the subjects get older, LINE-1 methylation did not change with age. This data proposes that genome-wide losses of methylation may be responsible for the increase in rate of common diseases with aging. Also, there is evidence that tissue-specific differences in DNA methylation with age[18] and DNA methylation profiles can predict age of multiple human cells and tissues.[19,20]

Three studies that applied genome scale DNA methylation profiling approaches to IPF lungs revealed extensive changes in methylation patterns. Rabinovich *et al.*, identified 625 differentially methylated CpG islands between IPF and healthy individuals using DNA immunoprecipitation and Agilent CpG island arrays. The authors also compared methylation profiles of IPF, lung cancer and controls, illustrating an intermediate methylation pattern in IPF lungs somewhat similar to lung cancer with an overlap of 402 differentially methylated CpG islands.[21] This study is of particular interest given the fact that cancer and IPF are both diseases of aging and also because trends of global hypomethylation and promoter hypermethylation found in cancer have also been observed in normal tissues with aging[12] suggesting a relationship between CpG island methylation and aging in IPF. Sanders *et al.* identified 870 differentially methylated DNA regions when comparing IPF and controls by using the Illumina Human Methylation 27 BeadChip and found an overlap of 35 genes from DNA methylation and RNA gene expression, of which 16 genes had inverse DNA methylation and RNA expression.[22] Yang *et al.*, performed the most extensive study so far. By applying comprehensive high throughput arrays for relative methylation arrays

(CHARM) and gene expression microarrays to lung samples obtained from 94 IPF and 67 control lungs they identified 2130 differentially methylated regions. Inverse relationship between DNA methylation and RNA expression was found in 738 of these regions, some of which including genes such as TOLLIP, NOTCH1 and FBXO32 that could be implicated in IPF pathogenesis.

One of the limitations of the aforementioned studies is that they focused on lung tissue lysates and not in specific cell subtypes, which can differ in methylation profiles. As an example, Sanders *et al.*, demonstrated hypermethylation of the promoter of Thy-1, an anti-fibrotic gene, in lung fibroblasts.[23] Methylation of the Thy-1 promoter induced by hypoxia led to suppressed Thy-1 expression and activation of a myofibroblast phenotype.[24] These observations demonstrate the importance of studying cell specific methylation patterns; they also demonstrate the difference between changes in the methylation of specific promoters and global changes in methylation. Although DNA methylation changes have been associated with aging, we have still to demonstrate whether the changes are similar in IPF and aging.

The role of histone modifications as a key contributor of senescence has been reported. A study in human fibroblasts has shown that histone deacetylase inhibitors induce a senescence-like state raising the possibility that epigenetic changes play a role in aging.[25] In contrast, another study revealed that global and chromatin-specific histone modifications led to an imbalance in the Bcl-2:Bax gene expression (high levels of the anti-apoptotic gene Bcl2 and low levels of the pro-apoptotic Bax gene) contributing to apoptosis-resistant phenotype in senescent fibroblasts.[26] These findings suggest a strong connection between histone modifications and the aging process, yet the direct effect of histone modifications in IPF and aging has not been defined. In a murine model, histone modifications (increased histone deacelylases) seemed to be responsible for decreased Fas expression, a cell death receptor, and to resistance to apoptosis in fibrotic lung fibroblasts,[27] suggesting a potential mechanism in disease pathogenesis.

There is growing literature about the function of microRNAs in many biological processes including senescence. Identification of several microRNAs that target genes implicated in age-associated signaling pathways, such as insulin/IGF signaling and TOR signaling, have been associated with human age-related disorders including cardiovascular and neurodegenerative disease.[28] The microRNAs known to participate in cellular senescence are the members of the mir-34 family, especially mir-34a[29] targeting the p53/RB pathway, mir-17-92 cluster through PTEN resulting in suppression of the insulin/IGF-1 pathway,[30] and the upregulation of let-7[31] and mir-21.[32] MicroRNA expression studies have revealed that microRNAs are differentially expressed in IPF and they are thought to play an important role in IPF pathogenesis. Mir-34a[33] and mir-21[34] are upregulated both in IPF and aging. Similarly, the mir 17–92 cluster is downregulated in both IPF and aging.[35] In contrast, let-7[36] as well as mir-29 and mir-30,[37] are increased in aging but decreased in IPF.[38] As the mechanistic roles of microRNAs in IPF are being revealed, their relative contribution to aging and *vice versa* will need to be systematically dissected.

More recently, emerging interest in the study of lncRNAs have uncovered their role in gene expression regulation,[39] diverse biological processes and human diseases. Many lncRNAs modulate several cellular processes well-known as the hallmark of aging, such as telomere attrition, epigenetic regulation, proteostasis, intercellular communication, stem cell function and cell proliferation.[40] In this context it is important to note that many telomerase pathway components are lncRNAs. The best-known scaffold lncRNA is probably TERC, the RNA subunit of the Telomerase[41] and TERRA is an important component of Telomerase heterochromatin[42] suggesting that both have significant roles in aging. The potential role of telomerase mutations (including TERC) in IPF is discussed below.

2.3. *Telomere attrition*

Telomere shortening, another hallmark of aging, has been repeatedly observed in IPF. Telomeres are regions of noncoding DNA sequences at the end of the chromosomes, whose function is essential to maintain chromosomal stability, therefore preventing deterioration or fusion with other chromosomes. Some forms of familial pulmonary fibrosis are caused by mutations in telomerase maintaining genes such as TERT, hTR, TERC[43,44] and RTEL1.[45] Also, short telomeres without telomerase mutations have been described in sporadic cases of IPF.[46,47] Genome Wide Association Studies (GWAS) demonstrated associations of single-nucleotide polymorphisms (SNPs) in the TERT, TERC and OBFC1, genes that maintain the integrity of the telomeres length, also with sporadic IPF. The first GWAS study found a significant association of a SNP in intron 2 of the TERT gene (rs2736100) with IPF.[48] The second, more recent and larger GWAS, identified common variants in TERT, TERC and OBFC1 in a large population of individuals with fibrotic interstitial pneumonias.[11] Interestingly, cigarette smoking, an important risk factor for IPF[49] and other age-related diseases, has been linked to shortened telomere length in a dose-dependent fashion.[50] This finding may suggest that tobacco exposure may be a potential link between the fibrotic response in IPF and accelerated aging.

2.4. *Loss of proteostasis*

The proteostasis network consists of molecular chaperones, stress-response transcription factors, and intracellular protein degradation that sense and respond to proteotoxic stress and protein misfolding to ensure cell viability.[51] The loss of proteostasis has been previously linked with aging[52] by the accumulation of unfolded or misfolded proteins in age-related disorders including Alzheimer and Parkinson's disease.[52] In the case of IPF, different abnormal proteostasis mechanisms such as endoplasmic reticulum stress[53] and unfolded protein response[54] have been proposed. ER stress facilitates fibrotic remodeling through activation of pro-apoptotic pathways, changes in epithelial cell phenotype, and promotion of remodeling. In fact, some of the genetic mutations that lead to pulmonary fibrosis, such as mutations in surfactant proteins lead to expression of ER stress markers in lung epithelial cells.[55] Tanjore *et al.* developed mice that expressed the human SFTPC mutation in type II alveolar epithelial cells. This expression led ER stress in the cells but not to development of lung fibrosis. However, the mice were more sensitive to fibrosis when exposed to bleomycin. Similarly, intratracheal administration of tunicamycin, an agent that causes ER stress, increased the sensitivity of the mice to lung fibrosis.[56] These findings suggest that in mice, and maybe humans, ER stress can enhance a predisposition to fibrosis caused by environmental agents.

2.5. *Deregulated nutrient sensing*

The Insulin and IGF signaling (ISS) pathway and its targets, the FOXO family of transcription factors and the mTOR multiprotein complex are the most conserved aging-controlling pathways in evolution. Several studies have demonstrated the relevance of the ISS signaling pathway as a critical regulator of aging in several experimental models. In yeast, flies and worms, disruption of the insulin/IGF-1 signaling has been shown to increase lifespan[57–59] and reduced IGF-1 levels are associated with prolonged longevity in dwarf mice.[60] Similarly, individuals with mutations in the growth hormone receptor that leads to marked IGF-1 deficiency have decreased prevalence of age-related disorders such as cancer and diabetes.[61]

The relevance of the IGF1 pathway in lung fibrosis has been demonstrated in animal models of lung fibrosis and *in vitro*.[62] Mice with IGF1 receptor blockade demonstrated improved survival after bleomycin injury compared with control mice and treatment of fibroblasts with an IGF1 receptor antagonist resulted in increased fibroblast apoptosis. In humans, microarray studies have shown that IGF-1 is overexpressed in the fibrotic lung tissue when compared to lung tissue from healthy controls.[63] While there is clear evidence for increased IGF-1 signaling in IPF lungs, it's role in the context of aging mechanisms in lung fibrosis is unclear nor is the direct pathogenic role of this pathway.

Another relationship between the IGF-1 pathway, IPF pathogenesis and aging comes from the observation from microarray studies that Insulin Growth Factor Binding Proteins (IGFBP), which serve as carries for IGF-1,[64] are also overexpressed in lung tissue from IPF patients[65] and in fibroblast cell lines from subjects with IPF.[66] IGFBP5, one of the overexpressed IGFBPs in IPF, also causes pulmonary fibrosis in mice and induces migration of primary human lung fibroblast *in vitro.* These findings are of particular interest since *in vitro* studies have also shown that IGFBPs are overexpressed in different models of senescence[67–69] suggesting a relationship between overexpression of IGF1 pathway members and aging in lung fibrosis.

2.6. *Mitochondrial dysfunction*

The link between mitochondrial dysfunction and aging has been extensively studied.[70] The initial premise postulated by Harman[71] was that reactive oxygen species (ROS) excess, produced by mitochondria, had deleterious effects on various cell components and induced cell damage. Albeit appealing, this hypothesis has been challenged by a series of studies showing that mice with increased mitochondrial ROS and oxidative damage do not age prematurely[72,73] and also by the fact that increases in ROS appears to prolong lifespan in C. elegans.[74,75] An alternative hypothesis suggests that mitochondrial dysfunction, independent of ROS, can be associated with aging. This observation comes from the fact that mitochondrial DNA (mtDNA) mutations in somatic stem cells drive progeroid phenotypes without increasing oxidative stress in mtDNA mutated mice, thus indicating that bioenergentic deficiency resulting from mtDNA mutated is an important driver in the aging process.[76]

In IPF, a recent report by Bueno *et al.*[77] demonstrated that alveolar epithelial cells of patients with IPF had accumulation of dysmorphic and dysfunctional mitochondria and these mitochondria were associated with markers of ER stress. The investigators also found a significant decrease in expression of PTEN-induced putative kinase 1 (PINK1) in lungs of IPF patients when compared to healthy control as well as a significant correlation between PINK1 expression with pro-apoptotic pathways in lung tissue from IPF patients. Interestingly, young PINK1-deficient mice developed dysfunctional mitochondria and alveolar epithelial cell apoptosis suggesting a relationship between mitochondrial dysfunction and age in pulmonary fibrosis.

Shuang Huang *et al.*[78] also explored the role of mitochondrial function in IPF pathogenesis by studying the expression of lysocardiolipin acyltransferase (LYCAT), a cardiolipin-remodeling enzyme necessary for maintaining normal mitochondrial function, in lung tissue and peripheral blood mononuclear cells (PBMCs) from patients with IPF. The investigators identified significant LYCAT underexpression in lung tissue from IPF patients as well as significant correlation between LYCAT expression in PBMCs and carbon monoxide diffusion capacity (DLCO) as well as patient survival. Moreover, in two mice models of lung fibrosis (bleomycin and radiation induced lung fibrosis), LYCAT overexpression reduced lung fibrosis whereas LYCAT silencing increased fibrosis. *In vitro* experiments demonstrated that LYCAT provided protection against apoptosis of alveolar epithelial cells. While this study did not look at the association between LYCAT expression and age in IPF, it did suggest the potential role of mitochondrial function in IPF pathogenesis and progression. In the context of genomics, all of these observations were, supported by transcriptomic profiling of human IPF lungs.

2.7. *Stem cell exhaustion*

Stem cell exhaustion is characterized by deterioration in the regenerative capacity of cells and tissues. Type II alveolar epithelial cells (AEC) are thought to be progenitor cells in IPF.[79] The abnormal re-epithelization of type II AEC results in stem cell exhaustion possibly due to premature cell senescence as a result of genetic mutations (telomerase mutations and abnormal surfactant proteins) and environmental exposures (cigarette smoking, pollution, toxic substances and infections).[79,80]

Evidence of altered gene expression profiles associated with abnormal re-epithelization has been shown in IPF patients with acute exacerbations. Acute exacerbations of IPF (IPF-AEx) are clinically significant deteriorations of unidentifiable cause in patients with IPF[81] associated with the pathological pattern of diffuse alveolar damage superimposed on the underlying usual interstitial pneumonia (UIP). Konishi *et al.* studied gene expression profiles in lungs of IPF patients with acute exacerbation (IPF-AEx) and compared them to stable IPF.[63] A signature of 579 differentially expressed genes was identified between both groups with no indication of an infectious or inflammatory etiology. Interestingly, the authors found increased expression of cyclinA2 (CCNA2, a cell-cycle regulator), as well as alveolar epithelial cell apoptosis by tunnel staining. The concomitant presence of apoptosis and markers of accelerated epithelial cell proliferation in patients with IPF-AEx could represent a compensatory response to injury and epithelial cell exhaustion suggesting the importance of epithelial cell exhaustion in IPF progression.

2.8. *Altered intercellular communication*

Alterations at the level of cellular communication have been associated with aging as a consequence of a proinflammatory state[82] which could potentially lead to abnormal autophagy[83] and cellular senescence.[84] This hypothesis, is based on a series of observations including a meta-analysis of gene expression profiles of 27 different microarray datasets in aging human, mice and rats which demonstrated that age-related changes across species were associated with a constant overexpression of inflammatory and immune response genes as well as lysosome-associated genes[85], a phenomenon described as "inflamm-aging".

While there is no evidence of how "inflamm-aging" directly affects IPF, one can hypothesize that recurrent antigenic exposure and stress, such as cigarette smoking, viruses or microaspirations, can lead to a pro-inflammatory state resulting in altered cross-talk between alveolar epithelial cells and fibroblasts leading to the aberrant wound healing response that is characteristic of IPF. However, the lack of benefit from anti-inflammatory and immunosuppressive agents in IPF suggests that inflammation does not play a central role in IPF pathogenesis.

2.9. *Cellular senescence*

Cellular senescence is defined as a permanent arrest of the cell cycle[86] that results from DNA damage, telomere shortening or replicative senescence, stress and oncogene activation. The complexity of cellular senescence in humans was demonstrated by Zhang *et al.*[87] who performed genome-scale transcript profiling in human fibroblasts cell lines and mammary epithelial cells. The investigators demonstrated that replicative senescence changes in gene expression differed greatly in fibroblast and mammary epithelial cells suggesting that cell senescence is a complex process that varies in different cell lines and tissues. Acknowledging this complexity is essential to understand that in IPF, the process of senescence in different cell lines (i.e. alveolar epithelial cells, fibroblast, immune cells) may contribute differently to disease pathogenesis and progression.

It is generally accepted that the ability to mount an immune response declines as the individual grows older. The process by which the host innate and adaptive immune response deteriorate with age is called immunosenescence,[88] which increases the susceptibility for infectious diseases and cancer. Age-related changes include an decrease of the naïve CD4 *T* cells with an expansion of the memory CD4 *T* cells,[89] changes in the *T* cell receptor signal transduction,[90] low IL-2 production[91] and loss of CD28 in CD4 and CD8 *T* cells.[92] Studies of gene expression in peripheral blood mononuclear cells (PMBCs) in IPF have demonstrated that low levels of CD28 have a strong correlation with outcome. Gilani *et al.*, demonstrated that the down-regulation of CD28 on circulating CD24 *T* cells was correlated with poor outcomes in patients with IPF.[93] Herazo-Maya *et al.* performed gene expression microarrays on PBMCs obtained from patients with IPF.[94] They identified a signature of 52 genes associated with decreased transplant-free survival in two independent cohorts. Notably the downregulation of genes belonging to the "costimulatory signal during *T* cell activation" Biocarta pathway was associated with poor outcome in IPF suggesting that immunosenescence might be important in the disease.

3. Conclusions

IPF is an age-related disease of unknown etiology with a progressive and lethal course. Results from genome-scale transcript profiling studies have elicited new insights and better understanding of the biological processes involved in IPF pathogenesis and their relationship with the aging process. The evidence presented in this chapter indicate that while some pathways related to aging seem to be active in IPF, others are not. Because of the complexity of the pathways and cellular populations that eventually lead to the lung phenotype in IPF it is clear that more detailed studies that dissect cell, genotype, environment and matrix interactions in the context of aging are required.

References

1. Selman M, Pardo A. (2002) Idiopathic pulmonary fibrosis: An epithelial/fibroblastic cross-talk disorder. *Respir Res* **3**: 3.
2. Raghu G, Weycker D, Edelsberg J *et al.* (2006) Incidence and prevalence of idiopathic pulmonary fibrosis. *Am J Respir Critic Care Med* **174**: 810–816.
3. Lopez-Otin C, Blasco MA, Partridge L *et al.* (2013) The hallmarks of aging. *Cell* **153**: 1194–1217.
4. Erol A. (2011) Deciphering the intricate regulatory mechanisms for the cellular choice between cell repair, apoptosis or senescence in response to damaging signals. *Cellular Signal* **23**: 1076–1081.
5. Moskalev AA, Shaposhnikov MV, Plyusnina EN *et al.* (2013) The role of DNA damage and repair in aging through the prism of Koch-like criteria. *Ageing Res Rev* **12**: 661–684.
6. Burtner CR, Kennedy BK. (2010) Progeria syndromes and ageing: What is the connection? *Nature reviews. Mol Cell Biol* **11**: 567–578.
7. Puzianowska–Kuznicka, M, Kuznicki J. (2005) Genetic alterations in accelerated ageing syndromes. Do they play a role in natural ageing? *Int J Biochem Cell Biol* **37**: 947–960.
8. Vassilakis DA, Sourvinos G, Spandidos DA *et al.* (2000) Frequent genetic alterations at the microsatellite level in cytologic sputum samples of patients with idiopathic pulmonary fibrosis. *Am J Respir Critic Care Med* **162**: 1115–1119.

9. Korfei M, Schmitt S, Ruppert C *et al.* (2011) Comparative proteomic analysis of lung tissue from patients with idiopathic pulmonary fibrosis (IPF) and lung transplant donor lungs. *J Proteome Res* **10**: 2185–2205.
10. Kuwano K, Kunitake R, Kawasaki M *et al.* (1996) P21Waf1/Cip1/Sdi1 and p53 expression in association with DNA strand breaks in idiopathic pulmonary fibrosis. *Am J Respir Critic Care Med* **154**: 477–483.
11. Fingerlin TE, Murphy E, Zhang W *et al.* (2013) Genome-wide association study identifies multiple susceptibility loci for pulmonary fibrosis. *Nat Genet* **45**: 613–620.
12. Fraga MF, Esteller M. (2007) Epigenetics and aging: The targets and the marks. *Trends Genet* **23**: 413–418.
13. Han S, Brunet A. (2012) Histone methylation makes its mark on longevity. *Trends Cell Biol* **22**: 42–49.
14. Johnson AA, Akman K, Calimport SR *et al.* (2012) The role of DNA methylation in aging, rejuvenation, and age-related disease. *Rev Res* **15**: 483–494.
15. Bell JT, Tsai PC, Yang TP *et al.* (2012) Epigenome-wide scans identify differentially methylated regions for age and age-related phenotypes in a healthy ageing population. *PLoS genetics* **8**: e1002629.
16. Christensen BC, Houseman EA, Marsit CJ *et al.* (2009) Aging and environmental exposures alter tissue-specific DNA methylation dependent upon CpG island context. *PLoS genetics* **5**: e1000602.
17. Bollati V, Schwartz J, Wright R *et al.* (2009) Decline in genomic DNA methylation through aging in a cohort of elderly subjects. *Mechan Ageing Dev* **130**: 234–239.
18. Thompson RF, Atzmon G, Gheorghe C *et al.* (2010) Tissue-specific dysregulation of DNA methylation in aging. *Aging cell* **9**: 506–518.
19. Horvath S. (2013) DNA methylation age of human tissues and cell types. *Genome Biol* **14**: R115.
20. Hannum G, Guinney J, Zhao L *et al.* (2013) Genome-wide methylation profiles reveal quantitative views of human aging rates. *Mol Cell* **49**: 359–367.
21. Rabinovich EI, Kapetanaki MG, Steinfeld I *et al.* (2012) Global methylation patterns in idiopathic pulmonary fibrosis. *PloS one* **7**: e33770.
22. Sanders YY, Ambalavanan N, Halloran B *et al.* (2012) Altered DNA methylation profile in idiopathic pulmonary fibrosis. *Am J Respir Critic Care Med* **186**: 525–535.

23. Sanders YY, Pardo A, Selman M *et al.* (2008) Thy-1 promoter hypermethylation: A novel epigenetic pathogenic mechanism in pulmonary fibrosis. *Am J Respir Cell Mol Biol* **39**: 610–618.
24. Robinson CM, Neary R, Levendale A *et al.* (2012) Hypoxia-induced DNA hypermethylation in human pulmonary fibroblasts is associated with Thy-1 promoter methylation and the development of a pro-fibrotic phenotype. *Respir Res* **13**: 74.
25. Ogryzko VV, Hirai TH, Russanova VR *et al.* (1996) Human fibroblast commitment to a senescence-like state in response to histone deacetylase inhibitors is cell cycle dependent. *Mol Cell Biol* **16**: 5210–5218.
26. Sanders YY, Liu H, Zhang X *et al.* (2013) Histone modifications in senescence-associated resistance to apoptosis by oxidative stress. *Red Biol* **1**: 8–16.
27. Huang SK, Scruggs AM, Donaghy J *et al.* (2013) Histone modifications are responsible for decreased Fas expression and apoptosis resistance in fibrotic lung fibroblasts. *Cell Death Dis* **4**: e621.
28. Jung HJ, Suh Y. (2012) MicroRNA in aging: From discovery to biology. *Current Genom* **13**: 548–557.
29. Bommer GT, Gerin I, Feng Y *et al.* (2007) p53-mediated activation of miRNA34 candidate tumor-suppressor genes. *Curr Biol* **17**: 1298–1307.
30. Grillari J, Hackl M, Grillari-Voglauer R. (2010) miR-17-92 cluster: Ups and downs in cancer and aging. *Biogerontol* **11**: 501–506.
31. Johnson CD, Esquela-Kerscher A, Stefani G *et al.* (2007) The let-7 microRNA represses cell proliferation pathways in human cells. *Cancer Res* **67**: 7713–7722.
32. Dellago H, Preschitz-Kammerhofer B, Terlecki-Zaniewicz L *et al.* (2013) High levels of oncomiR-21 contribute to the senescence-induced growth arrest in normal human cells and its knock-down increases the replicative lifespan. *Aging Cell* **12**: 446–458.
33. Honeyman L, Bazett M, TomkoTG *et al.* (2013) MicroRNA profiling implicates the insulin-like growth factor pathway in bleomycin-induced pulmonary fibrosis in mice. *Fibrogenesis Tissue Repair* **6**: 16.
34. Liu G, Friggeri A, Yang Y *et al.* (2010) miR-21 mediates fibrogenic activation of pulmonary fibroblasts and lung fibrosis. *J Exp Med* **207**: 1589–1597.
35. Dakhlallah D, Batte K, Wang Y *et al.* (2013) Epigenetic regulation of miR-17-92 contributes to the pathogenesis of pulmonary fibrosis. *Am J Respir Critic Care Med* **187**: 397–405.

36. Overhoff MG, Garbe JC, Koh J *et al.* (2014) Cellular senescence mediated by p16INK4A-coupled miRNA pathways. *Nucleic Acids Research* **42**: 1606–1618.
37. Martinez I, Cazalla D, Almstead LL *et al.* (2011) miR-29 and miR-30 regulate B-Myb expression during cellular senescence. *Proc Natl Acad Sci USA* **108**: 522–527.
38. Pandit KV, Corcoran D, Yousef H *et al.* (2010) Inhibition and role of let-7d in idiopathic pulmonary fibrosis. *Am J Respir Critic Care Med* **182**: 220–229.
39. Khalil AM, Guttman M, Huarte M *et al.* (2009) Many human large intergenic noncoding RNAs associate with chromatin-modifying complexes and affect gene expression. *Proc Natl Acad Sci USA* **106**: 11667–11672.
40. Grammatikakis I, Panda AC, Abdelmohsen K *et al.* (2014) Long noncoding RNAs(lncRNAs) and the molecular hallmarks of aging. *Aging* **6**: 992–1009.
41. Samper E, Flores JM, Blasco MA. (2001) Restoration of telomerase activity rescues chromosomal instability and premature aging in Terc-/- mice with short telomeres. *EMBO Rep* **2**: 800–807.
42. Redon S, Reichenbach P, Lingner J. (2010) The non-coding RNA TERRA is a natural ligand and direct inhibitor of human telomerase. *Nucleic Acids Res* **38**: 5797–5806.
43. Armanios MY, Chen JJ, Cogan JD *et al.* (2007) Telomerase mutations in families with idiopathic pulmonary fibrosis. *New Engl J Med* **356**: 1317–1326.
44. Tsakiri KD, Cronkhite JT, Kuan PJ *et al.* (2007) Adult-onset pulmonary fibrosis caused by mutations in telomerase. *Proc Natl Acad Sci USA* **104**: 7552–7557.
45. Cogan JD, Kropski JA, Zhao M *et al.* (2015) Rare Variants in RTEL1 are Associated with Familial Interstitial Pneumonia. *Am J Respir Critic Care Med.*
46. Alder JK, Chen JJ, Lancaster L *et al.* (2008) Short telomeres are a risk factor for idiopathic pulmonary fibrosis. *Proc Natl Acad Sci USA* **105**: 13051–13056.
47. Cronkhite JT, Xing C, Raghu G *et al.* (2008) Telomere shortening in familial and sporadic pulmonary fibrosis. *Am J Respir Critic Care Med* **178**: 729–737.
48. Mushiroda T, Wattanapokayakit S, Takahashi A *et al.* (2008) A genome-wide association study identifies an association of a common variant in

TERT with susceptibility to idiopathic pulmonary fibrosis. *J Med Genet* **45**: 654–656.

49. Baumgartner KB, Samet JM, Stidley CA *et al.* (1997) Cigarette smoking: A risk factor for idiopathic pulmonary fibrosis. *Am J Respir Critic Care Med* **155**: 242–248.
50. Valdes AM, Andrew T, Gardner JP *et al.* (2005) Obesity, cigarette smoking, and telomere length in women. *Lancet* **366**: 662–664.
51. Labbadia J, Morimoto RI. (2014) Proteostasis and longevity: When does aging really begin? *F1000 prime reports* **6**: 7.
52. Powers ET, Morimoto RI, Dillin A *et al.* (2009) Biological and chemical approaches to diseases of proteostasis deficiency. *Ann Rev Biochem* **78**: 959–991.
53. Torres-Gonzalez E, Bueno M, Tanaka A *et al.* (2012) Role of endoplasmic reticulum stress in age-related susceptibility to lung fibrosis. *Am J Respir Cell Mol Biol* **46**: 748–756.
54. Tanjore H, Blackwell TS, Lawson WE. (2012) Emerging evidence for endoplasmic reticulum stress in the pathogenesis of idiopathic pulmonary fibrosis. *Am J Physiol. Lung Cell Mol Physiol* **302**: L721–L729.
55. Tanjore H, Lawson WE, Blackwell TS. (2013) Endoplasmic reticulum stress as a pro-fibrotic stimulus. *Biochimica et Biophysica Acta* **1832**: 940–947.
56. Lawson WE, Cheng DS, Degryse AL *et al.* (2011) Endoplasmic reticulum stress enhances fibrotic remodeling in the lungs. *Proc Natl Acad Sci USA* **108**: 10562–10567.
57. Vanfleteren JR, Braeckman BP. (1999) Mechanisms of life span determination in Caenorhabditis elegans. *Neurobiol Aging* **20**: 487–502.
58. Clancy DJ, Gems D, Harshman LG *et al.* (2001) Extension of life-span by loss of CHICO, a Drosophila insulin receptor substrate protein. *Sci* **292**: 104–106.
59. Tissenbaum HA, Ruvkun G. (1998) An insulin-like signaling pathway affects both longevity and reproduction in Caenorhabditis elegans. *Genet* **148**: 703–717.
60. Bartke A, Brown-Borg H. (2004) Life extension in the dwarf mouse. *Curr Topics Dev Biol* **63**: 189–225.
61. Guevara-Aguirre J, Balasubramanian P, Guevara-Aguirre M *et al.* (2011) Growth hormone receptor deficiency is associated with a major reduction in pro-aging signaling, cancer, and diabetes in humans. *Sci Transl Med* **3**: 70ra13.

62. Choi JE, Lee SS, Sunde DA *et al.* (2009) Insulin-like growth factor-I receptor blockade improves outcome in mouse model of lung injury. *Am J Respir Critic Care Med* **179**: 212–219.
63. Konishi K, Gibson KF, LindellK O *et al.* (2009) Gene expression profiles of acute exacerbations of idiopathic pulmonary fibrosis. *Am J Respir Critic Care Med* **180**: 167–175.
64. Stewart CE, Bates PC, Calder TA *et al.* (1993) Potentiation of insulin-like growth factor-I (IGF-I) activity by an antibody: Supportive evidence for enhancement of IGF-I bioavailability in vivo by IGF binding proteins. *Endocrinol* **133**: 1462–1465.
65. Selman M, Pardo A, Barrera L *et al.* (2006) Gene expression profiles distinguish idiopathic pulmonary fibrosis from hypersensitivity pneumonitis. *Am J Respir Critic Care Med* **173**: 188–198.
66. Pilewski JM, Liu L, Henry AC *et al.* (2005) Insulin-like growth factor binding proteins 3 and 5 are overexpressed in idiopathic pulmonary fibrosis and contribute to extracellular matrix deposition. *Am J Pathol* **166**: 399–407.
67. Yoon IK, Kim HK, Kim YK *et al.* (2004) Exploration of replicative senescence-associated genes in human dermal fibroblasts by cDNA microarray technology. *Exp Gerontol* **39**: 1369–1378.
68. Moerman EJ, Thweatt R, Moerman AM *et al.* (1993) Insulin-like growth factor binding protein-3 is overexpressed in senescent and quiescent human fibroblasts. *Exp Gerontol* **28**: 361–370.
69. Goldstein S, Moerman EJ, Baxter RC. (1993) Accumulation of insulin-like growth factor binding protein-3 in conditioned medium of human fibroblasts increases with chronologic age of donor and senescence in vitro. *J Cell Physiol* **156**: 294–302.
70. Bratic A, Larsson NG. (2013) The role of mitochondria in aging. *J Clin Invest* **123**: 951–957.
71. Harman D. (1965) The free radical theory of A-aging: Effect of age on serum copper levels. *J Gerontol* **20**: 151–153.
72. Van Remmen H, Ikeno Y, Hamilton M *et al.* (2003) Life-long reduction in MnSOD activity results in increased DNA damage and higher incidence of cancer but does not accelerate aging. *Physiol Genom* **16**: 29–37.
73. Zhang Y, Ikeno Y, Qi W *et al.* (2009) Mice deficient in both Mn superoxide dismutase and glutathione peroxidase-1 have increased oxidative damage and a greater incidence of pathology but no reduction in longevity. *J Gerontol A Biol Sci Med Sci* **64**: 1212–1220.

74. Mesquita A, Weinberger M, Silva A *et al.* (2010) Caloric restriction or catalase inactivation extends yeast chronological lifespan by inducing H2O2 and superoxide dismutase activity. *Proc Natl Acad Sci USA* **107**: 15123–15128.
75. Van Raamsdonk JM, Hekimi S. (2009) Deletion of the mitochondrial superoxide dismutase sod-2 extends lifespan in Caenorhabditis elegans. *PLoS Genet* **5**: e1000361.
76. Edgar D, Shabalina I, Camara Y *et al.* (2009) Random point mutations with major effects on protein-coding genes are the driving force behind premature aging in mtDNA mutator mice. *Cell Metabol* **10**: 131–138.
77. Bueno M, Lai YC, Romero Y *et al.* (2015) PINK1 deficiency impairs mitochondrial homeostasis and promotes lung fibrosis. *J Clin Invest* **125**: 521–538.
78. Huang LS, Mathew B, Li H *et al.* (2014) The mitochondrial cardiolipin remodeling enzyme lysocardiolipin acyltransferase is a novel target in pulmonary fibrosis. *Am J Respir Critic Care Med* **189**: 1402–1415.
79. Chilosi M, Doglioni C, Murer B *et al.* (2010) Epithelial stem cell exhaustion in the pathogenesis of idiopathic pulmonary fibrosis. *Sarcoidosis Vasc Diffuse Lung Dis* **27**: 7–18.
80. Chilosi M, Carloni A, Rossi A *et al.* (2013) Premature lung aging and cellular senescence in the pathogenesis of idiopathic pulmonary fibrosis and COPD/emphysema. *Transl Res* **162**: 156–173.
81. Collard HR, Moore BB, Flaherty KR *et al.* (2007) Acute exacerbations of idiopathic pulmonary fibrosis. *Am J Respir Critic Care Med* **176**: 636–643.
82. Franceschi C, Bonafe M, Valensin S *et al.* (2000) Inflamm-aging. An evolutionary perspective on immunosenescence. *Ann NY Acad Sci* **908**: 244–254.
83. Salminen A, Kaarniranta K, Kauppinen A. (2012) Inflammaging: Disturbed interplay between autophagy and inflammasomes. *Aging* **4**: 166–175.
84. Salvioli S, Monti D, Lanzarini C *et al.* (2013) Immune system, cell senescence, aging and longevity—inflamm-aging reappraised. *Curr Pharm Des* **19**: 1675–1679.
85. de Magalhaes JP, Curado J, Church GM. (2009) Meta-analysis of age-related gene expression profiles identifies common signatures of aging. *Bioinformatics* **25**: 875–881.

86. Campisi J, d'Adda di Fagagna F. (2007) Cellular senescence: When bad things happen to good cells. *Nat Rev Mol Cell Biol* **8**: 729–740.
87. Zhang H, Pan KH, and Cohen SN. (2003) Senescence-specific gene expression fingerprints reveal cell-type-dependent physical clustering of up-regulated chromosomal loci. *Proc Natl Acad Sci USA* **100**: 3251–3256.
88. Goronzy JJ, Weyand CM. (2013) Understanding immunosenescence to improve responses to vaccines. *Nat Immunol* **14**: 428–436.
89. Lee N, Shin MS, Kang I. (2012) T-cell biology in aging, with a focus on lung disease. *J Gerontol A Biol Sci Med Sci* **67**: 254–263.
90. Tamura T, Kunimatsu T, Yee ST *et al.* (2000) Molecular mechanism of the impairment in activation signal transduction in CD4(+) T cells from old mice. *Int Immunol* **12**: 1205–1215.
91. Caruso C, Candore G, Cigna D *et al.* (1996) Cytokine production pathway in the elderly. *Immunol Res* **15**: 84–90.
92. Czesnikiewicz-Guzik M, Lee WW, Cui, D *et al.* (2008) T cell subset-specific susceptibility to aging. *Clin Immunol* **127**: 107–118.
93. Gilani SR, Vuga LJ, Lindell KO *et al.* (2010) CD28 down-regulation on circulating CD4 T-cells is associated with poor prognoses of patients with idiopathic pulmonary fibrosis. *PloS one* **5**: e8959.
94. Herazo-Maya JD, Noth I, Duncan SR *et al.* (2013) Peripheral blood mononuclear cell gene expression profiles predict poor outcome in idiopathic pulmonary fibrosis. *Sci Transl Med* **5**: 205ra136.

Chapter 16

Potential Mechanistic Links Between Aging and IPF

Hongyi Pan*, Mridu Gulati*, and Erica L. Herzog*,†

1. Introduction

Idiopathic pulmonary fibrosis is a chronic and incurable fibrosing condition involving the progressive accumulation of scar tissue in the adult human lung that typically leads to death within approximately three years of diagnosis.[1] It is a discrete clinicopathologic entity characterized by the finding of radiographic and/or histopathologic changes consistent with usual interstitial pneumonia in the absence of occupational exposures or classical forms of autoimmunity.[1] While several pharmacologic agents have shown some benefit in stabilizing the decline in ventilatory function caused by this disease, the effects of these interventions are limited, heterogeneous and accompanied by significant toxicities.[2,3] Thus, further investigation of the mechanisms driving initiation, development, maintenance and potentially resolution of fibrotic responses remain an important area of investigation in the field of lung biology. Because IPF incidence and prevalence increase with age,[4] some authors have

*Department of Internal Medicine, Section of Pulmonary, Critical Care and Sleep Medicine, Yale School of Medicine, 300 cedar street TAC 4415, New Haven CT 06520-8057.

†Corresponding author: erica.herzog@yale.edu

suggested that the development of IPF may be a form of age-related tissue dysfunction.[5–7] The following chapter will present a critical review of the existing evidence supporting this concept.

2. Paradigms of Fibrosis

Current paradigms of fibrosis posit that following injurious stimuli the respiratory epithelium undergoes a variety of injury responses.[8] This process is accompanied by inflammatory cell recruitment, which though likely not required for the development of fibrosis appear to modulate existing fibroproliferative processes, as well as expansion and activation of fibroblasts and myofibroblasts that produce granulation tissue and exert traction forces to close the wound.[9] Successful healing also involves the resorption of granulation tissue and programmed cell death of myofibroblasts to result in normal tissue structure, anatomy and function.[10] In the lung, insufficient healing responses as seen in acute respiratory distress syndrome, are dominated by acute injury with tissue destruction and diffuse alveolar damage ensues.[11] In contrast, over exuberant healing responses shift the local milieu towards fibrosis and remodeling, and the pathologic finding of scar tissue is seen.[12] This paradigm is illustrated in Fig. 1. Age-related changes in any or all of these processes could contribute to the development, maintenance and perpetuation of fibrotic responses.

3. Epithelial Responses

3.1. *Epithelial: Fibroblast crosstalk*

Pulmonary epithelial cell death is well accepted as an inciting event in IPF. Low grade and/or repetitive injury may result from etiologies including but not limited to certain viral infections, toxic exposures, cigarette smoke, chronic microaspiration and even genetic abnormalities.[13,14] Some epithelial cells die, with others producing soluble mediators and transforming from passive bystanders into high engaged cells that directly participate in the fibrotic response.[15]

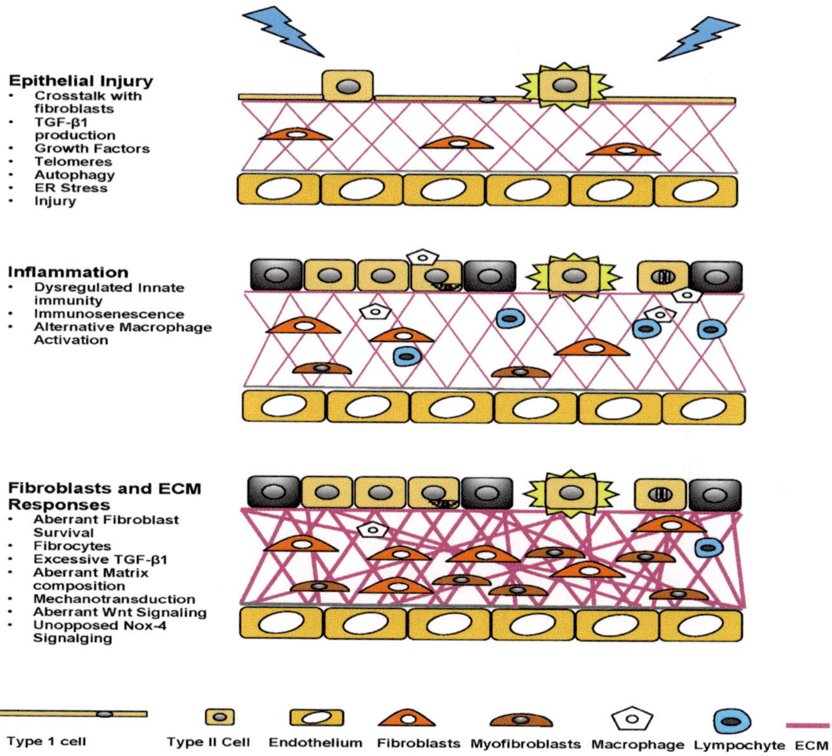

Fig. 1. Age-Related Changes Contributing to IPF.

In the top panel, age-related changes that may contribute to epithelial responses are shown. These include dysregulated communication with fibroblasts, excessive production of TGF-β1 and growth factors, and increased susceptibility to injury caused by shortened telomeres, abnormal autophagy, and ER stress. The middle panel includes the age related changes in immunity such as innate immune abnormalities, senescent lymphocytes, and alternatively activated macrophages, may amplify existing fibrotic pathways. The bottom panel shows age-related changes in fibroblast biology such as excessive survival and to initiate the fibrotic processes are shown. These include uncontrolled survival, the extrapulmonary origin of fibrocytes, aberrant production and activation of TGF-β1, production of abnormal ECM, mechanotransductive priming on excessively stiff surfaces, aberrant Wnt signaling, and unopposed Nox-4 signaling. Any or all of these pathways may contribute to the increased rates of IPF seen in the aged population.

The bulk of the data in this area comes from studies of the type II cell (AT2), which produce cytokines and chemokines such as TNF-α, IL-4 and IL-13[15,16] which modulate fibroblast phenotypes and induce production of ECM.[15,16] They secrete growth factors including EGF, PDGF and CTGF to induce migration, proliferation and activation of fibroblasts.[13] They also indirectly influence fibroblasts through their production of surfactant protein D, which stimulate TGF-β1 production by macrophages[17] in the bleomycin-challenged murine lung. AT2s themselves directly produce TGF-β1 to induce fibroblast activation and differentiation,[13] and they likely participate in TGF-β1 activation by producing the $\alpha v\beta 6$ integrin, an epithelial-specific integrin which mediates activation of latent TGF-β1 in the mesenchyme.[14,18] AT2s might also function to suppress myofibroblast transformation via their regulation of lung homeostasis. For example, animal modeling indicates that the AT2 anomalies seen in genetic syndromes such as Hermansky Pudlak Disease[19] or in animal models of inducible AT2 deletion[20] is sufficient to cause the accumulation of activated myofibroblasts and pulmonary fibrosis which may be due in part to the loss of AT2 fibroblast-suppressive functions. To date there exists little information regarding the development of age-related changes in epithelial-fibroblast crosstalk.

4. Epithelial Injury

4.1. *Telomeres*

A long and rich history of animal modeling indicates that loss of epithelial death responses are required for the development of experimentally induced fibrosis in mice.[8] While there are to date no animal data demonstrating that aged epithelial cells show increased vulnerability to injury, there exists a multitude of data from IPF patients suggesting this to be the case.[21] Several age related changes that would be expected to accompany increased epithelial death responses have been described in IPF. For example, GWAS studies have identified common variants in TERT and TERC in regions that are required for telomere homeostasis and shortened telomeres have been detected in cells of IPF patients with and without these mutations.[22–24] However, due to the difference between mouse and human telomere biology, animal modeling of telomerase biology has been difficult to interpret.[25,26]

4.2. *Autophagy*

Another homeostatic process that is thought to protect cells from age-related attrition is autophagy, a highly conserved process of cellular recycling in which damaged proteins and organelles are shuttled to lysosomes where toxic components are removed and alternate sources of cellular fuel are generated. Two recent studies demonstrate reduced detection of autophagy-associated markers in the IPF lung, and one of these studies went on to suggest that this finding may be mechanistically linked to the increased detection of p21 expressing senescent epithelial cells that has been reported in IPF.[27,28] In both of these studies, rapamycin treatment of bleomycin exposed mice led to impressive reductions in collagen content and in the histologic appearance of fibrosis, and though an epithelial-specific cytoprotective benefit has not been shown. Given the relationship between impaired autophagy and aging,[29] these studies support a potential mechanistic between these entities and the development of IPF.

4.3. *ER stress*

The enhanced epithelial cell injury that characterizes IPF may also result from endoplasmic reticulum stress and the unfolded protein response. In the normal setting this response occurs in the setting of many forms of cellular stress and functions to improve protein folding, thereby attenuating the retention of misfolded proteins and the resulting cell death response. Evidence of these responses is detected in AT2 cells that are resident in the IPF lung.[30] These findings may account for the increased propensity for AT2 cell death and pulmonary fibrosis that was seen in aged mice subject to MHV68 infection.[31] In fact, bleomycin administration to mice overexpressing a mutant form of surfactant leads to ER stress, worsened cell death and worsened fibrosis.[32] However, because other studies using the bleomycin model have found that aged mice sustain increased collagen accumulation in a manner that is independent of enhanced cell death responses,[33] the mechanism through which ER stress and UPR lead to fibrosis remains unclear. Nevertheless, given the relationship between ER stress and aging, this area remains an attractive and robust area of investigation in the field of IPF.

5. Immunologic Regulation

5.1. *Innate immunity*

A variety of age-related innate and adaptive immune responses have the potential to regulate fibrotic responses in the IPF lung. For example, recognition of pathogen-associated molecular patterns (PAMPs) by Toll-like receptors, which function abnormally in aged individuals,[34] show an increasingly recognized contribution to lung remodeling and fibrosis via the regulation of myofibroblast transformation. Specifically, Toll-like receptors 2 and 4 are associated with enhanced myofibroblast activation and fibrosis in the bleomycin model of lung fibrosis,[35] and fibroblasts obtained from the lungs of patients with rapidly progressive IPF express high levels of TLR9 that appear to mediate enhanced CpG island responses when compared to fibroblasts obtained from patients with more stable disease.[36] The relationship of these findings to age-related changes in innate immune signaling is unclear at this time but remains an important area of investigation.

5.2. *Lymphocyte mediated adaptive immune responses*

In terms of adaptive immune responses, the potential contribution of lymphocytes is an emerging area of investigation in IPF. This area remains controversial for several reasons with the most compelling being that lymphocytes are not required for the development of experimentally induced fibrosis in mouse models.[37] Additionally, IPF is not associated with classical immune responses and in the clinical setting in fact defined by its lack of autoimmunity.[1] Last, treatment of IPF patients with immunomodulatory agents that predominantly affect lymphocytes appears to worsen clinical outcomes.[38] When viewed in combination, these complex data could be explained by a unifying hypothesis in which non-classical immune responses participate in IPF by modulating existing fibrotic responses. For example, several Thelper populations could contribute to IPF immunopathogenesis. It remains noteworthy that substances produced by Th1 cells, such as interferon gamma, might be sufficient to induce structural cell injury and initiate fibrotic responses, but because Th1 cytokines exert suppressive effects on fibroblast proliferation and migration, Th1 cells would exert initiating effects on cells other than fibroblasts and would not directly influence myofibroblasts this model.[39] Th2 and Th17 cells are also recruited to the lung following epithelial injury where they produce IL-4, IL-13 and/or IL-17, which activate STAT6 signaling within fibroblasts to induce profibrotic gene programs.[9,40,41] Surprisingly, evidence gleaned from several animal models suggests that regulatory *T* cells, which are typically thought of as antifibrotic, may perpetuate fibrosis under certain circumstances.[42,43] Given the well described phenomenon of immunosenescence that characterizes lymphocyte responses in the elderly, further studies of adaptive immune responses may be of particular importance in IPF.

5.3. *Role of macrophages*

There exists a broad continuum of macrophage phenotypes arising in response to specific challenges. Among the best studied in the context of tissue remodeling and fibrosis are macrophages that are skewed towards classical ("M1") and alternative ("M2") activation. M1 macrophages are involved in the suppression of microbial infection via a variety of mechanisms including the production of proinflammatory cytokines such as TNF-α and IFN-γ, elaboration of reactive oxygen species and nitric oxide, induction of Th1 immune responses. M2 macrophages are more strongly associated with tissue remodeling and immunoregulation through their expression of scavenger receptors such as CD163, the expression of mannose receptors such as CD206, through the production of ornithine and through the secretion of cytokines and growth factors that suppress acute inflammatory responses and promote tissue repair (recently reviewed in Ref. 44). Functional polarization has in several experimental settings been found to be reversible,[45,46] though similar findings have yet to be shown in human pathology. If this type of reprogramming occurs in the setting of fibrosis, it is likely to be regulated by tissue specific factors that are known to regulate M1/M2 activation including but not limited to the presence of dying or apopotic cells,[47] the presence of ECM fragments,[48] and soluble mediators such as cytokines, chemokines and growth factors[44] and nonspecific mechanotransductive responses to local tissue stiffness[49] and even microbiome components.[50] Cell specific factors such as origin,[51] metabolic state[51] and epigenetic programming[52] could also play a role.

While the M1/M2 dichotomy is an overly simplified distillation of the manifold functions of macrophages, it is useful when considering general themes such as killing/destruction and healing. Many early studies of idiopathic pulmonary fibrosis that sought to attenuate potentially injurious immune responses using TNF-α inhibition[53] and immunosuppressants such as steroids and azathioprine[54] found no benefit of these agents and that in some situations their administration may be harmful. While these findings could suggest that the immune system is not involved in the regulation of fibrosis, a more accurate interpretation of the data may be that other forms of immune activation might be relevant in this disease. Therefore it is particularly relevant that a role for macrophages in the regulation of fibrosis was proposed nearly four decades ago in studies describing the ability of human alveolar macrophages to regulate fibroblast proliferation.[55,56] Further delineation of these findings determined that macrophages displaying properties of alternative activation in terms of expression of scavenger receptors and profibrotic soluble mediators may be influencing fibroblast activities.[12,57–59] Mechanistic studies performed in several animal models of fibrosis revealed that reduction in macrophage quantities[12,57,60] or shifting macrophage phenotypes away from alternative activation[60,61] attenuates both collagen accumulation and histologic evidence of lung remodeling and fibrosis. Based on these and other studies, most sources now agree that crosstalk between macrophages and fibroblasts might importantly regulate the maintenance and progression of existing fibrotic responses. Thus, it is of particular interest that age-related changes in macrophage polarization and function have been described in a variety of modeling systems[62] and in cells obtained from aged but otherwise healthy human subjects.[63]

6. Fibroblasts and Extracellular Matrix Responses

The fibroblast response to tissue damage involves a central role in repair and remodeling. In the healthy and injured lung, fibroblasts support lung architecture via the deposition and maintenance of extracellular matrix components such collagens I, III, IV, V, VI; and extracellular matrix-associated proteins such as glycoproteins and glycosaminoglycans[8,10] In addition to direct production of ECM, fibroblasts also participate in remodeling and fibrosis through their regulated transformation into activated myofibroblasts which, in addition to the above features, display the cytoskeletal characteristics of contractile smooth muscle cells including stress fibers and α-smooth muscle actin (α-SMA).[10] It is notable that both pirfenidone and nintedanib, which are the first agents to show efficacy in attenuating the decline in lung function seen in IPF, both are targeted towards fibroblast activation.[2,3] In fact, some of the most promising drugs in the IPF clinical pipeline target fibroblasts and matrix production. The available data regarding fibroblasts and ECM in the context of IPF and the potential relationship linking these entities with aging, are outlined below.

7. Aberrant Fibroblast Survival

Because the accumulation and activation of fibroblasts is believed to be the final common pathway of most fibrotic insults, it is of particular importance that fibroblasts and myofibroblasts obtained from the IPF lung demonstrate enhanced proliferation and survival compared to normal cells.[64–66] The possible mechanism(s) proposed for this observation include abnormalities in apoptotic pathways,[64–66] aberrant Wnt signaling,[67] defective autophagy[27] and more recently, unopposed Nox-4 signaling.[33] In some studies, these characteristics are accompanied by enhanced proliferation that might be related to alterations to the AKT inactivating transcription factor FOXO3a,[66] to integrin anomalies[68] or to abnormalities in Caveolin-1 and PTEN.[69] While these findings might suggest clonal proliferation, IPF fibroblasts lack classical signs of malignant transformation and do not seem to be polyclonal.[70] Nevertheless, studies employing newer profiling techniques have shown IPF fibroblasts to contain genome-wide aberrations in translational control similar to changes found in cancer cells.[71] Additional areas of interest include the potential contribution of epigenetic alterations including DNA methylation,[72] noncoding RNAs,[73,74] and histone modifications[75] though it is not known whether any of these findings contribute to fibrosis in the intact human lung. Nevertheless, because abnormalities in many of these pathways are also associated with aging, it is intriguing to speculate that age-associated alterations in epigenetic processes contribute to fibroblast activation in IPF.

8. Origin of Lung Fibroblasts

Another process contributing to fibroblast accumulation and fibroproliferation in IPF may involve the enhanced recruitment of myofibroblast precursors. While most sources agree that postembryonic lung fibrosis are the major source of myofibroblasts in IPF, additional sources have been proposed. Of these, the most extensively studied ARE epithelial-to-mesenchymal cell transition (EMT) and/or recruitment and maturation of circulating pluripotent mesenchymal progenitor cells called fibrocytes.[76]

The concept of EMT as a source of IPF is attractive given that this disease is believed to stem from aberrant fibroblast responses to epithelial injury. In fact, early studies of this process appeared promising when assessment of TGF-β1 stimulated alveolar type II cells revealed the seemingly regulated expression of fibroblast markers including α-SMA,[77] and several studies appeared to show the co-localization of AT2 and fibroblast markers in IPF lung tissue.[77,78] However, direct experimental evidence of this process contributing to mammalian lung fibrosis remains scarce, as mouse studies employing cell lineage tracking of AT2 cells in the bleomycin model do not demonstrate an AT2 origin of α-SMA-expressing myofibroblasts.[79] Thus, while it is widely believed that multiple stromal cell populations participate in pulmonary fibrosis, definitive evidence supporting a role for EMT as source of myofibroblasts remains elusive. Synthesis of the available data suggests that adoption of mesenchymal properties by AT2 cells is more likely to represent a response to injury rather than the regulated differentiation into bona fide myofibroblasts. A relationship between the aging lung and enhanced EMT has not been fully explored.

Fibroblasts might also derive from fibrocytes, a circulating leukocyte population with mesenchymal properties that was initially described in 1994.[80] Their identification in the peripheral blood is relatively straightforward and typically involves co-detection of hematopoietic markers such as CD45, and mesenchymal markers such as Pro-Collagen Iα1.[76,80] The understanding of the role that fibrocytes might play in inflammatory and fibrosing conditions continues to evolve. Fibrocytes are easily detected in the setting of experimentally induced lung fibrosis in mice[16,81,82] and in the lungs and circulation of patients with IPF.[21] However, definitive evidence of transformation into activated myofibroblasts has been more difficult to find.[76] Thus, more recent studies have focused on the role that fibrocytes might play in the regulation of evolving and established fibrotic responses.[76] Because increased levels of local and/or circulating fibrocytes have been detected in mouse models of accelerated aging[6] and in the blood of aged but otherwise healthy human volunteers,[63] further studies of this cell population might uncover additional insight into the relationship between aging and the development of IPF.

As has been proposed for other organs, additional sources of lung myofibroblasts in the fibrotic lung may exist. These include pericytes,[83,84] adipocytes,[85] bone marrow derived mesenchymal stem cells[86] and endothelial-to-mesenchymal transition.[87] To date these populations have been only minimally explored in IPF and/aging.

9. Interactions with Extracellular Matrix

While the above data might suggest that the excessive ECM that accumulates in IPF functions only as a product of activated myofibroblasts, recent evidence demonstrates that lung fibroblasts might also respond to biochemical and mechanical cues present in the disease local ECM. For example, relative to normal tissue, the ECM of the IPF lung is enriched for fibrillar Type I and III collagens, various glycoproteins, and proteoglycans.[88] While in normal repair responses fibrillar type I collagen functions dampens fibroblast proliferation via integrin-dependent mechanisms,[68,89,90] this interaction appears to be lacking in IPF. Glycoproteins such as alternatively spliced domain A containing fibronectin and periostin may also regulate myofibroblast differentiation in IPF.[91–94] Similarly, the proteoglycans hyaluronic acid (HA) (and HA fragments) are detected in human IPF where they seem to contribute to fibroblast invasiveness and ECM synthesis.[95] To date, there exists little to no information regarding how age-related differences in lung ECM influence the development and perpetuation of fibroproliferative responses in human IPF.

The normal and diseased human lung ECM also display mechanical abnormalities that could influence fibroblast phenotypes and the understanding of ECM mechanics in the fibrotic lung is expanding. The available data indicate that fibroblast function and differentiation into myofibroblasts are both enhanced on a stiff surface.[96] These findings might be parallel or in concert with classical profibrotic mediators such as TGFβ1.[97–99] Mechanically, the transmission of traction force from the cell to the ECM, and vice versa, occurs in focal adhesions (FA), which connect the cytoskeleton and ECM via integrins[100] which then activate a myriad of pathways including

Wnt/β-catenin,[101,102] Hippo,[103] and certain ion channels,[104] though other mechanisms are also involved. While aged tissue is known to be much stiffer than young tissue due in part to loss of normal elastic fibres,[105] a mechanical relationship between young and aging and the propensity to develop fibrosis has not been defined.

10. Conclusion

As can be seen, age-associated abnormalities in a variety of cellular compartments may contribute to the pathobiology of IPF. However, much uncertainty remains. Work in this field would be enhanced by a dedicated comparison of primary cells and tissues obtained from the young and aged lung. Development of improved *ex vivo* modeling systems to study cellular crosstalk and cell: matrix interactions are also needed. Last, advancements in animal modeling systems that could better simulate the complex environment of the aging, fibrotic lung would be of benefit as well. Accomplishment of these goals could cement the link between aging and fibrosis, and perhaps elucidate the mechanism(s) of other forms of age-related lung pathology as well.

References

1. Raghu G, Collard HR, Egan JJ *et al.* (2011) An official ATS/ERS/JRS/ALAT statement: Idiopathic pulmonary fibrosis: Evidence-based guidelines for diagnosis and management. *Am J Respir Crit Care Med* **183**: 788–824.
2. King TE, Jr., Bradford WZ, Castro-Bernardini S *et al.* (2014) A phase 3 trial of pirfenidone in patients with idiopathic pulmonary fibrosis. *N Engl J Med* **370**: 2083–2092.
3. Richeldi L, du Bois RM, Raghu G *et al.* (2014) Efficacy and safety of nintedanib in idiopathic pulmonary fibrosis. *N Engl J Med* **370**: 2071–2082.
4. Raghu G, Chen SY, Yeh WS *et al.* (2014) Idiopathic pulmonary fibrosis in US Medicare beneficiaries aged 65 years and older: Incidence, prevalence, and survival, 2001–2011. *Lancet Respir Med* **2**: 566–572.

5. Selman M, Pardo A. (2014) Revealing the pathogenic and aging-related mechanisms of the enigmatic idiopathic pulmonary fibrosis. An integral model. *Am J Respir Crit Care Med* **189**: 1161–1172.
6. Sueblinvong V, Neveu WA, Neujahr DC *et al.* (2014) Aging promotes pro-fibrotic matrix production and increases fibrocyte recruitment during acute lung injury. *Adv Biosci Biotechnol* **5**: 19–30.
7. Thannickal VJ, Murthy M, Balch WE *et al.* (2015) Blue Journal Conference: Aging and the Susceptibility to Lung Disease. *Am J Respir Crit Care Med.*
8. Blackwell TS, Tager AM, Borok Z *et al.* (2014) Future directions in idiopathic pulmonary fibrosis research. An NHLBI workshop report. *Am J Respir Crit Care Med* **189**: 214–222.
9. Homer RJ, Elias JA, Lee CG *et al.* (2011) Modern concepts on the role of inflammation in pulmonary fibrosis. *Arch Pathol Lab Med* **135**: 780–788.
10. Klingberg F, Hinz B, White ES. (2013) The myofibroblast matrix: Implications for tissue repair and fibrosis. *J Pathol* **229**: 298–309.
11. Ware LB, Bastarache JA, Calfee CS. (2014) ARDS: New Mechanistic Insights, New Therapeutic Directions. *Clin Chest Med* **35**: 15–16.
12. Zhou Y, Peng H, Sun H *et al.* (2014) Chitinase 3-like 1 suppresses injury and promotes fibroproliferative responses in Mammalian lung fibrosis. *Sci Transl Med* **6**: 240ra7.
13. Selman M, Pardo A. (2006) Role of epithelial cells in idiopathic pulmonary fibrosis: From innocent targets to serial killers. *Proc Am Thorac Soc* **3**: 364–372.
14. Noble PW, Barkauskas CE, Jiang D. (2012) Pulmonary fibrosis: Patterns and perpetrators. *J Clin Invest* **122**: 2756–2762.
15. Chapman HA. (2011) Epithelial-mesenchymal interactions in pulmonary fibrosis. *Annu Rev Physiol* **73**: 413–435.
16. Garibaldi BT, D'Alessio FR, Mock JR *et al.* (2013) Regulatory T cells reduce acute lung injury fibroproliferation by decreasing fibrocyte recruitment. *Am J Respir Cell Mol Biol* **48**: 35–43.
17. Aono Y, Ledford JG, Mukherjee S *et al.* (2012) Surfactant protein-D regulates effector cell function and fibrotic lung remodeling in response to bleomycin injury. *Am J Respir Crit Care Med* **185**: 525–536.
18. Munger JS, Huang X, Kawakatsu H *et al.* (1999) The integrin alpha v beta 6 binds and activates latent TGF beta 1: A mechanism for regulating pulmonary inflammation and fibrosis. *Cell* **96**: 319–328.

19. Young LR, Gulleman PM, Bridges JP *et al.* (2012) The alveolar epithelium determines susceptibility to lung fibrosis in Hermansky-Pudlak syndrome. *Am J Respir Crit Care Med* **186**: 1014–1024.
20. Sisson TH, Mendez M, Choi K *et al.* (2010) Targeted injury of type II alveolar epithelial cells induces pulmonary fibrosis. *Am J Respir Crit Care Med* **181**: 254–263.
21. Peng X, Mathai SK, Murray LA *et al.* (2011) Local apoptosis promotes collagen production by monocyte-derived cells in transforming growth factor beta1-induced lung fibrosis. *Fibrogenesis Tissue Repair* **4**: 12.
22. Liu T, Ullenbruch M, Young Choi Y *et al.* (2013) Telomerase and telomere length in pulmonary fibrosis. *Am J Respir Cell Mol Biol* **49**: 260–268.
23. Armanios MY, Chen JJ, Cogan JD *et al.* (2007) Telomerase mutations in families with idiopathic pulmonary fibrosis. *N Engl J Med* **356**: 1317–1326.
24. Tsakiri KD, Cronkhite JT, Kuan PJ *et al.* (2007) Adult-onset pulmonary fibrosis caused by mutations in telomerase. *Proc Natl Acad Sci USA* **104**: 7552–7557.
25. Degryse AL, Xu XC, Newman JL *et al.* (2012) Telomerase deficiency does not alter bleomycin-induced fibrosis in mice. *Exp Lung Res* **38**: 124–134.
26. Liu T, Chung MJ, Ullenbruch M *et al.* (2007) Telomerase activity is required for bleomycin-induced pulmonary fibrosis in mice. *J Clin Invest* **117**: 3800–3809.
27. Patel AS, Lin L, Geyer A *et al.* (2012) Autophagy in idiopathic pulmonary fibrosis. *PLoS One* **7**: e41394.
28. Araya J, Kojima J, Takasaka N *et al.* (2013) Insufficient autophagy in idiopathic pulmonary fibrosis. *Am J Physiol Lung Cell Mol Physiol* **304**: L56–L69.
29. Rubinsztein DC, Marino G, Kroemer G. (2011) Autophagy and aging. *Cell* **146**: 682–695.
30. Lawson WE, Crossno PF, Polosukhin VV *et al.* (2008) Endoplasmic reticulum stress in alveolar epithelial cells is prominent in IPF: Association with altered surfactant protein processing and herpesvirus infection. *Am J Physiol Lung Cell Mol Physiol* **294**: L1119–L1126.
31. Torres-Gonzalez E, Bueno M, Tanaka A *et al.* (2012) Role of endoplasmic reticulum stress in age-related susceptibility to lung fibrosis. *Am J Respir Cell Mol Biol* **46**: 748–756.

32. Lawson WE, Cheng DS, Degryse AL *et al.* (2011) Endoplasmic reticulum stress enhances fibrotic remodeling in the lungs. *Proc Natl Acad Sci USA* **108**: 10562–10567.
33. Hecker L, Logsdon NJ, Kurundkar D *et al.* (2014) Reversal of persistent fibrosis in aging by targeting Nox4-Nrf2 redox imbalance. *Sci Transl Med* **6**: 231ra47.
34. Shaw AC, Panda A, Joshi SR *et al.* (2011) Dysregulation of human Toll-like receptor function in aging. *Ageing Res Rev* **10**: 346–353.
35. Jiang D, Liang J, Fan J *et al.* (2005) Regulation of lung injury and repair by Toll-like receptors and hyaluronan. *Nat Med* **11**: 1173–1179.
36. Trujillo G, Meneghin A, Flaherty KR *et al.* (2010) TLR9 differentiates rapidly from slowly progressing forms of idiopathic pulmonary fibrosis. *Sci Transl Med* **2**: 57ra82.
37. Helene M, Lake-Bullock V, Zhu J *et al.* (1999) T cell independence of bleomycin-induced pulmonary fibrosis. *J Leukoc Biol* **65**: 187–195.
38. Raghu G, Anstrom KJ, King TE, Jr. *et al.* (2012) Prednisone, azathioprine, and N-acetylcysteine for pulmonary fibrosis. *N Engl J Med* **366**: 1968–1977.
39. Wynn TA. (2004) Fibrotic disease and the T(H)1/T(H)2 paradigm. *Nat Rev Immunol* **4**: 583–594.
40. Sivakumar P, Ntolios P, Jenkins G *et al.* (2012) Into the matrix: Targeting fibroblasts in pulmonary fibrosis. *Curr Opin Pulm Med* **18**: 462–469.
41. Wilson MS, Madala SK, Ramalingam TR *et al.* (2010) Bleomycin and IL-1beta-mediated pulmonary fibrosis is IL-17A dependent. *J Exp Med* **207**: 535–552.
42. Reilkoff RA, Peng H, Murray LA *et al.* (2013) Semaphorin 7a+ regulatory T cells are associated with progressive idiopathic pulmonary fibrosis and are implicated in transforming growth factor-beta1-induced pulmonary fibrosis. *Am J Respir Crit Care Med* **187**: 180–188.
43. Lo Re S, Lecocq M, Uwambayinema F *et al.* (2011) Platelet-derived growth factor-producing CD4+ Foxp3+ regulatory T lymphocytes promote lung fibrosis. *Am J Respir Crit Care Med* **184**: 1270–1281.
44. Sica A, Mantovani A. (2012) Macrophage plasticity and polarization: In vivo veritas. *J Clin Invest* **122**: 787–795.
45. Okabe Y, Medzhitov R. (2014) Tissue-specific signals control reversible program of localization and functional polarization of macrophages. *Cell* **157**: 832–844.

46. Cassol E, Cassetta L, Rizzi C *et al.* (2009) M1 and M2a polarization of human monocyte-derived macrophages inhibits HIV-1 replication by distinct mechanisms. *J Immunol* **182**: 6237–6246.
47. Weigert A, Tzieply N, von Knethen A *et al.* (2007) Tumor cell apoptosis polarizes macrophages role of sphingosine-1-phosphate. *Mol Biol Cell* **18**: 3810–3819.
48. Stahl M, Schupp J, Jager B *et al.* (2013) Lung collagens perpetuate pulmonary fibrosis via CD204 and M2 macrophage activation. *PLoS One* **8**: e81382.
49. Wong VW, Rustad KC, Akaishi S *et al.* (2012) Focal adhesion kinase links mechanical force to skin fibrosis via inflammatory signaling. *Nat Med* **18**: 148–152.
50. Kau AL, Ahern PP, Griffin NW *et al.* (2011) Human nutrition, the gut microbiome and the immune system. *Nature* **474**: 327–336.
51. Blagih J, Jones RG. (2012) Polarizing macrophages through reprogramming of glucose metabolism. *Cell Metab* **15**: 793–795.
52. Bowdridge S, Gause WC. (2010) Regulation of alternative macrophage activation by chromatin remodeling. *Nat Immunol* **11**: 879–881.
53. Raghu G, Brown KK, Costabel U *et al.* (2008) Treatment of idiopathic pulmonary fibrosis with etanercept: An exploratory, placebo-controlled trial. *Am J Respir Crit Care Med* **178**: 948–955.
54. Idiopathic Pulmonary Fibrosis Clinical Research N, Raghu G, Anstrom KJ *et al.* (2012) Prednisone, azathioprine, and N-acetylcysteine for pulmonary fibrosis. *N Engl J Med* **366**: 1968–1977.
55. Bitterman PB, Wewers MD, Rennard SI *et al.* (1986) Modulation of alveolar macrophage-driven fibroblast proliferation by alternative macrophage mediators. *J Clin Invest* **77**: 700–708.
56. Bitterman PB, Adelberg S, Crystal RG. (1983) Mechanisms of pulmonary fibrosis. Spontaneous release of the alveolar macrophage-derived growth factor in the interstitial lung disorders. *J Clin Invest* **72**: 1801–1813.
57. Gibbons MA, MacKinnon AC, Ramachandran P *et al.* (2011) Ly6Chi monocytes direct alternatively activated profibrotic macrophage regulation of lung fibrosis. *Am J Respir Crit Care Med* **184**: 569–581.
58. Karo-Atar D, Moshkovits I, Eickelberg O *et al.* (2013) Paired immunoglobulin-like receptor-B inhibits pulmonary fibrosis by suppressing profibrogenic properties of alveolar macrophages. *Am J Respir Cell Mol Biol* **48**: 456–464.

59. Wynn TA, Barron L. (2010) Macrophages: Master regulators of inflammation and fibrosis. *Semin Liver Dis* **30**: 245–257.
60. Murray LA, Chen Q, Kramer MS *et al.* (2011) TGF-beta driven lung fibrosis is macrophage dependent and blocked by Serum amyloid P. *Int J Biochem Cell Biol* **43**: 154–1562.
61. Murray LA, Rosada R, Moreira AP *et al.* (2010) Serum amyloid P therapeutically attenuates murine bleomycin-induced pulmonary fibrosis via its effects on macrophages. *PLoS One* **5**: e9683.
62. Mahbub S, Deburghgraeve CR, Kovacs EJ. (2012) Advanced age impairs macrophage polarization. *J Interferon Cytokine Res* **32**: 18–26.
63. Mathai SK, Gulati M, Peng X *et al.* (2010) Circulating monocytes from systemic sclerosis patients with interstitial lung disease show an enhanced profibrotic phenotype. *Lab Invest* **90**: 812–823.
64. Maher TM, Evans IC, Bottoms SE *et al.* (2010) Diminished prostaglandin E2 contributes to the apoptosis paradox in idiopathic pulmonary fibrosis. *Am J Respir Crit Care Med* **182**: 73–82.
65. Nho RS, Peterson M, Hergert P *et al.* (2013) FoxO3a (Forkhead Box O3a) Deficiency Protects Idiopathic Pulmonary Fibrosis (IPF) Fibroblasts from Type I Polymerized Collagen Matrix-Induced Apoptosis via Caveolin-1 (cav-1) and Fas. *PLoS One* **8**: e61017.
66. Nho RS, Hergert P, Kahm J *et al.* (2011) Pathological alteration of FoxO3a activity promotes idiopathic pulmonary fibrosis fibroblast proliferation on type i collagen matrix. *Am J Pathol* **179**: 2420–2430.
67. Chang W, Wei K, Jacobs SS *et al.* (2010) SPARC suppresses apoptosis of idiopathic pulmonary fibrosis fibroblasts through constitutive activation of beta-catenin. *J Biol Chem* **285**: 8196–8206.
68. Xia H, Seeman J, Hong J *et al.* (2012) Low alpha(2)beta(1) integrin function enhances the proliferation of fibroblasts from patients with idiopathic pulmonary fibrosis by activation of the beta-catenin pathway. *Am J Pathol* **181**: 222–233.
69. Xia H, Khalil W, Kahm J *et al.* (2010) Pathologic caveolin-1 regulation of PTEN in idiopathic pulmonary fibrosis. *Am J Pathol* **176**: 2626–2637.
70. Mio T, Nagai S, Kitaichi M *et al.* (1992) Proliferative characteristics of fibroblast lines derived from open lung biopsy specimens of patients with IPF (UIP). *Chest* **102**: 832–837.
71. Larsson O, Diebold D, Fan D *et al.* (2008) Fibrotic myofibroblasts manifest genome-wide derangements of translational control. *PLoS One* **3**: e3220.

72. Cisneros J, Hagood J, Checa M *et al.* (2012) Hypermethylation-mediated silencing of p14(ARF) in fibroblasts from idiopathic pulmonary fibrosis. *Am J Physiol Lung Cell Mol Physiol* **303**: L295–L303.
73. Milosevic J, Pandit K, Magister M *et al.* (2012) Profibrotic role of miR-154 in pulmonary fibrosis. *Am J Respir Cell Mol Biol* **47**: 879–887.
74. Yang S, Cui H, Xie N *et al.* (2013) miR-145 regulates myofibroblast differentiation and lung fibrosis. *FASEB J.*
75. Huang SK, Scruggs AM, Donaghy J *et al.* (2013) Histone modifications are responsible for decreased Fas expression and apoptosis resistance in fibrotic lung fibroblasts. *Cell Death Dis* **4**: e621.
76. Reilkoff RA, Bucala R, Herzog EL. (2011) Fibrocytes: Emerging effector cells in chronic inflammation. *Nat Rev Immunol* **11**: 427–435.
77. Willis BC, Liebler JM, Luby-Phelps K *et al.* (2005) Induction of epithelial-mesenchymal transition in alveolar epithelial cells by transforming growth factor-beta1: potential role in idiopathic pulmonary fibrosis. *Am J Pathol* **166**: 1321–1332.
78. Yamada M, Kuwano K, Maeyama T *et al.* (2008) Dual-immunohistochemistry provides little evidence for epithelial-mesenchymal transition in pulmonary fibrosis. *Histochem Cell Biol* **129**: 453–462.
79. Rock JR, Barkauskas CE, Cronce MJ *et al.* (2011) Multiple stromal populations contribute to pulmonary fibrosis without evidence for epithelial to mesenchymal transition. *Proc Natl Acad Sci USA* **108**: E1475–E1483.
80. Bucala R, Spiegel L, Chesney J *et al.* (1994) Circulating fibrocytes define a new leukocyte subpopulation that mediates tissue repair. *Mol Med* **1**: 71.
81. Hashimoto N, Jin H, Liu T *et al.* (2004) Bone marrow-derived progenitor cells in pulmonary fibrosis. *J Clin Invest* **113**: 243–252.
82. Moore BB, Murray L, Das A *et al.* (2006) The role of CCL12 in the recruitment of fibrocytes and lung fibrosis. *Am J Respir Cell Mol Biol* **35**: 175–181.
83. Humphreys BD, Lin SL, Kobayashi A *et al.* (2010) Fate tracing reveals the pericyte and not epithelial origin of myofibroblasts in kidney fibrosis. *Am J Pathol* **176**: 85–97.
84. Hung C, Linn G, Chow YH *et al.* (2013) Role of lung pericytes and resident fibroblasts in the pathogenesis of pulmonary fibrosis. *Am J Respir Crit Care Med* **188**: 820–830.

85. Uezumi A, Ito T, Morikawa D *et al.* (2011) Fibrosis and adipogenesis originate from a common mesenchymal progenitor in skeletal muscle. *J Cell Sci* **124**: 3654–3664.
86. Ueno T, Nakashima A, Doi S *et al.* (2013) Mesenchymal stem cells ameliorate experimental peritoneal fibrosis by suppressing inflammation and inhibiting TGF-beta1 signaling. *Kidney Int.*
87. Hashimoto N, Phan SH, Imaizumi K *et al.* (2010) Endothelial-mesenchymal transition in bleomycin-induced pulmonary fibrosis. *Am J Respir Cell Mol Biol* **43**: 161–172.
88. Booth AJ, Hadley R, Cornett AM *et al.* (2012) Acellular normal and fibrotic human lung matrices as a culture system for *in vitro* investigation. *Am J Respir Crit Care Med* **186**: 866–876.
89. Koyama H, Raines EW, Bornfeldt KE *et al.* (1996) Fibrillar collagen inhibits arterial smooth muscle proliferation through regulation of Cdk2 inhibitors. *Cell* **87**: 1069–1078.
90. Ivaska J, Nissinen L, Immonen N *et al.* (2002) Integrin alpha 2 beta 1 promotes activation of protein phosphatase 2A and dephosphorylation of Akt and glycogen synthase kinase 3 beta. *Mol Cell Biol* **22**: 1352–1359.
91. Serini G, Bochaton-Piallat ML, Ropraz P *et al.* (1998) The fibronectin domain ED-A is crucial for myofibroblastic phenotype induction by transforming growth factor-beta1. *J Cell Biol* **142**: 873–881.
92. Olsen AL, Sackey BK, Marcinkiewicz C *et al.* (2012) Fibronectin extra domain-A promotes hepatic stellate cell motility but not differentiation into myofibroblasts. *Gastroenterol* **142**: 928–937 e3.
93. Kohan M, Muro AF, White ES *et al.* (2010) EDA-containing cellular fibronectin induces fibroblast differentiation through binding to alpha4beta7 integrin receptor and MAPK/Erk 1/2-dependent signaling. *FASEB J* **24**: 4503–4512.
94. Naik PK, Bozyk PD, Bentley JK *et al.* (2012) Periostin promotes fibrosis and predicts progression in patients with idiopathic pulmonary fibrosis. *Am J Physiol Lung Cell Mol Physiol* **303**: L1046–L156.
95. Li Y, Jiang D, Liang J *et al.* (2011) Severe lung fibrosis requires an invasive fibroblast phenotype regulated by hyaluronan and CD44. *J Exp Med* **208**: 1459–1471.
96. Zhou Y, Huang X, Hecker L *et al.* (2013) Inhibition of mechanosensitive signaling in myofibroblasts ameliorates experimental pulmonary fibrosis. *J Clin Invest* **123**: 1096–1108.

97. Li Z, Dranoff JA, Chan EP *et al.* (2007) Transforming growth factor-beta and substrate stiffness regulate portal fibroblast activation in culture. *Hepatology* **46**: 1246–1256.
98. Liu F, Mih JD, Shea BS *et al.* (2010) Feedback amplification of fibrosis through matrix stiffening and COX-2 suppression. *J Cell Biol* **190**: 693–706.
99. Huang X, Yang N, Fiore VF *et al.* (2012) Matrix stiffness-induced myofibroblast differentiation is mediated by intrinsic mechanotransduction. *Am J Respir Cell Mol Biol* **47**: 340–348.
100. Goldmann WH. (2012) Mechanotransduction and focal adhesions. *Cell Biol Int* **36**: 649–652.
101. Samuel MS, Lopez JI, McGhee EJ *et al.* (2011) Actomyosin-mediated cellular tension drives increased tissue stiffness and beta-catenin activation to induce epidermal hyperplasia and tumor growth. *Cancer Cell* **19**: 776–791.
102. Charbonney E, Speight P, Masszi A *et al.* (2011) beta-catenin and Smad3 regulate the activity and stability of myocardin-related transcription factor during epithelial-myofibroblast transition. *Mol Biol Cell* **22**: 4472–4485.
103. Dupont S, Morsut L, Aragona M *et al.* (2011) Role of YAP/TAZ in mechanotransduction. *Nature* **474**: 179–183.
104. Sukharev S and Sachs F. (2012) Molecular force transduction by ion channels: Diversity and unifying principles. *J Cell Sci* **125**: 3075–3083.
105. Sherratt MJ. (2009) Tissue elasticity and the ageing elastic fibre. *Age (Dordr)* **31**: 305–325.

Chapter 17

Telomeres and Telomerase

Mary Armanios*

1. Preface

Telomere shortening is perhaps the best characterized molecular mechanism of cellular aging.[1] Telomeres define and protect chromosome ends; they are thus essential for genomic integrity. In humans and other vertebrates, they are made up of tandem TTAGGG nucleotide repeats and are bound by specialized proteins known as shelterin.[1] Because the DNA replication machinery incompletely copies the ends, telomeres shorten with each cell division.[2] Ultimately telomere length reaches a critically short threshold, and activates a DNA damage response that provokes programs of apoptosis and/or cellular senescence.[3] As this chapter will summarize, the last decade has uncovered several discoveries that link telomere defects intimately to the genetics and biology of age-related disease in the lung.[4–7] These connections establish telomere dysfunction as underlying the etiology of idiopathic pulmonary fibrosis (IPF) in a majority of cases. There is also emerging evidence that telomere dysfunction is a determinant of emphysema susceptibility, and rivals alpha-1 antitrypsin deficiency in its contribution.[5] This chapter aims to summarize the current and emerging knowledge in this area.

*Department of Oncology and Institute of Genetic Medicine; Johns Hopkins University School of Medicine, 733 N Broadway, Baltimore, MD 21205, USA, E-mail: marmani1@jhmi.edu

2. The Telomerase Enzyme

Telomerase is a remarkable enzyme that synthesizes new telomeres.[8–10] It is an RNA-dependent DNA polymerase that adds new telomere repeats onto the 3' ends of chromosomes. As such, it functions to offset the telomere shortening that normally occurs during DNA replication. The telomerase enzyme has two essential components. The telomerase reverse transcriptase, TERT, shares homology with other reverse transcriptases, and uses a template within TR, the telomerase RNA, for telomere repeat addition.[11,12] As will be discussed later, mutations in the *TERT* gene are the most common identifiable cause of familial forms of pulmonary fibrosis.

3. Telomeres as A "Molecular Clock"

Multiple pieces of evidence have long pointed to telomere shortening as a mechanism of cellular aging. Telomere length shortens in humans as they age, and it predicts the onset of senescence in cultured primary cells.[3] In clinical settings, telomere length measurement using flow cytometry-based techniques is useful in the diagnosis of bone marrow and lung disorders.[13] The application of telomere length measurement from in vitro studies to clinical settings in bone marrow and lung disease underscores how this mechanism of cellular aging has emerged as relevant for clinical care.[13]

4. How Studies in Protozoa Informed the Pathogenesis of Idiopathic Lung Disease

The role of telomere and telomerase biology in the context of lung disease exemplifies how basic science can inform clinical paradigms. Telomerase and telomeres were first discovered in *Tetrahymena thermophila*, a protozoan that is particularly amenable to the study of chromosomes and nuclear contents because it has an abundance of them.[14] Scientists who worked in this area initially aimed to understand how genomes are maintained given the so-called 'end-replication problem.'[14] In recognition of the discovery of telomeres and telomerase, Elizabeth Blackburn, Carol Greider and Jack Szostak, were awarded the Nobel Prize in Physiology or Medicine in 2009 for the discovery of telomerase and telomeres. Based on the prevalence of genetic abnormalities in patients with idiopathic pulmonary fibrosis and emphysema, telomere biology biology may have its greatest clinical implications in the area of age-related lung disease.

5. The Telomerase Knockout Mouse and the Consequences of Telomere Dysfunction

Telomere dysfunction in mammals was first studied in mice long before telomere shortening was appreciated to cause human disease. The telomerase knockout mouse ($mTR^{-/-}$) was engineered in 1997 and it was noted early on that it is phenotypically intact.[15] Only after multiple generations of $mTR^{-/-}$ breeding did telomere-mediated phenotypes appear.[15] This genetic anticipation phenomenon, the worsening of phenotypes with each generation, was related to the successive shortening of telomere length.[16] Mice with short telomeres develop several degenerative phenotypes. These include low blood counts, enteropathy, delayed wound healing and increased apoptosis in germ cells that leads to infertility.[17–19] As will be outlined below, similar to these mice, the genetic anticipation and all these degenerative phenotype have now been documented in humans with mutant telomerase genes.[20,21] These murine studies have been valuable in establishing telomere length as a predictor of disease severity.[1] The mouse pulmonary phenotype will be further discussed below in a dedicated section.

6. Telomere Defects in the Rare Disorder Dyskeratosis Congenita

Disease associated with telomerase mutations was first identified in the premature aging syndrome dyskeratosis congenita.[22] It has an estimated prevalence of 1 per 1 million and is defined by a mucocutaneous triad: Skin hyperpigmentation, oral leukoplakia and nail dystrophy.[23] Dyskeratosis congenita patients uniformly have abnormally short telomeres compared to age-matched controls.[1] Around 90% of dyskeratosis congenita patients develop bone marrow failure by the age of 20.[24] In some cases, dyskeratosis congenita patients may develop pulmonary disease as a first presentation.[24] More commonly, pulmonary fibrosis follows the onset of bone marrow failure by years to decades. Historically, pulmonary fibrosis was a serious and often fatal complication soon after bone marrow transplantation when conventional transplant preparative regimens were used.[25] In recent years, with expanding implementation of pre-transplant telomere length screening, as well as non-myeloablative regimens, bone marrow transplant outcomes have improved and lung disease is delayed.[13,26] As further discussed below, the dyskeratosis congenita clinical criteria identify only a small subset of patients with telomere and telomerase defects and adult-onset lung disease presentation account for more than 90% of individuals with germline defects in telomerase and telomere genes.

7. Telomerase Mutations in Familial Pulmonary Fibrosis

Pulmonary disease is the most common manifestation of telomere-mediated disease in adults.[27] Mutations in telomerase and telomere genes are the most common identifiable cause of familial forms of pulmonary fibrosis and account for nearly one-fourth of all cases (Fig. 1a). Mutations in *TERT* and *TR* mutations underlie the inheritance in 10–18% of all familial cases.[4,6,28] This discovery followed the report of autosomal dominant inheritance of IPF in a three-generation family with a *TERT* mutation.[20] The IPF phenotype in this family showed an earlier and more severe onset with each generation and this was associated with successive telomere shortening.[20] In families with *TERT* and *TR* mutations, heterozygous mutations cause telomerase loss-of-function and haploinsufficiency.[20,27] In addition to *TERT* and *TR*, mutations in three other telomerase and telomere genes have also been linked to familial

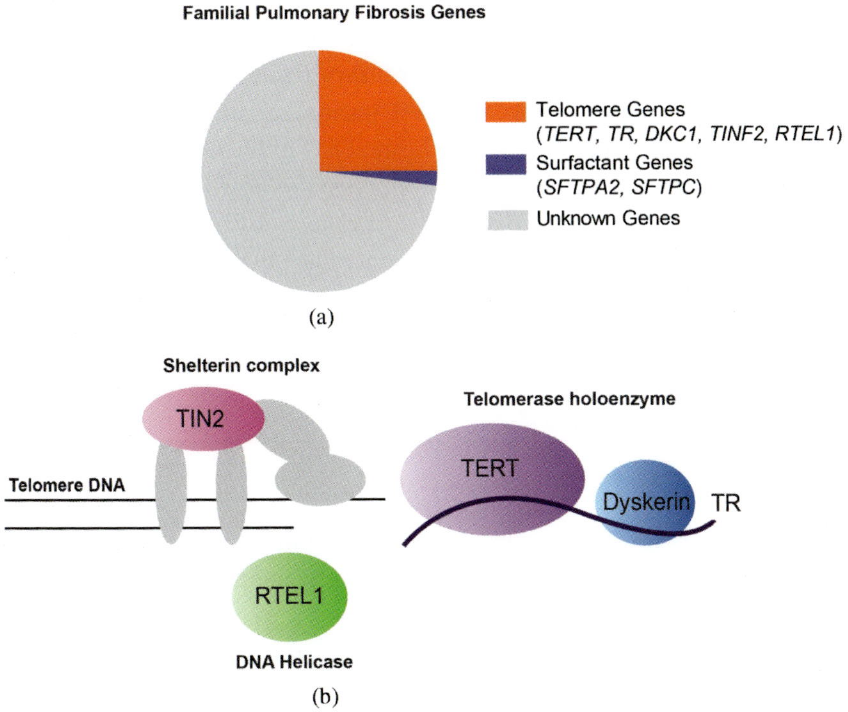

Fig. 1. The role of telomerase and telomere gene mutations in familial pulmonary fibrosis. (a) Percentage of families with known telomerase or telomere gene mutation relative to other causes such as surfactant mutations. (b) Simple schema showing function of the five telomere genes implicated in familial pulmonary fibrosis. Mutations in the telomerase holoenzyme complex, specifically in TERT, are the most common cause and explain approxiamtely 15% of cases. Fig. 1b is modified from Stanley *et al. AJRCCM* 2015.

pulmonary fibrosis, albeit at lower frequency. Mutations in the telomerase holoenzyme dyskerin, which is encoded by *DKC1,* cause X-linked inheritance.[29,30] Mutations in the shelterin component TRF1-interacting factor 2, *TINF2,* and the regulator of telomere length 1 gene, *RTEL1,* are genetic risk factors for autosomal dominant pulmonary fibrosis.[31,32] Beyond these five telomerase and telomere genes (Fig. 1b), it is predicted that mutations in other components of the pathway will be identified in families with pulmonary fibrosis.

8. The Extrapulmonary Telomere Syndrome Manifestations

Studies of telomere-mediated pulmonary disease have highlighted extrapulmonary disease in affected patients and these reflect the systemic short telomere defect (Table 1). Their co-occurrence represents a form of adult-onset telomere syndromes.[1] Telomere syndrome patients with lung disease most commonly have hematologic abnormalities including long-standing macrocytosis and are prone

Table 1. Pulmonary pathology and extrapulmonary telomere-mediated disease documented in telomerase mutation carriers.*

Pulmonary Disease
IPF (~65% of cases)
Non-specific interstitial pneumonitis (NSIP)
Bronchiolitis obliterans organizing pneumonia
Chronic hypersensitivity pneumonitis
Interstitial fibrosis, non-classifiable histology
Emphysema alone or combined with pulmonary fibrosis
Bone Marrow Failure
Macrocytosis
Cytopenias
Bone marrow hypoplasia or aplasia
Myelodysplastic syndromes
Acute myeloid leukemia
Liver Disease
Mild elevations in transaminases
Nodular regenerative hyperplasia
Cryptogenic cirrhosis
Enteropathy
Intestinal villous atrophy
Mycophenolate-related enteropathy
Failure to thrive

to develop aplastic anemia and myelodysplastic syndrome.[33,34] In some cases, acute myeloid leukemia may develop *de novo*.[35] Less commonly, telomere syndromes may manifest in concurrent cryptogenic liver disease and enteropathies; the latter may resemble the presentation of celiac disease.[34,36] An increased incidence of male and female infertility has also been reported to predate the diagnosis of telomere-associated pulmonary fibrosis in 10% of cases.[31] In the lung transplant setting, severe cytopenias increase the transfusion requirements and the risk of infection.[37] There is also a propensity to gastrointestinal bleeding and renal failure.[37] Awareness of these recurrent complications has the potential to inform management in several settings including in the pre-transplant workup as well as the post-transplant management. Considering pre-transplant genetic evaluation and an individualized management approach in the transplant setting may help avert some of these complications.[37]

9. Heterogeneous Histologies in Telomere–Mediated Lung Disease

Although mutations in telomerase provide a genetic explanation for the inheritance in families, it is clear that the histopathologies are heterogeneous even when a single mutation is shared. In a review of more than 150 published cases, the usual interstitial pneumonia histopathology was found in two-thirds of cases[27] (Table 1). In the remainder, diverse idiopathic interstitial pneumonia patterns including non-specific interstitial pneumonitis, hypersensitivity pneumonitis and others have been documented. Since the underlying driving molecular mechanism is shared amongst individuals, the heterogeneity in histopathologies raises the possibility that a molecular, rather than pathologic classification, may be more predictive of a more uniform natural history. Patients with telomere-mediated lung disease will share similar risks for comorbidities and likely similar responses to treatment; their collective molecular grouping may thus be more clinically informative.

10. Telomere Defects in Sporadic Forms of Pulmonary Fibrosis

While the evidence of a role for telomere dysfunction is most clear in families, there is evidence it extends to the more common sporadic form of IPF.[27] Eighty percent of cases have no family history of IPF; however even in these individuals, severe telomere shortening may be seen in at least in half the cases.[38] The telomere shortening is of biological significance because its magnitude is similar to that seen in telomerase mutation carriers, and it appears to be constitutional, seen not only in leukocyte lineages but also in alveolar epithelial cells.[38] Similar extrapulmonary manifestations of telomere-mediated disease have also been documented in these patients with short telomeres including bone marrow failure and liver disease.[38] These observations have suggested that short telomeres may be a risk factor for IPF and likely contributes to its age-dependent onset.[38] Beyond explaining its genetic origins, a recent study has suggested that short telomeres may also be associated with shorter survival and time-to-transplant in IPF.[39] The reasons for this remain unclear but it may be that telomere-mediated IPF may have an intrinsically more accelerated course or that the telomere-associated comorbidities complicate the natural history.[7] Efforts to further delineate the significance of short telomeres in sporadic IPF are ongoing.

11. Telomere Dysfunction and Mechanisms of Lung Disease

The genetic clues linking telomerase and telomere defects to IPF pathogenesis have raised important questions as to how telomere shortening may cause lung disease. Interestingly, although mice with short telomeres recapitulate many of the features of human telomere-mediated disease, they develop no *de novo* lung disease.[40] However, when exposed chronically to cigarette smoke, telomerase null mice with short telomeres are susceptible and develop emphysema.[40] The telomere-mediated emphysema in mice is associated with cumulative damage in epithelial cells and is not related to inflammation.[40] These studies have raised the possibility that telomere dysfunction in epithelial cells are a primary driver of telomere-mediated lung disease.[4,13,27] "The Current model posits that, in the lung, which is a slow turnover tissue, cigarette smoke exposure provokes a "second hit." The cumulative effect with this environmental injury, along with the genetically determined telomere defect, provokes alveolar damage.[13] Understanding the mechanisms underlying telomere-mediated lung disease is the focus of ongoing research, and the hope is that new insights born out of the genetic clues will translate into more effective therapies.

12. Inherited Telomerase Mutations Causing Emphysema

There is emerging evidence that the role of telomerase mutations in lung disease genetics extends to emphysema.[5] These build on the observation in mice that short telomeres increase the susceptibility to emphysema after cigarette smoke exposure.[40] Using a candidate gene approach and examining well-characterized COPDGene and Lung Health Study subjects, deleterious mutations in *TERT* were found in 1% of cases.[5] This frequency is comparable to that of alpha-1 antitrypsin deficiency in this population. Interestingly, a majority of telomerase mutation carriers were women, suggesting a sex specific predilection.[5] In families, pulmonary fibrosis and emphysema showed autosomal dominant inheritance along with other telomere syndrome features.[5] Smoking was a required second hit for emphysema to develop.[5] These discoveries highlight the shared genetic susceptibility of emphysema with pulmonary fibrosis, and indicate telomerase genetics may explain the increased susceptibility to cigarette smoke in certain populations, in particular women.[5]

13. Outlook for the Future

The study of aging biology may at times have as its focus finding "a fountain of youth." However, in pulmonary medicine, telomere biology has shed direct light on the etiology and biology of devastating disorders. The clues from telomere biology provide a window from which understanding how molecular aging contributes to lung disease has the potential to advance patient care.

Acknowledgement

I am grateful to Susan E. Stanley for help with the figures.

References

1. Armanios M , Blackburn EH. (2012) The telomere syndromes. *Nature Revs Genet* **13**(10): 693–704.
2. Greider CW. (1998) Telomeres and senescence: The history, the experiment, the future. *Curr Biol* **8**(5): R178–R181.
3. Harley CB, Futcher AB, Greider CW. (1990) Telomeres shorten during ageing of human fibroblasts. *Nature* **345**(6274): 458–460.
4. Armanios MY *et al.* (2007) Telomerase mutations in families with idiopathic pulmonary fibrosis. *N Engl J Med* **356**(13): 1317–1326.
5. Stanley SE *et al.* (2014) Telomerase mutations in smokers with severe emphysema. *J Clin Invest.*
6. Tsakiri KD *et al.* (2007) Adult-onset pulmonary fibrosis caused by mutations in telomerase. *Proc Natl Acad Sci USA* **104**(18): 7552–7557.
7. Stanley SE, Armanios M. (2014) Short telomeres: A repeat offender in IPF. *The Lancet Respir Med* **2**(7): 513–514.
8. Greider CW, Blackburn EH. (1985) Identification of a specific telomere terminal transferase activity in Tetrahymena extracts. *Cell* **43** (2): 405–413.
9. Greider CW, Blackburn EH. (1987) The telomere terminal transferase of Tetrahymena is a ribonucleoprotein enzyme with two kinds of primer specificity. *Cell* **51**(6): 887–898.
10. Greider CW, Blackburn EH. (1989) A telomeric sequence in the RNA of Tetrahymena telomerase required for telomere repeat synthesis. *Nature* **337**(6205): 331–337.
11. Nakamura TM *et al.* (1997) Telomerase catalytic subunit homologs from fission yeast and human. *Science* **277**(5328): 955–959.
12. Feng J *et al.* (1995) The RNA component of human telomerase. *Science* **269**(5228): 1236–1241.
13. Armanios M. (2013) Telomeres and age-related disease: How telomere biology informs clinical paradigms. *J Clin Invest* **123**(3): 996–1002.

14. Blackburn EH, Greider CW, Szostak JW. (2006) Telomeres and telomerase: The path from maize, Tetrahymena and yeast to human cancer and aging. *Nat Med* **12**(10): 1133–1138.
15. Blasco MA *et al.* (1997) Telomere shortening and tumor formation by mouse cells lacking telomerase RNA. *Cell* **91**(1): 25–34.
16. Rudolph KL *et al.* (1999) Longevity, stress response, and cancer in aging telomerase-deficient mice. *Cell* **96**(5): 701–712.
17. Lee HW *et al.* (1998) Essential role of mouse telomerase in highly proliferative organs. *Nature* **392**(6676): 569–574.
18. Hao LY *et al.* (2005) Short telomeres, even in the presence of telomerase, limit tissue renewal capacity. *Cell* **123**(6): 1121–1131.
19. Armanios M *et al.* (2009) Short telomeres are sufficient to cause the degenerative defects associated with aging. *Am J Hum Genet* **85**(6): 823–832.
20. Armanios M *et al.* (2005) Haploinsufficiency of telomerase reverse transcriptase leads to anticipation in autosomal dominant dyskeratosis congenita. *Proc Natl Acad Sci USA* **102**(44): 15960–15964.
21. Vulliamy T *et al.* (2004) Disease anticipation is associated with progressive telomere shortening in families with dyskeratosis congenita due to mutations in TERC. *Nat Genet.*
22. Dokal I. (2001) Dyskeratosis congenita. A disease of premature ageing. *Lancet* **358** :S27.
23. Dokal I. (2000) Dyskeratosis congenita in all its forms. *Br J Haematol* **110**(4): 768–779.
24. Knight S *et al.* (1998) Dyskeratosis Congenita (DC) Registry: Identification of new features of DC. *Br J Haematol* **103**(4): 990–996.
25. de la Fuente J, Dokal I. (2007) Dyskeratosis congenita: Advances in the understanding of the telomerase defect and the role of stem cell transplantation. *Pediatr Transplant* **11**(6): 584–594.
26. Dietz AC *et al.* (2010) Disease-specific hematopoietic cell transplantation: Nonmyeloablative conditioning regimen for dyskeratosis congenita. *Bone Marrow Transplant.*
27. Armanios M. (2012) Telomerase and idiopathic pulmonary fibrosis. *Mutation Res* **730**(1–2): 52–58.
28. Diaz de Leon A *et al.* (2010) Telomere lengths, pulmonary fibrosis and telomerase (TERT) mutations. *PLoS One* **5**(5):e10680.
29. Alder JK *et al.* (2013) Telomere Phenotypes in Females with Heterozygous Mutations in the Dyskeratosis Congenita 1 (DKC1) Gene. *Hum Mutat.*

30. Kropski JA *et al.* (2014) A novel dyskerin (DKC1) mutation is associated with Familial Interstitial Pneumonia. *Chest.*
31. Alder JK *et al.* (2014) Exome sequencing identifies mutant TINF2 in a family with pulmonary fibrosis. *Chest.*
32. Cogan JD *et al.* (2015) Rare Variants in RTEL1 are Associated with Familial Interstitial Pneumonia. *Am J Respir Crit Care Med.*
33. Parry EM, Alder JK, Qi X *et al.* (2011) Syndrome complex of bone marrow failure and pulmonary fibrosis predicts germline defects in telomerase. *Blood* **117**(21): 5607–5611.
34. Armanios M. (2009) Syndromes of telomere shortening. *Annu Rev Genomics Hum Genet* 10: 45–61.
35. Kirwan M *et al.* (2009) Defining the pathogenic role of telomerase mutations in myelodysplastic syndrome and acute myeloid leukemia. *Hum Mutat* **30**(11): 1567–1573.
36. Jonassaint NL, Guo N, Califano JA *et al.* (2013) The gastrointestinal manifestations of telomere-mediated disease. *Aging cell* **12**(2): 319–323.
37. Silhan LL *et al.* (2014) Lung transplantation in telomerase mutation carriers with pulmonary fibrosis. *Eur Respir J* **44**(1): 178–187.
38. Alder JK *et al.* (2008) Short telomeres are a risk factor for idiopathic pulmonary fibrosis. *Proc Natl Acad Sci USA* **105**(35): 13051–13056.
39. Stuart BD *et al.* (2014) Effect of telomere length on survival in patients with idiopathic pulmonary fibrosis: An observational cohort study with independent validation. *The Lancet Respir Med* **2**(7): 557–565.
40. Alder JK *et al.* (2011) Telomere length is a determinant of emphysema susceptibility. *Am J Respir Crit Care Med* **184**(8): 904–912.

Chapter 18
Endoplasmic Reticulum Stress

Marta Bueno*,† and Ana L. Mora*,†,‡

1. Summary

With the expected rapid growth of the aging population, there is a clear need to understand the complex process of aging and senescence and their impact in the pathogenesis of age-related diseases. The endoplasmic reticulum (ER) is critical to maintain proteostasis, the control of protein folding and protein quality in the cell. Protein folding abnormalities activate the adaptive unfolded protein responses (UPR) to halt protein production and facilitate protein folding by increasing chaperone synthesis. In the presence of chronic ER stress and/or insufficient UPR the proteostasis balance is not recovered and the UPR pro-apoptotic responses are activated. It is known that the function of the ER declines with age. Several defects in the chaperoning system have been reported, causing aggregation of insoluble proteins and increased inflammation and apoptotic responses. This patho-mechanism is common to several age-related diseases including neurodegenerative diseases, diabetes type 2 and inflammatory bowel disease among others. Similarly, in the lung, persistent ER stress has been associated with the pathogenesis of Idiopathic Pulmonary Fibrosis (IPF), a lung disease that predominantly affects

* Heart, Lung, and Blood Vascular Medicine Institute, University of Pittsburgh, USA
† Division of Pulmonary, Allergy and Critical Care Medicine. University of Pittsburgh, USA
‡ Corresponding author.

older adults. Markers of ER stress have been found abundantly expressed in type II alveolar epithelial cells from familial and sporadic forms of pulmonary fibrosis. In familial pulmonary fibrosis ER stress has been linked to mutations in the surfactant protein; whereas aging and environmental exposures (like herpesvirus infection and cigarette smoke) are believed to contribute to the persistent activation of ER stress in sporadic IPF.

2. ER, Protein Folding and Protein Quality Control

Proteins are fascinating macromolecules with structural, signaling or catalytic functions. But none of these functions can be achieved without a proper tridimensional structure, without a correct folding (already imprinted in the primary sequence of the aminoacid polypeptide[1]). This folded or native state is usually a low energy state reached spontaneously such so proteins don't expend much time navigating the conformational space leading to non-productive folding variants.[2] In the cell, proteins are synthesized and folded in an extremely crowded environment from which, they emerge from the ribosome and are exposed to potentially harmful interactions. Nature devised several mechanisms to facilitate *in vivo* folding as, for example, compartmentalization,[3] the assistance of molecular chaperones,[4] the presence of disulfide isomerases or the participation of other enzymes regulating post-translational modifications. All this machinery ensures a fast and proper folding, however it is tightly regulated to avoid unwanted products like macromolecular aggregates that can lead to diseases.[5] The cell needs to be able to control not only the protein synthesis but also their trafficking and degradation, thus establishing protein homeostasis. Only when all this mechanisms function simultaneously, the biochemical network that supports life can be established and living organisms can properly function.

Protein biosynthesis is prone to errors, while waiting to be fold proteins can expose hydrophobic surfaces making them vulnerable to aggregation. Also, unusual post-translational modifications and/or addition of disulfide bonds (usually outside the cytosol, in the

ERlumen) can lead to non-native proteins that need to be eliminated. Even well-folded active proteins can be irreversibly modified (and inactivated) by other modifications driven by reactive metabolic by-products, such as reactive oxygen and nitrogen species. So, it is easy to imagine that cells evolved two different ways to deal with protein damage in order to survive: (a) the quality control response and (b) the stress responses. When there is an accumulation of acute damaged proteins, they have to be either repaired or eliminated by protein quality control networks. First, the action of molecular chaperones is required to try to refold and repair, however when damage is irreparable, a proteolityc system is deployed. In eukaryotes, these ill-damaged proteins are eliminated by the ubiquitin proteasome system (UPS) or by macroautophagy. In both cases, proteins need to be ubiquitinated by an ATP-consuming process.[6]

In the stress response, protein damage induces adaptive responses that decrease global protein synthesis while increase the abundance of chaperones and proteolytic systems. There are two main adaptive responses, the heat shock response (HSR) in the cytosol and the UPR in the ER. HSR is mediated by the heat shock transcription factor HSF1, which exists as a monomer (bound to Hsp90) in the cytosol but under stress conditions (when Hsp90 is needed elsewhere) oligomerizes and, as a trimer can be relocated to the nucleus to activate the expression of HSR target genes.[7] Accumulation of damaged proteins in the ER induces the UPR though the activation of ER-membrane stress transducers that initiate a cascade of signals leading to the transcription of proteins containing the unfolded protein response element (UPRE).[8] Using these pathways, cells are able to reduce the load of damaged proteins at the same time that the amount of endangered new proteins is decreased.

3. ER Stress and UPR

Almost a third of the proteins synthetized by the cell need to be imported to the ER for further post-translational modification and trafficking to the secretory pathways or the plasma membrane. Proteostasis in the ER is maintained by a tight balance of two mechanisms, the ER-assisted folding (ERAF) and the ER-associated degradation (ERAD).[9] Nascent polypeptides translocate from the closest ribosomes into the ER lumen, where they interact with a group or resident chaperones to facilitate their proper folding (ERAF pathway). Then, these native three-dimensional active conformers are ready to be pack in vesicles for further trafficking to other cellular organelles or to finally localize in the plasma membrane. However, sometimes proteins do not achieve their correct fold. If that is the case, they are recognized by members of the ERAD pathway and translocated back to the cytosol where they will be degraded by the cytosolic proteasome.

When the balance between misfolding and degradation is broken (so-called ER stress), the ER triggers the UPR, which is aimed to restore ER proteostasis, but can eventually lead to apoptosis if the ER dysfunction is persistent or severe. Three distinct UPR signaling pathways exist in mammalian cells, including the inositol-requiring protein 1 (IRE1), the pancreatic ER kinase (PERK) and the activating transcription factor 6 (ATF6). These three proteins act as sensors of the ER proteostasis environment (Fig. 1). Under healthy (non-stress) conditions, the chaperone BiP (binding immunoglobulin protein) is bound to the ER-lumen side of the receptors. When misfolded proteins accumulate (due to environmental, genetic, developmental or aging-related stress), BiP dissociate from the receptors to cope with the increased exposure of nascent protein hydrophobic regions allowing the receptors to activate. ATF6 expose a Golgi translocation signal, where it is translocated and processed to a smaller active transcription factor ($ATF6^{NT}$) that will activate the transcription of other chaperones. PERK oligomerize and undergoes autophosphorylation, causing the phosphorylation of eiF2alpha and attenuating global translation. Finally, IRE1 activates itself by homodimerization and transautophosphorylation, causing the activation of its cytosolic endoribonuclease domain able to splice the transcription factor XBP1 (Xbox binding protein) mRNA by cleavage and removal of a 252bp intron. The activated transcription factor (XBP1s) up-regulates UPRE genes, increasing ERAF and ERAD. IRE-1 decreases also the production of new proteins in the ER by degradation of ER-target mRNAs.[10]

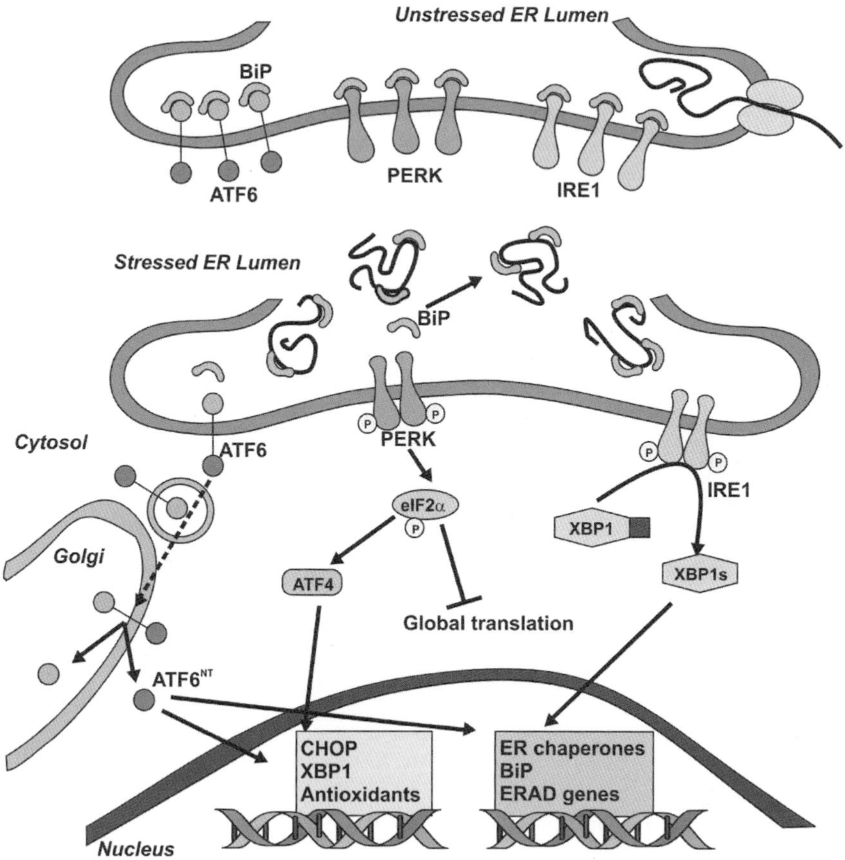

Fig 1. UPR Pathways.

On ER stress, BiP dissociates from three ER stress transmembrane sensors (PERK, IRE1 and ATF6) allowing their activation. When activated, PERK phosphorylates eiF2alpha to upregulate the selective translation of the transcriptional factor ATF4 to induce the UPR-target genes. ATF6 translocates from the endoplasmic reticulum to the Golgi, in which ATF6 cleavage produces a transcriptionally active cytosolic fragment ($ATF6^{NT}$). $ATF6^{NT}$ activates a subset of UPR- and non-UPR-target genes, including XBP1. During ER stress, activation of IRE1 elicits an endo ribonuclease activity that specifically cleaves the mRNA encoding the transcriptional factor XBP1. This unconventional splicing reaction is required for translation of transcriptionally active XBP1s to induce UPR- and non–UPR-target genes.

As we mentioned above, in many circumstances, the protective pathways of the UPR could be insufficient or fail to restore the folding capacity with the subsequent activation of intrinsic and extrinsic apoptotic pathways (Fig. 2). The initiation of apoptotic responses by

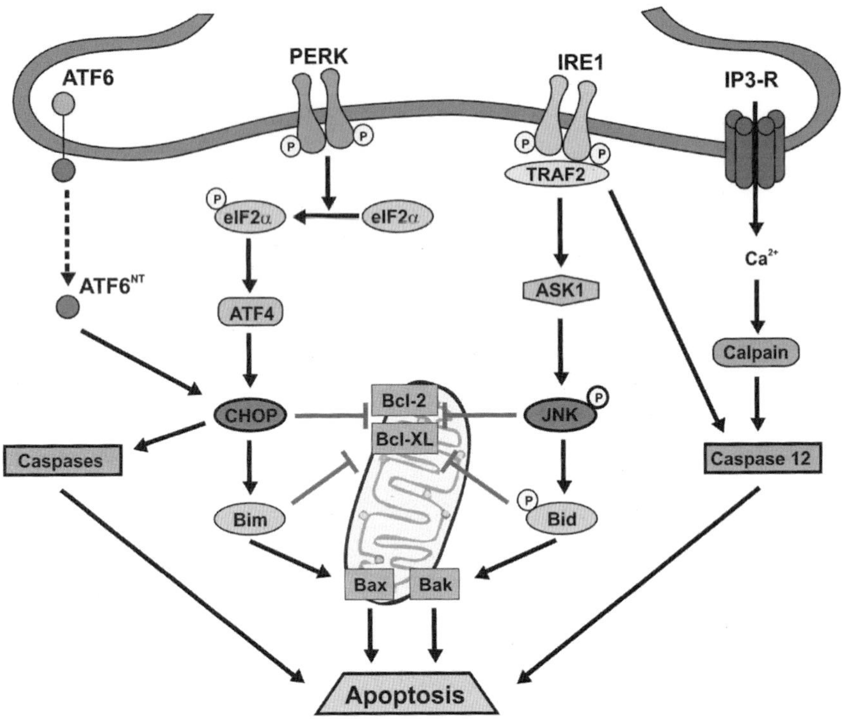

Fig 2. Cell Death Signaling by the ER Stress Response/UPR.

In case of severe and sustained ER stress, a number of pro-apoptotic events begin to dominate and lead to apoptosis. Transcription factors ATF4 and $ATF6^{NT}$ stimulate CHOP expression. CHOP inhibits antiapoptotic proteins of the Bcl-2 family and stimulates pro-apoptotic Bim, altogether leading to heterodimerization and activation of pro-apoptotic Bax and Bak. CHOP also sensitizes cells to pro-apoptotic stimuli involving caspase-pathways. Similarly, association of TRAF2 with activated IRE1 leads to activation of caspase 12 and the activation of ASK1, now able to phosphorylate and activate JNK. Calcium release from the ER via IP3 receptors can activate calpains, which further stimulate caspase 12 activation via proteolytic cleavage of its inactive procaspase precursor.

prolonged or chronic ER stress activates downstream molecules such as CHOP, JNK and members of the Bcl2 family proteins. IRE-1 triggers apoptotic responses by two different signaling pathways. First, by upregulation of c/EBP homologous protein (CHOP), a nuclear transcription factor that represses the promoter of the anti-apoptotic molecule Bcl2.[11] Additionally, IRE-1 can induce apoptotic cell death by the recruitment of the adaptor molecule TNF-receptor associated factor 2 (TRAF2). The IRE-1-TRAF2 complex can recruit the apoptosis-signal-regulating kinase (ASK1), which activates JNK (c-Jun NH-terminal kinase) downstream. JNK regulates the phosphorylation of Bcl2 at the ER, blocking its anti-apoptotic activity. JNK also phosphorylate BH3-only members of the Bcl2 family, such as BAD (Bcl2-associated death promoter protein) and BIM (Bcl2-like 11), enhancing their pro-apoptotic activity. High levels of BH3-only proteins have been implicated in the mobilization of ER Ca^{2+} stores that sensitizes mitochondria to undergo apoptosis, as well as Ca^{2+} independent apoptotic pathways like the activation of caspases located in the ER including procaspase-12. Independently of the pathway apoptotic, cell death is executed via the activation of different caspase cascades.[12]

4. ER Stress and Hormetic Regulation of the Aging Process: Chaperones, XBP-1 and Apoptosis

The capacity to adapt to intrinsic and environmental stress seems to be strongly associated to aging (Fig. 3). At this respect, the phenomenon of hormesis describes a dose-dependent response to stress, where mild stress induces tolerance and increase longevity while severe stress aggravates the aging process.[13–15] In congruency with the concept of hormesis, ER stress transducers identify the intensity of stress and induce dose-dependent responses that mediate adaptation, stress resistance and survival or trigger apoptosis.[16,17] Thus, for instance a common signature response in prolonged ER stress and aging is inflammation.[18] The sensitivity of the UPR system seems to decline with age, e.g. a decline has been observed in the levels of eIF2alpha phosphorylation and the expression levels of ATF4 and XBP1,[19,20] that might result in a decay in the expression of PERK and IRE1.

Chaperones are key folding sensors in the ER and include BiP (also known as glucose regulated protein 78 or GRP78), GRP94, calnexin, calreticulin, thiol-distulfide oxidoreductases, protein disulfide isomerase (PDI) among others (Table 1). Aging is linked

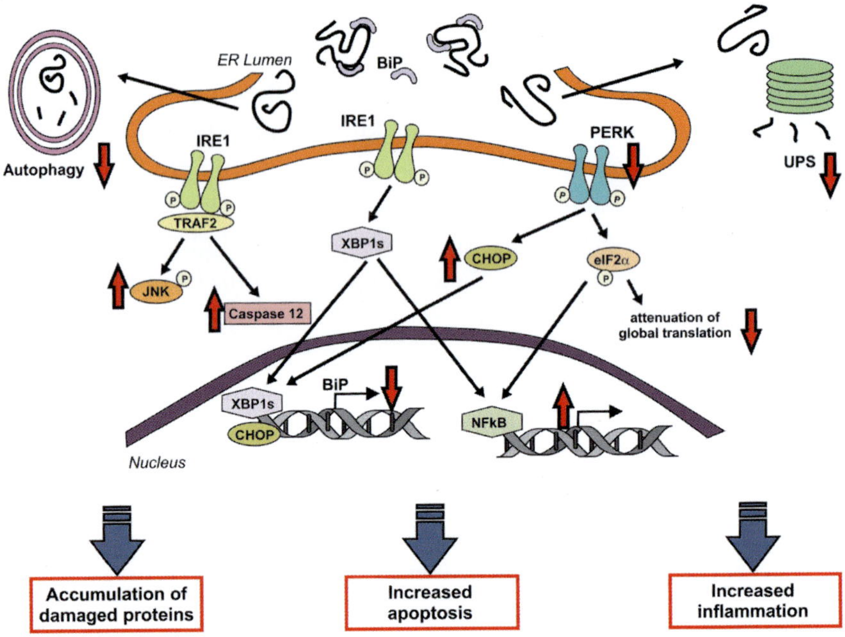

Fig 3. General and Organelle-Specific Stress Response Pathways Influenced by the Aging Process.

Depending on the type of macromolecule and the site of damage, distinct stress response pathways, such as autophagy, HSP or UPR are initiated. Aging broadly affects stress response pathways in multiple steps (denoted by red arrows). An attenuation of autophagy mechanisms and protesome activity, in combination with an impaired ER stress response leads to accumulation of damaged proteins with increased apoptosis and inflammation.

to chaperones oxidation reducing their enzymatic activity.[21] For example, significant reduction of BiP expression levels has been found in cerebral cortex of aging mice,[22] hippocampus of rats[19] and in peripheral tissue of rats including lung, liver, kidney, heart and spleen.[20] Additionally, age has been related with an increase in the heat shock proteins (HSP) expression but also is responsible for a diminished heat shock protein response.[23]

Furthermore, aging cells show an increased tendency to pro-apoptotic responses under ER stress conditions. A potential explanation is that the expression of CHOP, one of the major apoptotic inducer during ER stress and caspase 12 are increased in aging

Table 1. Alterations of different chaperones with age.

Protein	Alteration	Reference
HSF	Reduced DNA binding activity Reduced transcriptional activity	Heydari 2000[117] Choi 1990[118] Morimoto 2002[119]
Cytosolic chaperones	Elevated chaperone levels Decreased chaperone activity in cytosol Decreased chaperon function	Zou 1998[120] Soti 2002[121] Nardai 2002[122] Csermely 2001[123]
BiP	Decreased basal expression Oxidative damage	Naidoo 2008[22] Paz Gavilan 2006[19] Hussain 2007[20] Erickson 2006[124]
PDI	Reduced enzyme activity Oxidative damage	Nuss 2008[21] Van der Vlies 2002[125] Rabek 2003[126]
Calnexin	Decreased levels Oxidative damage	Erickson 2006[124] Paz Gavilan 2006[19] Van der Vlies 2002[125]
Calreticulin	Oxidative damage	Rabek 2003[126]

cells.[19,20,24] Additionally, JNK phosphorylation and JNK kinases have also found upregulated during aging.[25] On contrary, young cells have a more efficient UPR response preventing pro-apoptotic responses by activation of the PERK/eIF2alpha and IRE-1 pathway. In summary, with age, the efficiency of the UPR response decreases resulting in low protein quality control, increasing pro-apoptotic responses and higher susceptibility to ER stress-induced pathology.

5. Proteostasis and Aging

Proteostasis is the quality control system that regulates folding, misfolding, unfolding and degradation of proteins. The efficiency of proteostasis declines with age, in parallel to changes in protein structure secondary to oxidative modification, missense mutations and defective translation. Alteration in proteostasis results in insufficient functional proteins, accumulation of toxic proteins and/or aggregation of misfolded proteins. This is a very active cell process since around 30% of the newly synthesized proteins are targeted for immediate degradation because inadequate folding. Moreover, misfolding and aggregation of a metastable protein might cause a general impairment in proteostasis[26,27] and globally inhibit the ubiquitin proteosome system.[28]

Genetic mutations can cause protein misfolding with severe consequences for proteostasis and the normal function of the cell. Examples of lung pathologies associated with genetic mutation and altered proteostasis are: Cystic fibrosis (CF; alterations of the cystic fibrosis transmembrane conductance regulator, CFTR), pulmonary fibrosis (surfactant proteins) and Hemansky-Pudlak syndrome. In addition, recent studies show that genetic alterations outside the coding region of MUC5B can alter mucin 5B protein (muc5B) secretion and contribute to cell stress in IPF, CF and chronic obstructive pulmonary disease (COPD). Mutations or alterations in the normal function of the UPR, the ubiquitin proteosome system, or the autophagy-lysosome pathway can increase the pathology caused by impaired proteostasis. For instance, autophagy plays a critical role antagonizing proteostatic stress by allowing cellular reorganization and remodeling required for tissue repair. The details of the molecular mechanisms associated with the age-related modifications in proteostasis are not well understood yet, but it is known that younger individuals can enhance proteostasis to compensate for some protein misfolding mutations. In high contrast, with advanced age there is an accumulation of cell stress due to environmental exposures such as infections, cigarette smoke, or co-morbidities (including metabolic syndrome and sleep deprivation) that might have a negative impact in proteostasis and activate UPR responses in the ER. In addition, it seems that defects in the proteostasis process can have an impact in longevity. Studies in *C. elegans* show that impaired proteostasis and aging are both related with accumulation of aggregated proteins and activation of HSP and UPR.[26,29] Additionally, manipulations that extended lifespan by mild stresses (including downregulation of insulin/IGF-1 signaling or induction of HSP) restored proteostasis in aging worms.[30]

6. Diseases Linked to ER Stress and Aging

ER stress has been known to be involved in the pathogenesis of various diseases, predominantly neurodegenerative disorders. The pathogenesis of many of these diseases is linked to abnormal protein processing, protein aggregation, ER stress, and sustained activation of the UPR leading to neuronal apoptotic cell death (review by Johnson *et al.*).[31] These diseases include Alzheimer's disease (AD), Parkinson's disease (PD), amyotrophic lateral sclerosis (ALS) and Huntington's disease (HD). Markers of UPR activation and ER stress-induced cell death have been found in neurons of AD patients (including XBP1 splicing, expression of CHOP and activation of caspase-3, 4 and 12).[32] Activation of the PERK-eIF2alpha pathway has been also found in dopaminergic neurons in the substantia nigra of PD patients.[33] In addition, loss of Parkin function, a ubiquitin protein ligase whose mutations are associated with PD, result in the misfolding and accumulation of Parkin-associated endothelin receptor-like receptor (Pael-R), an ER stress inducer and causative factor of familial PD.[34] Aging has been also linked to disruption of normal sleep patterns in animals with increased basal levels ER stress markers in brain cortex.[22] Also, several studies in animals have demonstrated that sleep deprivation causes ER stress with upregulation of BiP and activation of PERK in the brain.[35,36] After sleep recovery BiP expression return to baseline levels.[37]

ER stress is also linked to several chronic diseases characterized by inflammation.[38–40] Good examples of this group of entities are arthritis, neuromuscular inflammation and inflammatory bowel disease.[41–44] It is not clear whether ER stress triggers the disease or it is activated by inflammatory responses. In the case of inflammatory bowel disease, secretory cells from the intestine mucosa are at high risk of ER stress by misfolding of the high molecular weight cysteine rich mucin that they produce.[45] Another disease whose pathogenesis maybe linked to ER stress and inflammation is metabolic syndrome. Metabolic syndrome is a disorder of energy utilization and storage associated with insulin resistance, reduced glucose utilization, type 2 diabetes, UPR chronic activation and subsequent activation of inflammation and pro-apoptotic pathways.[46] Similarly, vascular inflammation during atherosclerosis is also associated with ER stress and activation of the UPR response.[47,48] It is believed that the ER senses dysfunctional lipid biosynthesis and lipid exposure and mediates activation of inflammation and apoptotic pathways in the vasculature.[49]

The incidence of cancer also increases with age.[50] ER stress and UPR markers are elevated in several tumor types and a relation is found with cancer cell survival and resistance to anti-cancer treatments.[51] Cancer cells are under physiological ER stress due to their high proliferation rate and high demand of protein synthesis, folding and transport. With tumor growth, cancer cells are exposed to deprivation of nutrients and hypoxia, resulting in protein misfolding, ER stress and UPR activation. Moreover, tumor cells activate selectively UPR responses that mediate survival and suppress pathways that mediate apoptosis. For instance BiP has been found upregulated in several cancers[52] and its expression levels correlate directly with malignancy and resistance to chemotherapy.[52–55] XBP1 also seems to be essential for tumor growth. Studies in human tumor xenograft models show that the IRE-1-XBP1 pathway is essential to stimulate angiogenesis and tumor development.[56] Taken together, these studies show that malfunction of ER stress with age predispose to chronic activation of the UPR with increased inflammation and apoptotic cell death with a higher predisposition to several age-related diseases.

7. Lung: ER Stress in Familial and Sporadic IPF

Markers of ER stress are found in lungs of COPD,[57] ARDS (acute respiratory distress syndrome)[58] and IPF patients. ER stress, especially in PBMC (lymphocytes, monocytes and macrophages), is associated with activation of NF-kB pathway and inflammation in patients with ARDS and animal models of asthma[59] and LPS induced lung injury. On the contrary, presence of ER stress markers in IPF and COPD lungs have been associated with cytopathic effects in lung epithelial cells. For instance, higher levels of phosphorylated eIF2alpha and CHOP are observed in lung tissue of COPD patients in concordance with disease severity and activation of the caspase pathway. The role of ER stress in the pathogenesis of a lung disease has been studied in deep in IPF (Fig. 4). IPF is the most common of the idiopathic interstitial pneumonia, characterized by progressive fibrosis, respiratory failure with an average life expectancy of 2–5 years from the initial diagnosis.[60,61] IPF prevalence dramatically increases with age, from 0.8/100,000 in patients younger than

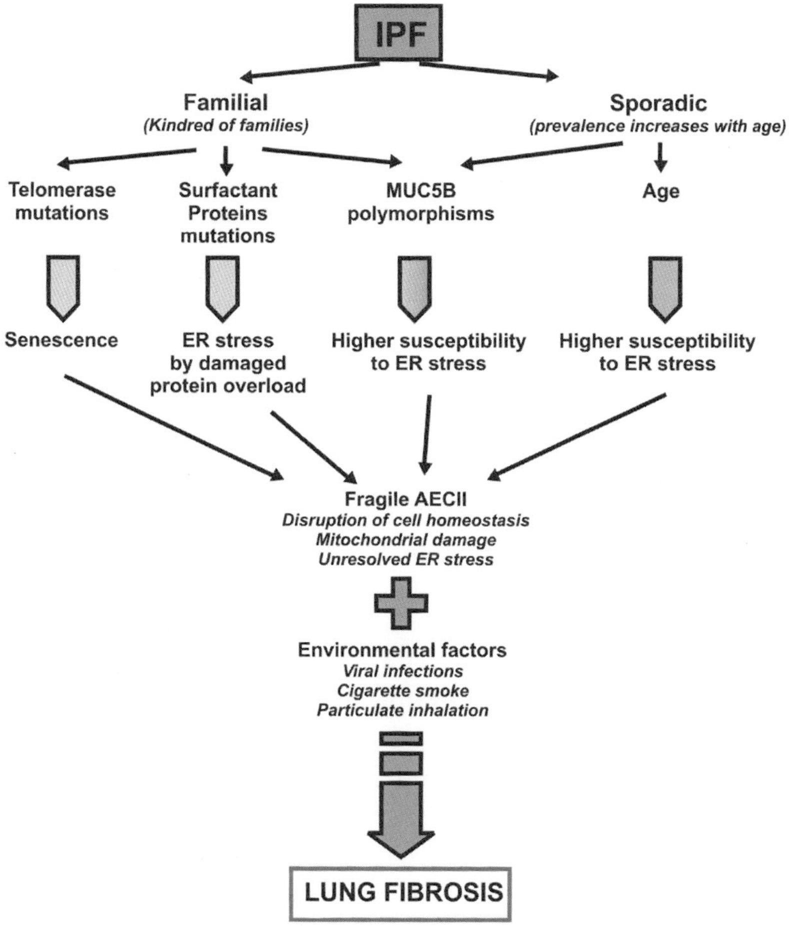

Fig 4. Similarities and Differences in the Etiology of Familiar and Sporadic IPF.

35 years old to 65/100,000 in individuals older than 75.[62] Important data support the concept that ER stress and apoptosis of the alveolar type II epithelial cells contribute to the pathogenesis of IPF. Apoptotic and hyperplasic alveolar type II cells are a common finding in IPF lungs adjacent to fibrotic foci where active collagen deposition occurs. Studies in animal models of bleomycin induced lung fibrosis have shown type II cell apoptosis and attenuation of fibrosis by treatment with caspase inhibitors.[63] Additionally, targeted injury of alveolar type II cells by SP-C driven expression of diphtheria toxin was sufficient to induce pulmonary fibrosis.[64]

Although the majority of the IPF cases are sporadic, 5–20% of the pulmonary fibrosis cases are presented in kindred of families.[65–68] This hereditable pulmonary fibrosis is called familial interstitial pneumonia (FIP). Several mutations in surfactant protein C and A have been linked to FIP.[69–73] Surfactant protein C (SP-C) is a hydrophobic protein produced by alveolar type II epithelial cells. SP-C secretion requires folding and multiple proteolytic cleavages. Around 50 mutations have been described for pro-SP-C gene, the majority of them in the C-terminus where the linker and BRICHOS domain are located.[74] The BRICHOS domain has been found in 12 protein families[75] and function as a chaperone domain that binds to precursor protein regions with high β-sheet propensity preventing the formation of amyloid fibers.[76] Amyloid formation has been associated with several diseases including lung fibrosis, AD and PD. These mutations can be spontaneous or inherited and all of them are found only in one allele. The most common SP-C mutation, I173T, is located in the linker region of the protein, triggering impaired trafficking and processing of the precursor pro-SP-C.[77,78] Two mutations have been found in the BRICHOS domain of SP-C linked to FIP. The first one is the exon4 deletion (Δexon4), which causes impaired processing and secretion of pro-SP-C with the subsequent ER stress, activation of the UPR and apoptotic cell death.[69,79–81] Lungs of patients with Δexon4 have low levels of mature SP-C and present abnormal lung morphology.[69] Bridges *et al.* has also reported abnormal lung morphogenesis and fetal death in transgenic mice expressing Δexon4 pro-SP-C mutation.[79] The second mutation in the BRICHOS domain is L188Q. This mutation has been analyzed in a transgenic mouse that uses the tet-on system to induce conditional overexpression of the L188Q mutant in type II alveolar epithelial cells. This L188Q overexpression causes ER stress but not spontaneous fibrosis. However, when transgenic mice are exposed to a second hit injury such as bleomycin, mice develop enhanced alveolar epithelial cell apoptosis and lung fibrosis.[82]

Familial and sporadic IPF have also been related to mutations in the telomerase genes TERC and TERT.[83,84] Around 8–15% of the familiar pulmonary fibrosis and 1–3% of sporadic IPF are associated with germline mutation in telomerase genes.[85] The loss of telomerase function causes shortening of telomeres and induction of senescence (which normally occurs with age). Telomere shortening is a common finding in patients with IPF, even in the absence of telomerase gene mutations. The molecular mechanisms linking telomerase genetic defects and the development of lung fibrosis are not yet well understood. It is postulated that these telomerase mutations could cause senescence of type II epithelial cells affecting directly their regeneration capacity increasing the susceptibility to lung injury. Recently, another genetic alteration has been found to increase the susceptibility to lung fibrosis. Polymorphisms of the promoter of MUC5B gene have been found in 34% of the familial pulmonary fibrosis and 38% of the sporadic IPF.[86,87] Exaggerated mucin expression by the secretory intestinal goblet cells has been linked to ER stress and the development of inflammatory bowel disease. Mucin are prone to folding errors in the ER because their size and complex structure. Ectopic expression of MUC5B has been found in epithelial cells from bronchiolised distal airspaces in IPF patients.[88] The high expression of MUC5B was not associated with the normal goblet cell transcription factor SPDEF, that drives the expression of mucin and molecules required for mucin biosynthesis, increasing the risk for misfolding of MUC5B, ER stress and activation of UPR.

Studies have also shown strong evidence of ER stress in lungs from sporadic IPF patients.[89,90] Analyses of IPF lysates from whole lung and isolated alveolar type II epithelial cells show high expression of ER stress markers such as processed ATF-6, ATF-4, BiP, CHOP and spliced XBP1. Particularly, type II epithelial cells from the zones with dense fibrosis and fibroblasts foci have the highest expression of ER stress markers that co-localize with markers of apoptosis. The cause of ER stress in sporadic IPF is not well understood. Some of the potential factors involved in the induction of ER stress in lung epithelium, which have been previously associated with IPF, are herpesvirus infection and exposure to cigarette smoke.[91,92] Several studies have shown positive detection of herpesvirus (Epstein Barr virus-EBV, Cytomegalovirus, Kaposi sarcoma virus, herpesvirus saimiri) antigens and DNA in lungs of IPF patients but not in control lungs.[93–96] Especially, alveolar type II cells lining the dense fibrotic areas show expression of herpesvirus protein markers.[89] Supporting a potential role of herpesvirus in the induction of ER stress and the development of lung fibrosis, our studies using the murine gammaherpesvirus 68 (MHV68, a murine homologous of EBV and Kaposi sarcoma virus) have shown to induce ER stress, alveolar epithelial cell death and spontaneous fibrosis in susceptible hosts (IFN-γR KO and wild type aged mice).[25,97] In addition, we have demonstrated that virus reactivation and establishment of latency are required for the development of MHV68-induced lung fibrosis.[98,99] Studies by Lok and McMillan also shown that gammaherpesvirus infection can exacerbate established lung fibrosis.[100,101] During gammaherpesvirus lytic replication there is a high demand for protein synthesis and folding, leading to ER stress and initiation of the compensatory UPR. During the latent phase, gammaherpesvirus (like EVB) express latent membrane protein 1 (LMP1) that induces PERK activation and XBP1 splicing. XBP-1 initiates transcription of viral genes required for productive lytic virus leading to persistent infection;[102] whereas PERK induces transcription of LMP1, perpetuating the UPR activation and leading to apoptosis.[91] The role of cigarette smoke exposure in ER stress induction has been analyzed *in vitro* and *in vivo*. A549 cells exposed to cigarette smoke show high expression of BiP and total and phosphorylated eIF2alpha, indicating induction of ER stress and UPR activation.[92]

More relevant, proteomic analyses of lung samples from chronic cigarette smokers show upregulation of several UPR proteins compared to non-smokers (including BiP, foldase and calreticulin).[103] Further studies are required to determine the relevance of these environmental factors in the induction of ER stress and activation of pro-fibrotic responses in the lung.

8. ER Stress and Lung and Age-Related Susceptibility to Lung Fibrosis

As we mentioned above, aging is an important risk factor for the development of IPF.[104,105] Our group is pioneer to demonstrate, in experimental models, that aging lungs are highly susceptible to injury, disrepair and fibrosis.[106,107] Studies using the mouse model of herpesvirus induced lung fibrosis have shown that individuals with advanced age respond differently to this injury stimuli.[25] In sharp contrast with young mice infected with MHV68 (which resolve rapidly virus induced pneumonitis), old mice develop increased inflammatory and fibrotic responses after infection. Moreover, we were able to show that lung pathology was linked with increase and persistent activation of UPR measured by expression of BiP and splicing of XBP1. The chronic ER stress in the aging lung by MHV68 infection led to preferential apoptosis of type II lung epithelial cell and activation of pro-fibrotic pathways.[25] ER stress also influences mitochondria function and mitochondria dysfunction is a common finding in aging cells. Accumulated evidence shows that ER and mitochondria have structural and functional communication.[108,109] The outer mitochondria membrane and the ER are joined by tethers allowing ER proteins to associate directly with proteins and lipids of the mitochondria membrane. It is known that ER stress disrupts mitochondria Ca^{2+} homeostasis contributing to apoptosis. How this crosstalk between ER and mitochondria influences the susceptibility to age-related lung diseases is still unknown. Our studies indicate that ER stress in alveolar type II cells can influence mitochondria function, dynamics and mitophagy.[110] Aging mitochondria are notably susceptible to ER stress stimulation. Further investigations are required in this field to establish the role of ER — mitochondria crosstalk in the development of age-related diseases in the lung.

9. Therapeutic Interventions

Since ER stress is involved in the pathogenesis of numerous diseases there are efforts underway to ameliorate ER stress as a therapeutic approach. There are two main approaches to targeting ER stress. The first strategy is to decrease the stress by activation of the adaptive pathway of the UPR. The second approach is to shut off the apoptotic pathways of UPR. Several compounds have been identified that can work as chaperones or improve their folding activity. One of these compounds is the chemical chaperone 4-PBA (phenyl butyric acid), which can stabilize proteins in their native conformation and rescue mutant protein folding and trafficking defects. PBA is clinically used to treat patients with defects in the urea cycle and ALS. Additionally PBA has been tested in models of diabetes type 2, deficiency of α1antitrypsine and CF.[111,112] *In vitro* and *in vivo* studies have shown that 4-PBA is effective in the lung reducing expression of ER stress markers induced by LPS.[58] Additionally, 4-PBA is reported to improve lung function in the bleomycin lung fibrosis models with decrease expression of ER stress markers and collagen deposition.[113] Because PBA has already been approved clinically, its translational potential in ER stress-related lung diseases is promising. Other compounds clinically approved and identified with the capacity to reduce or protect against ER stress (particularly in neural cells) are lithium and valproate, two commonly used mood stabilizers. Both of these compounds have shown to mediate protection against cytotoxicity induced by ER stress.[114] The protective effect of these drugs is associated with increased expression of chaperone BiP, GRP94 and calreticulin, as well as, upregulation of the antiapoptotic molecule Bcl-2.[115] Psychoactive drugs such as benzodiazepines have also been identified as compounds able to rescue ER stress-induced cell death. Studies of their mechanisms of action suggest that these compounds mediate suppression of the IRE-1/ASK1 pathway activation.[116] Although targeting the ER stress responses seems promising as future therapies for lung diseases, there is limited knowledge how UPR pathways like IRE1a and PERK activate both pro-survival adaptive responses and cell death. Future research needs to address the molecular mechanisms of UPR in lung diseases to identify targets for therapeutic interventions.

10. Conclusions

Similar to the hormetic regulation, the adaptive responses to ER stress are dose-dependent. Low doses help to maintain the protein homeostasis but chronic or strong stimuli induce cell death and disease. With age, there is defective activation of the survival UPR pathways with a higher susceptibility to apoptosis and inflammation. The aging lung and especially the alveolar epithelial type II are low resistance to ER stress. As a consequence, aging lungs exposed to extrinsic ER stress stimuli have severe apoptosis of type II epithelial cells leading to low epithelial regeneration and higher propensity to disrepair and fibrosis. Therapeutic approaches that look for a decrease of the ER stress by promoting proteostasis could be useful of age-related diseases associated with sustained activation of the UPR.

References

1. Epstein CJ, Goldberger RF, Anfinsen CB. (1963) Genetic Control of Tertiary Protein Stucture — Studies with Model Systems. *Cold Spring Harb Sym* **28**: 439&.
2. Wolynes PG, Onuchic JN, Thirumalai D. (1995) Navigating the Folding Routes. *Science* **267**: 1619–1620.
3. Gidalevitz T, Stevens F, Argon Y. (2013) Orchestration of secretory protein folding by ER chaperones. *Bba-Mol Cell Res* **1833**: 2410–2424.
4. Kim YE, Hipp MS, Bracher A *et al.* (2013) Molecular Chaperone Functions in Protein Folding and Proteostasis. *Annu Rev Biochem* **82**: 323–355.

5. Vendruscolo M, Knowles TPJ, Dobson CM. (2011) Protein Solubility and Protein Homeostasis: A Generic View of Protein Misfolding Disorders. *Csh Perspect Biol* **3**:
6. Hochstrasser M. (1996) Ubiquitin-dependent protein degradation. *Annu Rev Genet* **30**: 405–439.
7. Akerfelt M, Morimoto RI, Sistonen L. (2010) Heat shock factors: Integrators of cell stress, development and lifespan. *Nat Revs Mol Cell Biol* **11**: 545–555.
8. Ron D, Walter P. (2007) Signal integration in the endoplasmic reticulum unfolded protein response. *Nat Revs Mol Cell Biol* **8**: 519–529.
9. Guerriero CJ, Brodsky JL. (2012) The delicate balance between secreted protein folding and endoplasmic reticulum-associated degradation in human physiology. *Physiol Rev* **92**: 537–576.
10. Hollien J, Weissman JS. (2006) Decay of endoplasmic reticulum-localized mRNAs during the unfolded protein response. *Science* **313**: 104–107.
11. McCullough KD, Martindale JL, Klotz LO *et al.* (2001) Gadd153 sensitizes cells to endoplasmic reticulum stress by down-regulating Bcl2 and perturbing the cellular redox state. *Mol Cell Biol* **21**: 1249–1259.
12. Zhivotovsky B. (2003) Caspases: The enzymes of death. *Essays Biochem* **39**: 25–40.
13. Gems D, Partridge L. (2008) Stress-response hormesis and aging: That which does not kill us makes us stronger. *Cell Metabol* **7**: 200–203.
14. Mattson MP. (2008) Hormesis defined. *Ageing Research Revs* **7**: 1–7.
15. Rattan SI. (2008) Hormesis in aging. *Ageing Research Revs* **7**: 63–78.
16. Szegezdi E, Logue SE, Gorman AM *et al.* (2006) Mediators of endoplasmic reticulum stress-induced apoptosis. *EMBO reports* **7**: 880–885.
17. Hetz CA. (2007) ER stress signaling and the BCL-2 family of proteins: From adaptation to irreversible cellular damage. *Antioxid Redox Sign* **9**: 2345–2355.
18. de Magalhaes JP, Curado J, Church GM. (2009) Meta-analysis of age-related gene expression profiles identifies common signatures of aging. *Bioinformatics* **25**: 875–881.
19. Paz Gavilan M, Vela J, Castano A *et al.* (2006) Cellular environment facilitates protein accumulation in aged rat hippocampus. *Neurobiol Aging* **27**: 973–982.

20. Hussain SG, Ramaiah KV. (2007) Reduced eIF2alpha phosphorylation and increased proapoptotic proteins in aging. *Biochem Biophys Res Commun* **355**: 365–370.
21. Nuss JE, Choksi KB, DeFord JH *et al.* (2008) Decreased enzyme activities of chaperones PDI and BiP in aged mouse livers. *Biochem Biophys Res Commun* **365**: 355–361.
22. Naidoo N, Ferber M, Master M *et al.* (2008) Aging impairs the unfolded protein response to sleep deprivation and leads to proapoptotic signaling. *J Neurosci* **28**: 6539–6548.
23. Kourtis N, Tavernarakis N. (2011) Cellular stress response pathways and ageing: Intricate molecular relationships. *The EMBO journal* **30**: 2520–2531.
24. Li J, Holbrook NJ. (2004) Elevated gadd153/chop expression and enhanced c-Jun N-terminal protein kinase activation sensitizes aged cells to ER stress. *Exp Gerontol* **39**: 735–744.
25. Torres-Gonzalez E, Bueno M, Tanaka A *et al.* (2012) Role of endoplasmic reticulum stress in age-related susceptibility to lung fibrosis. *Am J Respir Cell Mol Biol* **46**: 748–756.
26. David DC, Ollikainen N, Trinidad JC *et al.* (2010) Widespread protein aggregation as an inherent part of aging in C. elegans. *PLoS biology* **8**: e1000450.
27. Gidalevitz T, Ben-Zvi A, Ho KH *et al.* (2006) Progressive disruption of cellular protein folding in models of polyglutamine diseases. *Science* **311**: 1471–1474.
28. Bennett EJ, Shaler TA, Woodman B, *et al.* (2007) Global changes to the ubiquitin system in Huntington's disease. *Nature* **448**: 704–708.
29. Ben-Zvi A, Miller EA, Morimoto RI. (2009) Collapse of proteostasis represents an early molecular event in Caenorhabditis elegans aging. *Proc Natl Acad Sci USA* **106**: 14914–14919.
30. Olsen A, Vantipalli MC, Lithgow GJ. (2006) Lifespan extension of Caenorhabditis elegans following repeated mild hormetic heat treatments. *Biogerontol* **7**: 221–230.
31. Johnson JA, Johnson DA, Kraft AD*et al.* (2008) The Nrf2-ARE pathway: An indicator and modulator of oxidative stress in neurodegeneration. *Ann NY Acad Sci* **1147**: 61–69.
32. Lee JH, Won SM, Suh J *et al.* (2010) Induction of the unfolded protein response and cell death pathway in Alzheimer's disease, but not in aged Tg2576 mice. *Exp Mol Med* **42**: 386–394.

33. Hoozemans JJ, van Haastert ES, Eikelenboom P *et al.* (2007) Activation of the unfolded protein response in Parkinson's disease. *Biochem Biophys Res Commun* **354**: 707–711.
34. Omura T, Kaneko M, Okuma Y *et al.* (2013) Endoplasmic reticulum stress and Parkinson's disease: The role of HRD1 in averting apoptosis in neurodegenerative disease. *Oxid Med Cell Longevity* **2013**: 239854.
35. Naidoo N, Giang W, Galante RJ *et al.* (2005) Sleep deprivation induces the unfolded protein response in mouse cerebral cortex. *J neurochem* **92**: 1150–1157.
36. Mackiewicz M, Shockley KR, Romer MA *et al.* (2007) Macromolecule biosynthesis: A key function of sleep. *Physiol Genom* **31**: 441–457.
37. Naidoo N, Casiano V, Cater J *et al.* (2007) A role for the molecular chaperone protein BiP/GRP78 in Drosophila sleep homeostasis. *Sleep* **30**: 557–565.
38. Hotamisligil GS. (2010) Endoplasmic reticulum stress and atherosclerosis. *Nat Med* **16**: 396–399.
39. Hotamisligil GS. (2010) Endoplasmic reticulum stress and the inflammatory basis of metabolic disease. *Cell* **140**: 900–917.
40. Hasnain SZ, Lourie R, Das I *et al.* (2012) The interplay between endoplasmic reticulum stress and inflammation. *Immunol Cell Biol* **90**: 260–270.
41. Hybiske K, Fu Z, Schwarzer C *et al.* (2007) Effects of cystic fibrosis transmembrane conductance regulator and DeltaF508CFTR on inflammatory response, ER stress, and Ca2+ of airway epithelia. *Am J Physiol Lung Cell Mol Physiol* **293**: L1250–L1260.
42. Mhaille AN, McQuaid S, Windebank A *et al.* (2008) Increased expression of endoplasmic reticulum stress-related signaling pathway molecules in multiple sclerosis lesions. *J Neuropathol Exp Neurol* **67**: 200–211.
43. Colbert RA, DeLay ML, Klenk EI *et al.* (2010) From HLA-B27 to spondyloarthritis: A journey through the ER. *Immunol Revs* **233**: 181–202.
44. McGuckin MA, Eri RD, Das I *et al.* (2010) ER stress and the unfolded protein response in intestinal inflammation. *Am J Physiol Gastrointest Liver Physiol* **298**: G820–G832.
45. Heazlewood CK, Cook MC, Eri R *et al.* (2008) Aberrant mucin assembly in mice causes endoplasmic reticulum stress and spontaneous inflammation resembling ulcerative colitis. *PLoS medicine* **5**: e54.
46. Hotamisligil GS. (2006) Inflammation and metabolic disorders. *Nature* **444**: 860–867.

47. Zhang K, Kaufman RJ. (2008) From endoplasmic-reticulum stress to the inflammatory response. *Nature* **454**: 455–462.
48. Santos CX, Tanaka LY, Wosniak J *et al.* (2009) Mechanisms and implications of reactive oxygen species generation during the unfolded protein response: Roles of endoplasmic reticulum oxidoreductases, mitochondrial electron transport, and NADPH oxidase. *Antioxid Redox Sign* **11**: 2409–2427.
49. Tabas I. (2009) Macrophage apoptosis in atherosclerosis: Consequences on plaque progression and the role of endoplasmic reticulum stress. *Antioxid Redox Sign* **11**: 2333–2339.
50. Burkle A, Caselli G, Franceschi C*et al.* (2007) Pathophysiology of ageing, longevity and age related diseases. *Immun Ageing* **4**: 4.
51. Wang G, Yang ZQ, Zhang K. (2010) Endoplasmic reticulum stress response in cancer: Molecular mechanism and therapeutic potential. *Am J Transl Res* **2**: 65–74.
52. Zhang LH, Zhang X. (2010) Roles of GRP78 in physiology and cancer. *J Cell Biochem* **110**: 1299–1305.
53. Reddy RK, Mao C, Baumeister P *et al.* (2003) Endoplasmic reticulum chaperone protein GRP78 protects cells from apoptosis induced by topoisomerase inhibitors: Role of ATP binding site in suppression of caspase-7 activation. *J Biol Chem* **278**: 20915–20924.
54. Lee AS. (2007) GRP78 induction in cancer: Therapeutic and prognostic implications. *Cancer Res* **67**: 3496–3499.
55. Pyrko P, Schonthal AH, Hofman FM *et al.* (2007) The unfolded protein response regulator GRP78/BiP as a novel target for increasing chemosensitivity in malignant gliomas. *Cancer Research* **67**: 9809–9816.
56. Romero-Ramirez L, Cao H, Regalado MP *et al.* (2009) X box-binding protein 1 regulates angiogenesis in human pancreatic adenocarcinomas. *Transl Oncol* **2**: 31–38.
57. Malhotra D, Thimmulappa R, Vij N *et al.* (2009) Heightened endoplasmic reticulum stress in the lungs of patients with chronic obstructive pulmonary disease: The role of Nrf2-regulated proteasomal activity. *Am J Respir Critic Care Medicine* **180**: 1196–1207.
58. Kim HJ, Jeong JS, Kim SR *et al.* (2013) Inhibition of endoplasmic reticulum stress alleviates lipopolysaccharide-induced lung inflammation through modulation of NF-kappaB/HIF-1alpha signaling pathway. *Sci Rep* **3**: 1142.

59. Kim SR, Kim DI, Kang MR *et al.* (2013) Endoplasmic reticulum stress influences bronchial asthma pathogenesis by modulating nuclear factor kappa B activation. *J Allergy Clin Immunol* **132**: 1397–1408.
60. Kim DS, Collard HR, King TE, Jr. (2006) Classification and natural history of the idiopathic interstitial pneumonias. *Proc Am Thorac Soc* **3**: 285–292.
61. Raghu G, Collard HR, Egan JJ *et al.* (2011) An official ATS/ERS/JRS/ALAT statement: Idiopathic pulmonary fibrosis: Evidence-based guidelines for diagnosis and management. *Am J Respir Crit Care Med* **183**: 788–824.
62. Raghu G, Weycker D, Edelsberg J *et al.* (2006) Incidence and prevalence of idiopathic pulmonary fibrosis. *Am J Respir Crit Care Med* **174**: 810–816.
63. Kuwano K, Kunitake R, Maeyama T *et al.* (2001) Attenuation of bleomycin-induced pneumopathy in mice by a caspase inhibitor. *Am J Physiol Lung Cell Mol Physiol* **280**: L316–L325.
64. Osterholzer JJ, Christensen PJ, Lama V *et al.* (2012) PAI-1 promotes the accumulation of exudate macrophages and worsens pulmonary fibrosis following type II alveolar epithelial cell injury. *J Pathol* **228**: 170–180.
65. Marshall RP, Puddicombe A, Cookson WO *et al.* (2000) Adult familial cryptogenic fibrosing alveolitis in the United Kingdom. *Thorax* **55**: 143–146.
66. Hodgson U, Laitinen T, Tukiainen P. (2002) Nationwide prevalence of sporadic and familial idiopathic pulmonary fibrosis: Evidence of founder effect among multiplex families in Finland. *Thorax* **57**: 338–342.
67. Loyd JE. (2003) Pulmonary fibrosis in families. *Am J Respir Cell Mol Biol* **29**: S47–S50.
68. Garcia-Sancho C, Buendia-Roldan I, Fernandez-Plata MR *et al.* (2011) Familial pulmonary fibrosis is the strongest risk factor for idiopathic pulmonary fibrosis. *Respir Med* **105**: 1902–1907.
69. Nogee LM, Dunbar AE, 3rd, Wert SE *et al.* (2001) A mutation in the surfactant protein C gene associated with familial interstitial lung disease. *New Engl J Med* **344**: 573–579.
70. Thomas AQ, Lane K, Phillips J *et al.* (2002) Heterozygosity for a surfactant protein C gene mutation associated with usual interstitial pneumonitis and cellular nonspecific interstitial pneumonitis in one kindred. *Am J Respir Critic Care Medicine* **165**: 1322–1328.

71. van Moorsel CH, van Oosterhout MF, Barlo NP *et al.* (2010) Surfactant protein C mutations are the basis of a significant portion of adult familial pulmonary fibrosis in a dutch cohort. *Am J Respir Critic Care Medicine* **182**: 1419–1425.
72. Ono S, Tanaka T, Ishida M *et al.* (2011) Surfactant protein C G100S mutation causes familial pulmonary fibrosis in Japanese kindred. *Euro Respir J* **38**: 861–869.
73. Wang M, Bridges JP, Na CL *et al.* (2009) Meckel-Gruber syndrome protein MKS3 is required for endoplasmic reticulum-associated degradation of surfactant protein C. *J Biol Chem* **284**: 33377–33383.
74. Beers MF, Lomax CA, Russo SJ. (1998) Synthetic processing of surfactant protein C by alevolar epithelial cells. The COOH terminus of proSP-C is required for post-translational targeting and proteolysis. *J Biol Chem* **273**: 15287–15293.
75. Sanchez-Pulido L, Devos D, Valencia A. (2002) BRICHOS: A conserved domain in proteins associated with dementia, respiratory distress and cancer. *Trends Biochem Sci* **27**: 329–332.
76. Willander H, Hermansson E, Johansson J *et al.* (2011) BRICHOS domain associated with lung fibrosis, dementia and cancer — a chaperone that prevents amyloid fibril formation? *The FEBS journal* **278**: 3893–3904.
77. Brasch F, Griese M, Tredano M *et al.* (2004) Interstitial lung disease in a baby with a de novo mutation in the SFTPC gene. *Euro Respir J* **24**: 30–39.
78. Tredano M, Griese M, Brasch F *et al.* (2004) Mutation of SFTPC in infantile pulmonary alveolar proteinosis with or without fibrosing lung disease. *Am J Med Genet A* **126A**: 18–26.
79. Bridges JP, Wert SE, Nogee LM *et al.* (2003) Expression of a human surfactant protein C mutation associated with interstitial lung disease disrupts lung development in transgenic mice. *J Biol Chem* **278**: 52739–52746.
80. Wang WJ, Mulugeta S, Russo SJ *et al.* (2003) Deletion of exon 4 from human surfactant protein C results in aggresome formation and generation of a dominant negative. *J Cell Sci* **116**: 683–692.
81. Mulugeta S, Nguyen V, Russo SJ *et al.* (2005) A surfactant protein C precursor protein BRICHOS domain mutation causes endoplasmic reticulum stress, proteasome dysfunction, and caspase 3 activation. *Am J Respir Cell Mol Biol* **32**: 521–530.

82. Lawson WE, Cheng DS, Degryse AL *et al.* (2011) Endoplasmic reticulum stress enhances fibrotic remodeling in the lungs. *Proc Natl Acad Sci USA* **108**: 10562–10567.
83. Armanios MY, Chen JJ, Cogan JD *et al.* (2007) Telomerase mutations in families with idiopathic pulmonary fibrosis. *N Engl J Med* **356**: 1317–1326.
84. Lawson WE, Grant SW, Ambrosini V *et al.* (2004) Genetic mutations in surfactant protein C are a rare cause of sporadic cases of IPF. *Thorax* **59**: 977–980.
85. Armanios M. (2012) Telomerase and idiopathic pulmonary fibrosis. *Mutation Res* **730**: 52–58.
86. Seibold MA, Wise AL, Speer MC *et al.* (2011) A common MUC5B promoter polymorphism and pulmonary fibrosis. *New Engl J Med* **364**: 1503–1512.
87. Zhang GY, Liao T, Gao WY. (2011) MUC5B promoter polymorphism and pulmonary fibrosis. *New Engl J Med* **365**: 178–179.
88. Plantier L, Crestani B, Wert SE *et al.* (2011) Ectopic respiratory epithelial cell differentiation in bronchiolised distal airspaces in idiopathic pulmonary fibrosis. *Thorax* **66**: 651–657.
89. Lawson WE, Crossno PF, Polosukhin VV *et al.* (2008) Endoplasmic reticulum stress in alveolar epithelial cells is prominent in IPF: Association with altered surfactant protein processing and herpesvirus infection. *Am J Physiol Lung Cell Mol Physiol* **294**: L1119–L1126.
90. Korfei M, Ruppert C, Mahavadi P *et al.* (2008) Epithelial endoplasmic reticulum stress and apoptosis in sporadic idiopathic pulmonary fibrosis. *Am J Respir Crit Care Med* **178**: 838–846.
91. Lee DY, Sugden B. (2008) The LMP1 oncogene of EBV activates PERK and the unfolded protein response to drive its own synthesis. *Blood* **111**: 2280–2289.
92. Jorgensen E, Stinson A, Shan L. (2008) Cigarette smoke induces endoplasmic reticulum stress and the unfolded protein response in normal and malignant human lung cells. *BMC cancer* **8**: 229.
93. Tang YW, Johnson JE, Browning PJ *et al.* (2003) Herpesvirus DNA is consistently detected in lungs of patients with idiopathic pulmonary fibrosis. *J Clin Microbioly* **41**: 2633–2640.
94. Egan JJ, Stewart JP, Hasleton PS *et al.* (1995) Epstein-Barr virus replication within pulmonary epithelial cells in cryptogenic fibrosing alveolitis. *Thorax* **50**: 1234–1239.

95. Stewart JP, Egan JJ, Ross AJ *et al.* (1999) The detection of Epstein-Barr virus DNA in lung tissue from patients with idiopathic pulmonary fibrosis. *Am J Respir Critic Care Med* **159**: 1336–1341.
96. Folcik VA, Garofalo M, Coleman J *et al.* (2013) Idiopathic pulmonary fibrosis is strongly associated with productive infection by herpesvirus saimiri. *Modern Pathol.*
97. Mora AL, Woods CR, Garcia A *et al.* (2005) Lung infection with gamma-herpesvirus induces progressive pulmonary fibrosis in Th2-biased mice. *Am J Physiol Lung Cell Mol Physiol* **289**: L711–L721.
98. Krug LT, Torres-Gonzalez E, Q in Q *et al.* (2010) Inhibition of NF-kappaB signaling reduces virus load and gammaherpesvirus-induced pulmonary fibrosis. *Am J Pathol* **177**: 608–621.
99. Mora AL, Torres-Gonzalez E, Rojas M *et al.* (2007) Control of virus reactivation arrests pulmonary herpesvirus-induced fibrosis in IFN-gamma receptor-deficient mice. *Am J Respir Crit Care Med* **175**: 1139–1150.
100. Lok SS, Haider Y, Howell D *et al.* (2002) Murine gammaherpes virus as a cofactor in the development of pulmonary fibrosis in bleomycin resistant mice. *Euro Respir J* **20**: 1228–1232.
101. McMillan TR, Moore BB, Weinberg JB *et al.* (2008) Exacerbation of established pulmonary fibrosis in a murine model by gammaherpesvirus. *Am J Respir Critical Care Med* **177**: 771–780.
102. Sun CC, Thorley-Lawson DA. (2007) Plasma cell-specific transcription factor XBP-1s binds to and transactivates the Epstein-Barr virus BZLF1 promoter. *J Virol* **81**: 13566–13577.
103. Kelsen SG, Duan X, Ji R *et al.* (2008) Cigarette smoke induces an unfolded protein response in the human lung: A proteomic approach. *Am J Respir Cell Mol Biol* **38**: 541–550.
104. Selman M, Rojas M, Mora AL *et al.* (2010) Aging and interstitial lung diseases: Unraveling an old forgotten player in the pathogenesis of lung fibrosis. *Semin Respir Crit Care Med* **31**: 607–617.
105. Selman M, Pardo A. (2014) Revealing the pathogenic and aging-related mechanisms of the enigmatic idiopathic pulmonary fibrosis: An integral model. *Am J Respir Critic Care Med.*
106. Xu J, Gonzalez ET, Iyer SS *et al.* (2009) Use of senescence-accelerated mouse model in bleomycin-induced lung injury suggests that bone marrow-derived cells can alter the outcome of lung injury in aged mice. *J Gerontol A Biol Sci Med Sci* **64**: 731–739.

107. Sueblinvong V, Neujahr DC, Mills ST *et al.* (2012) Predisposition for disrepair in the aged lung. *Am J Med Sci* **344**: 41–51.
108. Giorgi C, De Stefani D, Bononi A *et al.* (2009) Structural and functional link between the mitochondrial network and the endoplasmic reticulum. *Int J Biochem Cell Biol* **41**: 1817–1827.
109. Csordas G, Hajnoczky G. (2009) SR/ER-mitochondrial local communication: Calcium and ROS. *Biochimica et Biophysica Acta* **1787**: 1352–1362.
110. Bueno M, Lai Yc, Romero Y *et al.* (2015) PINK, deficiency impairs mitochondrial homeostasis and promotes lung fibrosis. *J Clin Invest.* **125(2)**: 521–538.
111. Lee B, Rhead W, Diaz GA *et al.* (2010) Phase 2 comparison of a novel ammonia scavenging agent with sodium phenylbutyrate in patients with urea cycle disorders: Safety, pharmacokinetics and ammonia control. *Mol Genet Metabol* **100**: 221–228.
112. Cudkowicz ME, Andres PL, Macdonald SA *et al.* (2009) Phase 2 study of sodium phenylbutyrate in ALS. *Amyotrophic Lateral Sclerosis.* **10**: 99–106.
113. Ehab A, James W, Madelaine HL *et al.* (2013) 4-Phenylbutyrate Prevents UPR Activation And Myofibroblast Differentiation In Experimental Bleomycin-Induced Lung Fibrosis. In *D41. The Bleomycin Model Of Lung Fibrosis And Beyond,* American Thoracic Society. pp. A5657–A5657
114. Hiroi T, Wei H, Hough C *et al.* (2005) Protracted lithium treatment protects against the ER stress elicited by thapsigargin in rat PC12 cells: Roles of intracellular calcium, GRP78 and Bcl-2. *Pharmacogenom* J **5**: 102–111.
115. Shao L, Sun X, Xu L *et al.* (2006) Mood stabilizing drug lithium increases expression of endoplasmic reticulum stress proteins in primary cultured rat cerebral cortical cells. *Life sciences* **78**: 1317–1323.
116. Kim I, Shu CW, Xu W *et al.* (2009) Chemical biology investigation of cell death pathways activated by endoplasmic reticulum stress reveals cytoprotective modulators of ASK1. *JBiol Chem* **284**: 1593–1603.
117. Heydari AR, You S, Takahashi R *et al.* (2000) Age-related alterations in the activation of heat shock transcription factor 1 in rat hepatocytes. *Exp Cell Res* **256**: 83–93.
118. Choi HS, Lin Z, Li BS *et al.* (1990) Age-dependent decrease in the heat-inducible DNA sequence-specific binding activity in human diploid fibroblasts. *J Biol Chem* **265**: 18005–18011.

119. Morimoto RI. (2002) Dynamic remodeling of transcription complexes by molecular chaperones. *Cell* **110**: 281–284.
120. Zou J, Guo Y, Guettouche T *et al.* (1998) Repression of heat shock transcription factor HSF1 activation by HSP90 (HSP90 complex) that forms a stress-sensitive complex with HSF1. *Cell* **94**: 471–480.
121. Soti C, Csermely P. (2002) Chaperones come of age. *Cell Stress Chaperones* **7**: 186–190.
122. Nardai G, Csermely P, Soti C. (2002) Chaperone function and chaperone overload in the aged. A preliminary analysis. *Exp Gerontol* **37**: 1257–1262.
123. Csermely P. (2001) Chaperone overload is a possible contributor to 'civilization diseases'. *Trends Genet* **17**: 701–704.
124. Erickson RR, Dunning LM, Holtzman JL. (2006) The effect of aging on the chaperone concentrations in the hepatic, endoplasmic reticulum of male rats: The possible role of protein misfolding due to the loss of chaperones in the decline in physiological function seen with age. *J Gerontol. A Bioll Sci Med Sci* **61**: 435–443.
125. van der Vlies D, Pap EH, Post JA *et al.* (2002) Endoplasmic reticulum resident proteins of normal human dermal fibroblasts are the major targets for oxidative stress induced by hydrogen peroxide. *Biochem J* **366**: 825–830.
126. Rabek JP, Boylston WH, Papaconstantinou J. (2003) Carbonylation of ER chaperone proteins in aged mouse liver. *Biochem Biophys Res Commun* **305**: 566–572.

Chapter 19
Autophagy and Metabolism

Jaime L. Schneider* and Cecilia G. Sanchez†,‡

1. Introduction

Like other organs, the lung cannot escape from aging signatures such as defects in stress recognition, genomic instability, telomere attrition, epigenetic alterations, loss of proteostasis, defective nutrient sensing, mitochondrial dysfunction, cellular senescence, stem cell exhaustion and changes in intercellular communication.[1] The progressive loss of physiological integrity of the aging lung leads to impaired function, susceptibility to diseases and death.

Fortunately, an important characteristic of all living organisms is their capacity to respond, counteract and adapt quickly to disturbances. Mechanisms of the favorable biological response (hormesis) will be activated by cells, tissues and organs against internal or external sources of disturbances. Autophagy, the process by which intracellular components are degraded in lysosomes, represents an inducible adaptive response to lung injury resulting from exposure to stress agents, including hypoxia, oxidants, inflammation,

*Department of Developmental and Molecular Biology, Albert Einstein College of Medicine, Bronx, NY 10461, USA.

†Division of Lung Biology, Department of Medicine, Tulane University, New Orleans, LA, USA. Email:csanche3@tulane.edu

‡Corresponding author.

ischemia–reperfusion, endoplasmic reticulum (ER) stress and inhaled xenobiotics. An adequate autophagic response can facilitate cell survival, differentiation, repair, adaptation and remodeling.[2,3]

Unfortunately, stress recognition systems such as autophagy decline during aging.[4] As a consequence, most differentiated cells exhibit altered cellular homeostasis and accumulate damaged non-functional organelles and proteins, thus compromising their response to injury and promoting age-related lung diseases such as COPD, lung cancer and fibrosis.[5] Other functions of autophagy include mitigating the deleterious effects of oxidative stress through turnover of dysfunctional mitochondria, the engulfment of damaged ER and degradation of protein aggregates that may otherwise promote tissue degeneration. Failure of autophagy and increased ROS may overwhelm antioxidant defenses and contribute to chronic cellular stress as well as aberrant lung repair in the aging lung.[6,7] Efficient autophagy is also essential to limit DNA damage and genomic instability.[8] Substrates for autophagy not only include mitochondria protein aggregates and ER (reticulophagy/ER-phagy), but, also ribosomes (ribophagy) and peroxisomes (pexophagy), metals and particles, pathogens (xenophagy), RNA, and chromatin.[9–12] In addition, autophagy controls inflammation through regulatory interactions with innate immune signaling pathways and contributes to antigen presentation and to *T* cell activation, energy metabolism and survival.[13–15] Finally, autophagy dictates cellular bioenergetics and metabolism by degrading intracellular energy stores like glycogen and lipid droplets.[16,17] Due to the numerous functions, substrates and outputs, it is logical to conclude that an unbalanced autophagic response can have detrimental effects during lung aging. Since several diseases are associated with or causally linked to its deregulation, appropriate induction, control and execution of autophagy are necessary to maintain cellular homeostasis.[18,19,20]

Beyond the function of autophagy in individual cells or organs, it has been shown that autophagy plays an important role in determining life span.[21] For instance, studies in worms and flies have revealed that autophagy genes are required to attain maximal lifespan extension and that upregulation of macroautophagy has been observed in almost all experimental models of increased longevity.[22] Reduced autophagy can accelerate aging, whereas stimulation of autophagy has potent anti-aging effects.[23]

2. Autophagy: A Complex Process

The term Autophagy (defined as "self-eating") was coined by the Nobel laureate Christian de Duve in 1963 and refers to the degradation of cytoplasmic contents within the lysosome/vacuole. Autophagy is a catabolic process conserved from yeast to mammals and serves as a mechanism of stress recognition, response and hormesis. The basic research on autophagy is expanding and the knowledge about new proteins, complexes, the origin of the membranes involved, selectivity and substrates are in constant discovery, as are the interconnected pathways that regulate and are regulated by autophagy.[24] The ongoing molecular dissection of autophagy in a cell type-specific manner will help to reveal the role of this process in the maintenance of lung homeostasis and the progression of lung diseases.

The three major types of autophagy are Macroautophagy, Microautophagy and Chaperone-Mediated Autophagy (CMA) (Fig. 1). Macroautophagy refers to the multifaceted process of sequestering portions of the cytosol (including soluble proteins, organelles and aggregates) inside a forming autophagosomal membrane which ultimately seals and fuses with lysosomes for degradation of the entrapped cargo.[25] In the case of microautophagy, cytosolic content is internalized and degraded in lysosomes through invaginations of the lysosomal membrane.[26] Lastly, CMA is the autophagic pathway in which select substrate proteins translocate into the lysosome through the coordinated action of chaperones on the cytosolic and luminal sides of the lysosomal membrane.[27] Here, we will describe the relevance of two major types of autophagy, macroautophagy and CMA, in lung cell physiology and metabolism.

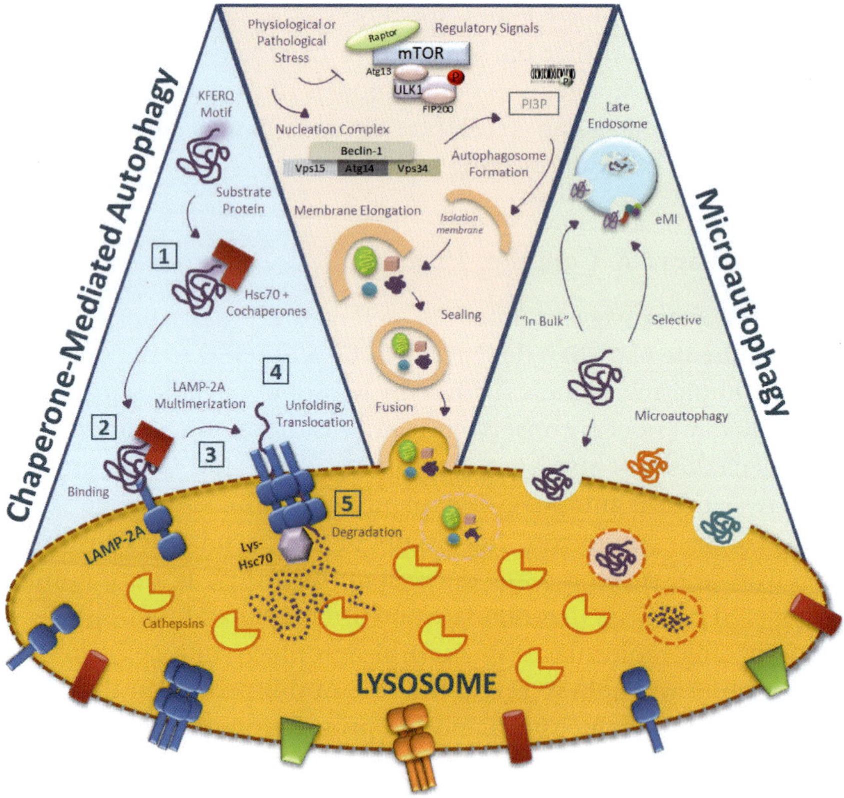

Fig. 1. Different autophagic pathways present in mammalian cells. *Left:* In Chaperone-Mediated Autophagy (CMA), cytosolic substrate proteins are recognized through their CMA targeting motif (a pentapeptide sequence biochemically related to KFERQ) by hsc70 and cochaperones (Step 1), followed by their delivery to lysosomes for binding to monomeric forms of the CMA receptor, LAMP-2A (Step 2). Binding of substrate proteins to the cytosolic tail of LAMP-2A induces its multimerization into a translocation complex (Step 3) so that unfolded proteins can be translocated across the lysosomal membrane (Step 4) into the lumen for degradation by resident cathepsins (Step 5). *Center:* Under different types of cellular stress (i.e. starvation), the activity of the nutrient-sensing kinase complex comprised of mTORC1 is suppressed, leading to the derepression and release of the autophagy complex, ULK1-FIP200-Atg13, that enables its relocation to the site of membrane formation. Nutrient deprivation also stimulates the activity of the nucleation complex composed of Beclin-1, Atg14, Vps15, and Vps34, a class III phosphatidylinosital-3-kinase that drives the formation of PI3P which promotes autophagosome membrane nucleation and formation of the isolation membrane. Several other factors contribute to the elongation of the isolation membrane,

Fig. 1. (*Continued*) which sequesters cargo for degradation, after which, it seals and fuses with the lysosome compartment so that the entrapped cargo can be degraded. *Right:* Microautophagy refers to the process by which cytosolic material is sequestered by invaginations in the lysosomal membrane that are pinched off into the lumen for degradation. A similar process has also been identified at late endosomes (eMI: endosomal microautophagy) where cargo can be internalized "in bulk" or selectively through a chaperone-cargo protein interaction.

2.1. *Macroautophagy, a picky eater?*

Macroautophagy is a central autophagy pathway in eukaryotic cells, consisting of unique double-membrane vesicles known as autophagosomes that engulf cellular material, fuse with lysosomes and promote degradation of their contents (Fig. 2).[28] This process can degrade cellular components in bulk as well in a substrate-specific manner.

mTORC1 and AMPK are nutrient sensors that regulate the downstream autophagy machinery. They control the activity of the Ulk1 complex through phosphorylation to modulate autophagy under nutrient deprivation, such as low amino acids, growth factors, oxygen and ATP (Fig. 1).[29,30] The inhibition of mTOR through nutrient depletion can be mimicked by mTOR inhibitor drugs like Rapamycin, Torin1 and Nelfinavir.[31–33] Rapamycin is the autophagy modulator most studied in the lung. It has been shown to attenuate pulmonary fibrosis and to inhibit mesenchymal cell proliferation in murine models of pulmonary fibrosis as well as pulmonary vascular remodeling in murine models of allergic vasculitis.[34–37] Rapamycin has also shown inhibitory effects on lung cancer through activation of autophagy.[36]

The formation and elongation of the autophagosomal double membrane is controlled by the coordinated actions of autophagy-regulated genes (Atgs).[38,39] These complexes initiate the formation and maturation of the isolation membrane, the precursor of the autophagosome.[40] The Atg5–Atg12–Atg16L1 complex and the LC3–PE conjugation complex promote the elongation and closure of the isolation membrane.[41] A double membrane will expand in

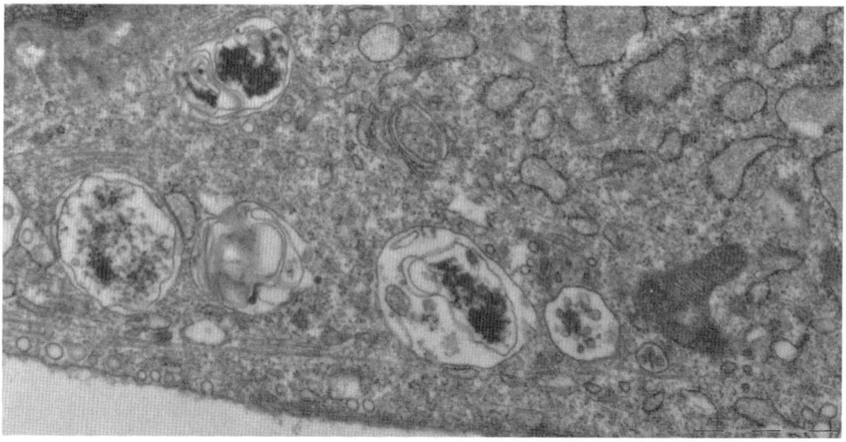

Fig. 2. Autophagy in human lung fibroblasts. Electron microscopy from human lung fibroblasts undergoing autophagy at different stages.

size to form an autophagosome with a diameter of 0.5–1.5 μm in mammalian cells. After autophagosome fusion with the lysosome, the cargo is degraded by hydrolases. This process can be done in bulk or can be highly selective[42–44] since receptors carrying LC3-interacting region (LIR) motifs[45–47] allows recruitment of the autophagic machinery to the site of the targeted substrate. Electron microscopy of human lung fibroblasts demonstrates the presence of autophagosomes and autophagolysosomes at different stages of degradation (Fig. 2).

2.2. *Selective receptors*

Sequestosome-1 (SQSTM1), also known as p62, was the first selective autophagy receptor to be identified.[6,45,48] p62/SQSTM1 associates with the autophagosome-localizing protein LC3 and with ubiquitinated proteins, damaged mitochondria or endosomes ruptured by invasive microbes.[44,49,50] In the presence of ubiquitinated cargo, p62 is phosphorylated, promoting the translocation of the ubiquitinated cargo into the autophagosome for degradation.[44,51]

*p*62 also interacts with the Keap1–Nrf2 system, regulating one of the major cellular defense mechanisms in oxidative stress and linking it with autophagy. This functional interaction regulates not only the oxidative-stress response but also metabolic pathways, and innate immunity. Loss of *p62* has been linked to accelerated aging and to age-related pathologies.[52] Deficiency of *p62* recapitulates all the characteristics of metabolic syndrome, including glucose intolerance, insulin resistance and systemic and adipose tissue-specific inflammation.[53]

Interestingly, *p62* regulates the abundance of Nrf2 and Nrf2-mediated induction of p62/SQSTM1, promoting a positive feedback loop.[54] Nrf2 activity inhibits lipogenesis, supports β-oxidation of fatty acids, facilitates flux through the pentose phosphate pathway and increases NADPH regeneration and purine biosynthesis (reviewed in[55]). Furthermore, Nrf2 controls the expression of transcription factors directly involved in metabolism and cell differentiation, including PPARγ, RXRα CCAAT/enhancer-binding protein (C/EBP)β.[56–58] Defective Nrf2 function has been linked to many aging-related lung diseases such as chronic obstructive pulmonary disease (COPD), vascular remodeling, pulmonary fibrosis and lung cancer.[59–63]

Taken together, p62/SQSTM1 has emerged as a key player in age-extending interventions and age-associated pathologies. Our recent studies have demonstrated that myofibroblast differentiation by TGFβ1 drives deregulation of *p62* gene expression and defective recruitment of damaged mitochondria to the autophagosome in human lung fibroblasts.[64] Treatment with hormetic compounds such as resveratrol promotes the transcriptional induction of *p62* and inhibits myofibroblast differentiation. Supporting these observations, other laboratories have reported a decrease in Nrf2 activity in primary fibroblasts isolated from Idiopathic Pulmonary Fibrosis (IPF) patients, while Nrf2 activation increases antioxidant defenses and myofibroblast de-differentiation.[65]

Bnip3 is another central player in autophagy signaling. It induces autophagy in many different cell types.[66,67] Bnip3 localizes to both mitochondria and ER and induces autophagic removal of ER (ER-phagy) and mitochondria (mitophagy). Briefly, LC3 binds to the LIR in the Bnip3 homodimer, promoting the removal of mitochondria and ER.[68] Compounds like arsenic trioxide protect the lung against bleomycin exposure in animal models of pulmonary fibrosis.[69] Interestingly, the same treatment induces autophagic cell death in malignant glioma cells by upregulation of Bnip3.[70]

Other autophagy receptors like NBR1, a related neighbor of BRCA1 gene 1, act as receptors for the sequestration and degradation of protein aggregates (aggrephagy).[71] The nuclear dot protein 52 *k*Da (NDP52) and optineurin are important for both aggrephagy and xenophagy.[72–74] Interestingly, NDP52 is also required for selective autophagy of DICER and AGO2, micro-RNA regulators.[75] Finally, SMAD-specific E3 ubiquitin protein ligase 1 (SMURF1) was recently identified as a receptor for both viral autophagy and mitophagy.[76,77]

2.3. *Mitophagy*

Mitochondria quality control ensures mitochondrial function through the lifetime of the cell.[78] The quality of mitochondria depends of the efficient turnover of mitochondrial DNA, proteins and lipids. Mitophagy is a hormetic system fine-tuned to maintain turnover and to selectively eliminate damaged or dysfunctional mitochondria. Short-term oxidative stress induces mitochondrial hormesis (mitohormesis) through autophagic degradation of mitochondria, promoting cell protection and contributing to lifespan extension.[79] However, excessive autophagy can result in cellular damage in certain cell types and contribute to premature cell death and accelerated aging.[80,81] Immunostainings to visualize mitophagy in lung tissues from bleomycin animal models of pulmonary fibrosis shows cell type-dependent differences in the levels of co- localization of LC3b (autophagosomal marker) with Tomm20 (mitochondria) (as presented in Fig. 3). The deterioration of mitochondrial turnover during lung aging could have detrimental consequences by promoting chronic oxidative stress and apoptosis and by exacerbating the susceptibility to injury and accelerating degeneration in the aging lung (Fig. 4). Defects in mitochondrial turnover correlate with late onset pathologies and accumulation of defective mitochondria

Lung-YoungBleoCQ

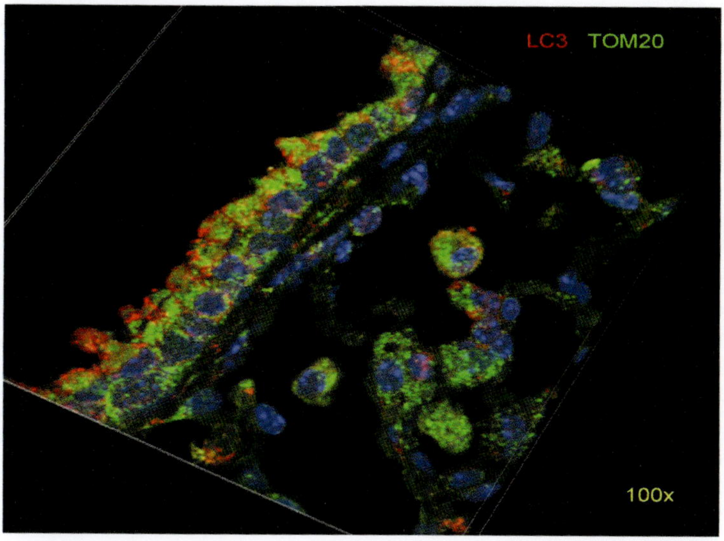

Fig. 3. Mitophagy in a bleomycin exposed lung. Mitophagy in the lung of 4 months animal model of pulmonary fibrosis. After 14 days of single dose Bleomycin-exposition, mice were treated for 4 hours (i.v) with lysosome inhibitor (Chloroquine, CQ) before tissue fixation. LC3 puncta(red)/Mitochondria TOMM20 (green). Colocalization (yellow) indicates autophagosomes containing mitochondria.

in aging tissues. This is demonstrated by reduced mitochondrial activity of complexes I–IV, affecting redox status, ATP production and mtDNA integrity in old mice. Induction of mitochondrial turnover and recycling through autophagy is thus a legitimate pharmacological target in age-related lung diseases. This is particularly important, considering that in cells like alveolar type II, mitochondria proliferation plays an important role to support surfactant metabolism and to maintain alveolar barrier integrity.[82]

Under stress, mitochondrial dysfunction induces ubiquitin-dependent responses that involve remodeling of the mitochondrial proteome resulting in organelle removal by mitophagy. PINK and Parkin are two Parkinson's Disease-linked genes known to be involved in the degradation of dysfunctional mitochondria. PINK1, a serine/threonine kinase, accumulates on depolarized mitochondria and

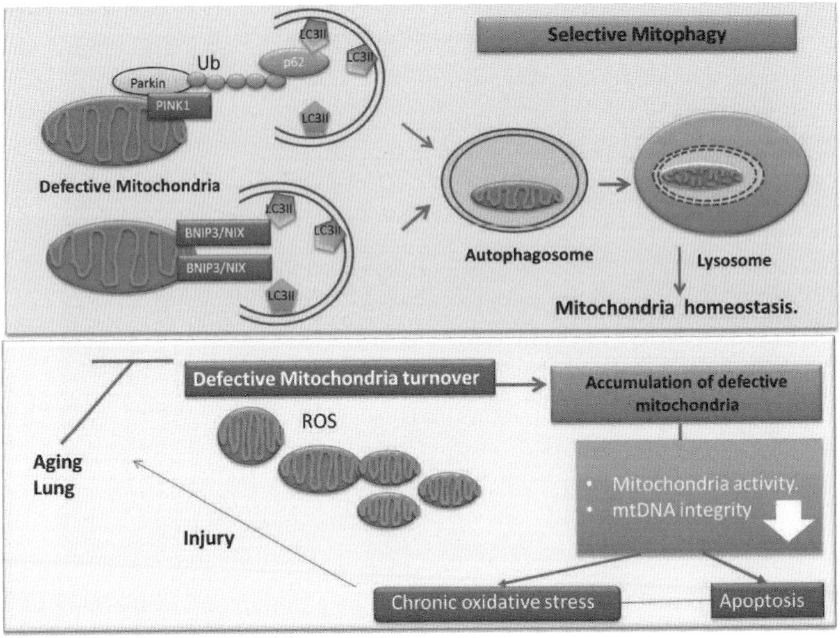

Fig. 4. Selective mitophagy. *Upper:* Selective recruitment of mitochondria through PINK/PARKIN pathway and specific receptors such as BNIP3/NIX which contain the LIR motif. Mitochondria sequestered in the autophagosome undergoes subsequent degradation in the lysosome. *Lower:* Proposed model representing the deterioration of mitochondrial turnover during lung aging and exacerbation of injury and tissue degeneration.

recruits Parkin. At the depolarized mitochondria, Parkin, an E3 ubiquitin ligase, catalyzes the polyubiquitination of several substrates, including mitofusins and VDACs, triggering the engulfment of mitochondria by the autophagosome-lysosome pathway through recruitment by *p*62 and several other factors.[48,83] Parkin is also known to promote innate immune defense against *M. tuberculosis* and other intracellular pathogens by promoting xenophagy.[84]

Mitochondria can also be cleared via direct binding of ATG8 family proteins to autophagy receptors on the mitochondria. This is the case with SMURF1, which binds membrane phospholipids and targets proteins to the plasma membrane and/or other subcellular membrane compartments.[85] SMURF1, as well as NIX and Bnip3, regulate the process of mitophagy by mediating the delivery of autophagic substrates to the new autophagosomes via their LIR motifs[76,9,116] In conclusion, multiple proteins can serve as autophagy receptors to ensure the removal of aberrant mitochondria (Fig. 4). It is likely that in the lung, there are cell type differences and redundancy in the mitophagy machinery that promote mitochondrial health, although further investigation is needed in this area.

2.4. *Lipophagy*

Lipophagy is another organelle-specific type of macroautophagy that refers to the sequestration of lipid droplets inside the autophagosomes (reviewed in[86]). Lipids droplets (LDs) store nutrients in the form of neutral lipids (triglycerides and cholesterol esters) in a membrane-enclosed organelle and help to maintain bioenergetics. LDs serve not only as an energy reservoir but also as signaling scaffolds, ligands for transcription factors and as a depots for sequestration of misfolded proteins.[87,88] The size, composition and function of LDs have been shown to change according to cell type and/or metabolic state.[89] More importantly, early studies of LDs with Nile red ratiometric measurements revealed a cell fate-dependent lipid composition of LDs that correlated with differences between proliferating and quiescent cells.[90]

Some degree of lipophagy may occur "in bulk," however under lipid challenges, a preferential sequestration of lipids in autophagosomes has been observed in order to facilitate the breakdown of triglycerides into free fatty acids for energy production. The determinants for autophagic initiation on the surface of LD are still unknown as well as the specific mechanisms by which the limiting autophagosome membrane grows around and sequesters the LDs (Fig. 5). However, it is known that membrane-type structures are present in the LDs core.[91] Interestingly, a recent study identified that LD-associated Proteins Perilipin 2nd Perilipin 3 undergo CMA-mediated degradation prior to lipolytic break down of fat stores. (Kaushik and cuervo, nature cell biology 2015, PMID: 25961502)

Elegant studies in the liver revealed that autophagy inhibition results in blocked lipolysis and consequent accumulation of LDs. On

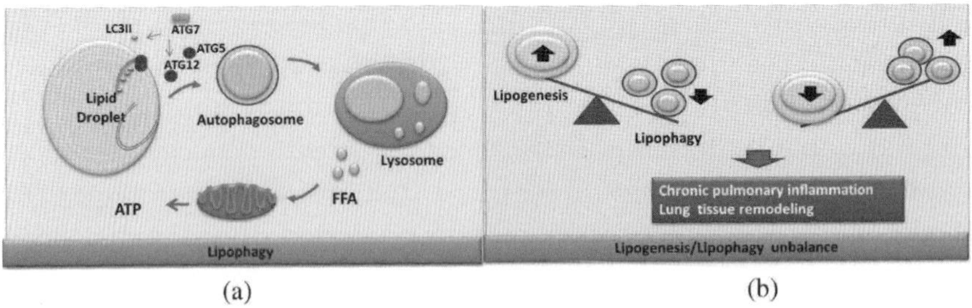

Fig. 5. Conceptual model of Lipophagy in normal lung and the consequence of unbalance lipolisis/lipophagy. (a) Squematic representation of theformation of vacuoles at the surface of an lipid droplet; Atg: autophagy related proteins. (b) Deregulation of the autophagic process can modify the Lypogenesis/Lipolytic balance with pathological consequences such as inflammation and fibrosis.

the other hand, treatment with rapamycin or lithium chloride, activators of autophagy, significantly decreases intracellular LDs and triglyceride stores in the presence of lipid stimuli by promoting lipophagy.[92] Failure to regulate lipid accumulation in hepatocytes promotes liver steatosis.[93] Interestingly, lipophagy has been observed in cell types not typically known to store fat such fibroblasts and *T* cells.[15,92,94,95] Accumulation of neutral lipids in type II epithelial cells, alveolar macrophages and alveoli are associated with chronic pulmonary inflammation and alveolar remodeling.[96] Based on these studies, it is reasonable to hypothesize that the deregulation of lipophagy could promote inflammation and tissue remodeling in the lung (Fig. 5), but autophagy-mediated breakdown of lipid stores in these pathological contexts has yet to be analyzed.

3. CMA: Another Route into Lysosomes

CMA is a type of autophagy in which a subset of cytosolic proteins bearing a targeting motif (biochemically related to the pentapeptide KFERQ) are recognized by the chaperone hsc70[97] and delivered to lysosomes one-by-one for degradation (Fig. 1).[27,98] CMA is distinct from other types of autophagy in that it does not require any type of vesicular compartmentalization such as the autophagosome (in macroautophagy) or the invagination of the lysosomal membrane (in microautophagy). Instead, a receptor protein embedded in the lysosomal membrane, LAMP-2A,[99] serves as the CMA receptor, to which substrate proteins bind, and as part of the translocation complex, by facilitating the transport of unfolded proteins from the cytosolic surface into the lumen of lysosomes.[100]

Sequence analysis of the proteome has revealed that approximately 30% of all soluble cytosolic proteins contain a KFERQ-like motif,[101] implying that CMA has the capability of regulating diverse cellular pathways. Validated CMA substrates include proteins involved in transcriptional regulation,[102] protein degradation,[103] neurologic function,[104,105] hypoxia,[106] oncogenesis[107] and metabolism.[108] Other substrates identified have cell-type specific functions that impact cellular physiology in a tissue-specific manner, including renal cell proflieration[109] and neuronal survival.[110] The contribution of CMA to the selective elimination of pulmonary-related proteins has yet to be elucidated.

CMA plays several important physiological roles in cells. True to its autophagic identity, CMA is robustly upregulated during times of nutrient deprivation.[111] Additionally, CMA serves as a type of stress-response pathway, as it is activated during conditions of oxidative stress[112] and proteotoxicity.[113] Reactive oxygen species that accumulate during times of oxidative damage enhance substrate degradation via CMA by improving the accessibility of the CMA targeting motif which increases the efficiency of substrate internalization and degradation in lysosomes.[114] Interestingly, most cells have basal levels of CMA activity which serve to continuously degrade substrates, even in the absence of stress, supporting a role for CMA in the maintenance of the cellular proteome even under normal conditions.[115]

Since CMA plays an important role in maintaining protein quality control as well as its newly identified function in the regulation of cellular metabolism, it is not surprising that CMA malfunction has been observed in variety of disease states, including cancer,[116] Parkinson's Disease (PD)[117], tauopathies[118], obesity,[119] hepatosteatosis[108] and myopathies.[120] In the case of neurodegenerative diseases, CMA dysfunction results from the impaired ability of the CMA receptor, LAMP-2A, to successfully translocate proteins into lysosomes for degradation. For example, mutant or dopamine-modified α-synuclein fails to undergo CMA-mediated degradation due to faulty translocation[121] while LRRK2, another PD-related protein, blocks the assembly of the CMA translocation complex at lysosomes, compromising its own degradation as well as the turnover of several other substrates.[117] In addition to the disease-related dysfunction of CMA, physiological aging in the absence of any type of compounding stress is sufficient to reduce CMA activity. Decreased levels of LAMP-2A at the lysosomal membrane are responsible for the age-dependent decline of this pathway, an effect observed both in aged rodents and cells isolated from elderly humans.[122–124] Intriguingly, genetic rescue of LAMP-2A using transgenic mouse models restored CMA activity in old mice and prevented the age-related functional decline of this organ in terms of stress resistance, oxidative damage and protein homeostasis.[125] Whether or not alterations in CMA activity contribute to the pathogenesis of pulmonary diseases is unknown and whether or not the decline of CMA with age contributes to the functional decline in lungs remains to be determined.

3.1. *CMA and the response to metabolic stress*

The earliest studies of CMA highlighted the robust activation of this pathway during nutrient deprivation. Whereas macroautophagy activity is responsive almost immediately after starvation, with an activation peak around six hours, CMA stimulation is evident by eight hours of starvation, reaching a plateau of maximal induction by 36 hrs.[111] Overlapping but temporal differences in the activation of each autophagic pathway implies a distinct role for the subtypes of autophagy. Furthermore, the selective nature of CMA combined with the requirement of a targeting motif embedded in a protein's amino acid sequence make it likely that a distinct subproteome undergoes regulated turnover through CMA. Together with macroautophagy, CMA contributes to the elimination of superfluous proteins during starvation so their amino acid constituents can be recycled and either utilized for anabolic purposes (gluconeogenesis,[126] *de novo* protein synthesis)[26] or catabolic pathways (TCA cycle entry, oxidative phosphorylation, ATP generation).[127,128] This starvation-induced stimulation of CMA activity appears to be cell- and tissue-specific in nature, as certain organs like the liver and heart demonstrate a more robust degradation fasting response of KFERQ-containing proteins compared to skeletal muscle.[129] More work is needed to analyze whether lung cells induce CMA during starvation or in the context of other types of stress conditions.

Mechanistically, changes in the lysosomal compartment can explain the sharp increase in CMA activity during nutrient depletion. The fraction of cellular lysosomes that are specifically active for CMA activity, as defined by those that contain lysosomal-hsc70 which is necessary for translocation of substrates,[97] expands. This amplification is poignantly observed in rat livers in which under basal conditions, twenty percent of cellular lysosomes contain lys-hsc70, whereas after prolonged nutrient deprivation, up to eighty percent of cellular lysosomes are CMA competent (Fig. 6).[130] This expansion of CMA-active lysosomes is paralleled by an increase in levels of LAMP-2A at the lysosomal membrane. Starvation-induced increase in LAMP-2A is not attained through transcriptional upregulation of the *lamp2* gene, but by a post-translational effect that results in decreased degradation of LAMP-2A and its augmented stabilization at the membrane.[131] During starvation, the amount of LAMP-2A continues to increase through the retrieval of a pool of intact LAMP-2A from vesicles inside the lysosomal lumen.[132]

In contrast to the upregulation of CMA during times of nutrient paucity, CMA activity is thwarted during conditions of excessive dietary lipid intake. Interestingly, CMA upregulation occurs early in response to lipid overload, but chronic exposure to dietary fat compromises CMA function, at least in the liver.[119] This is an example of how environmental stressors (like diet) can interfere with CMA function. More specifically, this effect of loss of CMA function is mediated by changes in the composition of the lysosomal membrane. Typically, there are discrete regions of the lysosomal membrane that are enriched in certain lipids and associate with the serine protease Cathepsin A.[133] Under normal dietary conditions, a small fraction of LAMP-2A localizes to these microdomain regions and undergoes regulated degradation, starting with cleavage by Cathepsin A (Fig. 6).[134] When mice are subjected to a high lipid

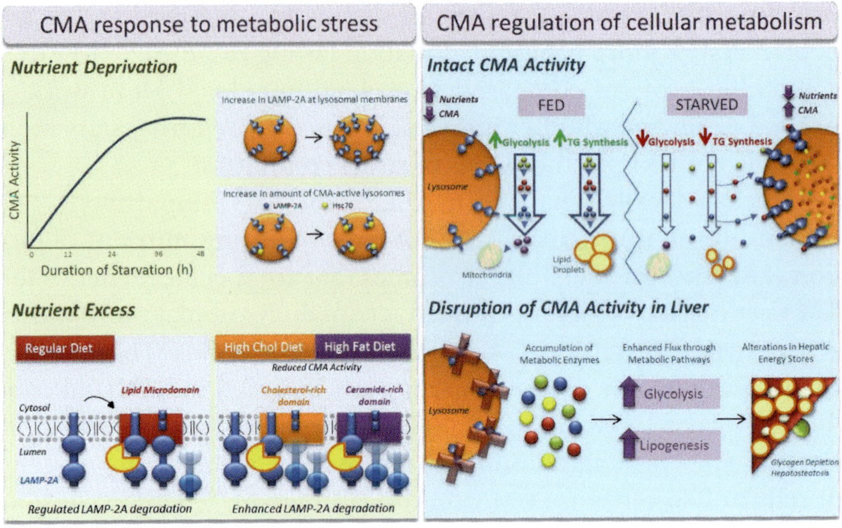

Fig. 6. CMA and Metabolism. *Left:* Prolonged nutrient deprivation is a robust activator of CMA. During starvation, there is an increase in the percentage of lysosomes active for CMA activity, as defined by those that contain lysosomal-hsc70 which is necessary for translocation of substrates. This expansion of CMA-competent lysosomes is paralleled by an increase in levels of LAMP-2A, the CMA receptor, present at the lysosomal membrane. The starvation-induced increase in LAMP-2A is not attained through *de novo* synthesis but by decreased degradation of this protein at lysosomes. In contrast, excessive nutrient intake enhances the degradation of LAMP-2A and has a negative effect on CMA activity. Under normal dietary conditions, a small fraction of LAMP-2A is recruited to discrete compartments of the lysosomal membrane (lipid microdomains) where it undergoes regulated degradation upon cleavage by Cathepsin A. A diet enriched in lipids increases the presence and changes the composition of these microdomains, resulting in a higher fraction of LAMP-2A degradation and reduced CMA activity. *Right:* Recently, CMA has been described to contribute to the regulation of cellular metabolism through the selective degradation of metabolic enzymes. During fed conditions, nutrients are abundant and CMA is active at a basal level. During starvation, CMA activity is induced and metabolic enzymes that participate in glycolysis and lipid synthesis are selectively turned over by CMA in an effort to downregulate flux through these pathways. When CMA activity is disrupted, in the case of genetic deletion of LAMP-2A, these enzymes accumulate inside cells which leads to abnormally enhanced glucose utilization and lipid synthesis, causing glycogen depletion, hepatosteatosis, and metabolic dysregulation.

content diet, the composition of the lysosomal microdomains changes, entrapping more LAMP-2A for degradation and thus impairing CMA activity due to a decrease in the presence of the CMA receptor and translocation complex.[119] Interestingly, the resulting changes in the lipid composition of the lysosomal membrane from a high-fat diet resemble the changes in the lipidomic profile that are observed with age, implying that the age-related functional decline of CMA activity can perhaps be accelerated by dietary-induced obesity. The bulk of these studies were performed in the liver but it is of interest to decipher whether acute and chronic lipid challenges impact CMA function in other tissues.

3.2. *CMA and the regulation of cellular metabolism*

In addition to the responsiveness of CMA to different nutritional cues, a new role has emerged for CMA in regulating different aspects of cellular metabolism. Some of the earliest identified CMA substrates were enzymes involved in glycolysis, including GAPDH and phosphoglucomutase.[135,136] Recently, studies in cancer cells have further uncovered a link between glycolysis and CMA, as failure to turnover PKM2 by CMA was shown to favor cancer cell profliferation.[137] Interestingly, blockage of CMA in different cancer cell lines and in solid tumors was sufficient to abrogate cellular proliferation and to reduce tumorigenesis.[116] Further analysis the metabolic profiles of cancer cells (including lung cancer lineages) upon CMA inhibition uncovered a severe energetic compromise due a reduction in glycolytic capacity, further supporting the connection between CMA and glycolysis in the context of carcinogenesis.

However, the *in vivo* physiological relevance of the nutrition-regulated degradation of metabolic enzymes by CMA was unknown until recent studies were performed using mouse models with a conditional deletion of the LAMP-2A gene, allowing the assessment of the impact of the malfunction of CMA on metabolic homeostasis. Liver-specific loss of CMA activity resulted in an impairment in lysosomal degradation of several metabolic enzymes involved in glycolysis and lipid synthesis.[108] These studies identified CMA a regulator of hepatic metabolism through its modulation of carbohydrate and lipid metabolism and furthermore, highlighted the necessity of CMA in helping cells adapt to dietary lipid challenges (Fig. 6). While livers with CMA failure exhibited a depletion in their glycogen stores and an accumulation of lipids, it remains to be seen whether other tissues have similar metabolic dysregulation in the face of CMA compromise. Additionally, the metabolic dysfunction observed upon CMA blockage suggests that the age-related decline of CMA may contribute to the energetic deficiencies and metabolic dysregulation observed in elderly populations.

4. Lung Bioenergetics and Autophagy

Autophagy has been shown to be critical for survival and to be an energy-generating process under conditions of nutrient limitation in mammalian cells.[138,139] For instance, macroautophagic activity promotes the degradation of protein and lipid stores, whose components are recycled and released from lysosomes as amino acids and free fatty acids. These substrates may be used for anabolic (protein synthesis) or catabolic (β-oxidation, ATP generation) purposes. Furthermore, the tightly controlled turnover of mitochondria by autophagic processes contributes to regulating cellular bioenergetics. Thus, it is important to understand the metabolic significance of the autophagic activity in a tissue-specific manner.

The lung is a highly metabolically active organ. It uses glucose from the circulation as primary fuel for its metabolic needs such as for maintenance, secretion and clearance. Glucose is catabolized in the lung by cytoplasmic and mitochondrial pathways.[140,141] In aging mice, lungs, like other tissues, have reduced mitochondrial activity of complex I–IV, affecting both redox status and ATP production. A decline in intracellular NAD+ levels and NAD:NADH ratio is also observed in middle-aged rats compared to young rodents and this changing metabolite phenotype is accompanied by alterations in lipid peroxidation, protein carbonylation and antioxidant capacity.[142] Whether a decline in autophagy is behind this changing metabolic profile remains to be determined.

It is also important to consider that there is a regulatory feedback effect between lipid composition and autophagy. While autophagy can modulate lipid metabolism, changes in lysosomal membrane lipid composition can alter autophagy flux, as is the case for both macroautophagy and CMA.[119,143,144] Defects in autophagy and intracellular lipid homeostasis have been linked to obesity, insulin resistance, diabetes, atherosclerosis and lipid-storage diseases.[93,143,145] More studies need to be conducted to understand the changes in lipid homeostasis in the aging lung.

Our studies demonstrate that basal autophagy (indicated by the number of LC3b-positive autophagosomes) does not change significantly between the lungs from young (4 months old) and middle-aged (14 months old) mice, but significant age-related differences are observed after bleomycin injury, as presented by the LC3b puncta (autophagosome) semi-quantification (Fig. 7). The consequences of this defective autophagic response to injury requires further characterization. Few cell-type-specific studies have been done in the lung to evaluate the relevance of the autophagic response in metabolic homeostasis. Nevertheless, recent analyses have demonstrated that liver-specific deficiency in autophagy is not fatal to fasted mice,[126,146] providing insights about the potential importance of active autophagy in tissues like the lung and its role in cell survival and glucose homeostasis.

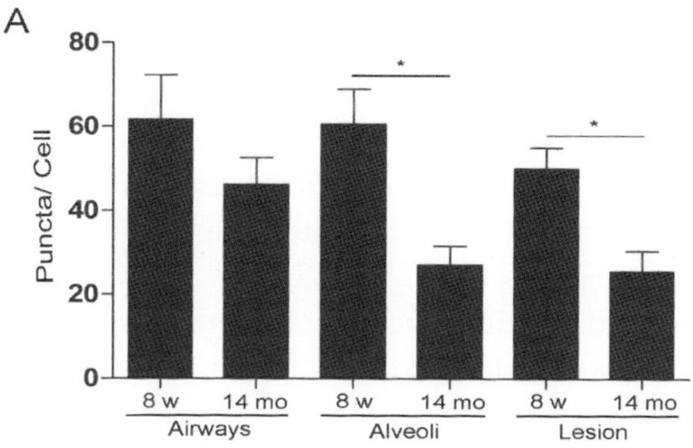

Fig 7. Deregulated autopagic response to injury in the lung of 14 months old mice. Analysis of LC3 puncta in 8 weeks old mice and 14 months old mice, 14 days after bleomycin exposure (oropharyngeal aspiration). ImageJ semiquantification was done for upper airways, alveoli areas and fibrotic lesions. (*) Statistical significance.

Multiple cells in the lung participate in iron homeostasis, where autophagy also plays a key role. Iron mishandling has detrimental consequences for tissue integrity, as iron is a redox active metal required for many vital cellular functions including oxygen transport and energy production.[147] Furthermore, iron is essential to the function of a wide range of cellular proteins. Lung cells store and export their excess of iron to prevent it from rising to toxic levels, as iron overload promotes oxidative stress, tissue inflammation, cellular injury and death.[147] Interestingly, iron homeostasis is found to be disrupted after acute and chronic lung injury.[148] The quantity of iron deposits and the percentage of iron-positive macrophages correlate with the severity of COPD and emphysema.[149] Lung epithelial cells and inflammatory cells express a variety of iron-associated molecules, including ferritin and transferrin, that are important for iron storage and transport. Selective autophagy has been shown to regulate ferritin and cellular transferrin receptor levels — and, consequently, iron storage and transport.[150–151] Unfortunately, the mechanisms underlying iron homeostasis and autophagy in the lung remain poorly understood.

5. Bioenergetic Sensors and Autophagy Modulators

Insulin and IGF1 signaling are the most conserved lifespan-controlling pathways in evolution. Their targets include the FOXO family of transcription factors and mTOR complexes. Longevity in humans and animal models have being linked to mutations in the key players of this pathway, such as IGF-1 receptors, insulin receptors or downstream effectors such as AKT, mTOR.[152,153] Conversely, dietary restriction, a condition in which signaling through these pathways is suppressed, increases lifespan in animal models, including nonhuman primates.[153–155]

One of the most important nutrient sensing systems is mTOR, which interconnects aging, autophagy, metabolism and age-related diseases.[156,157] mTOR can be activated by insulin, growth factors and nutrients. It promotes protein synthesis, ribosomal biogenesis, cell mass growth and growth factor secretion.[3,158,159] Inhibition of autophagy through mTOR induces accumulation of aggregation-prone proteins and defective organelles (reviewed in[160]). Thus, mTOR limits lifespan by accelerating age-related diseases.

The mTOR pathway is activated in lung aging-related pathologies such as chronic inflammation, cancer and pulmonary fibrosis.[161–163] mTOR activation disables autophagy in the early stages of lung oncogenesis, but interestingly, autophagy is reinstated at later states of tumor progression, allowing tumor cells to cope with endogenous stress and increase resistance to chemotherapy or radiotherapy.[164,166] Furthermore, mTOR activation and consequent blockage in autophagy promotes the initial cell fate changes to myofibroblasts, key players in the pathogenesis of pulmonary fibrosis[33,166] (Sousulski *et al.*, 2014 in submission). It is also suggested that insufficient autophagy underlies accelerated epithelial cell senescence, which is a promising clue for understanding the pathogenesis of age-related diseases such as IPF.[167] Interestingly, promotion of autophagy in human lung fibroblasts protects them from myofibroblast differentiation induced by TGFβ1 (Sousulski *et al.*, 2014 in submission).

Activation of AMPK through increasing concentrations of adenosine monophosphate (AMP)[168,169] also acts as a nutrient sensing system and is an upstream modulator of autophagy. AMPK activation inhibits protein synthesis and glycogen synthesis and promotes G1 cell cycle arrest, glucose uptake, glycolysis and fatty acid oxidation in order to conserve energy.[170,171] AMPK activates TSC2, inhibiting mTORC1 and consequently stimulates autophagy to catabolize organelles and to mobilize intracellular nutrients.[172,173]

Signaling pathways induced by hypoxia also modulate autophagy. Oxygen is essential for use in the mitochondrial respiratory chain, allowing the generation of ATP thorugh oxidative phosphorylation. Oxygen can also modulate autophagy through AMPK and mTOR. Hypoxia results in a reduction of ATP levels, activating AMPK and deactivating mTOR and shifts the cellular metabolic profile towards glycolysis and away from mitochondrial respiration.[174] The transcription factor HIF1α activates an array of genes that are involved in metabolic adaptation to hypoxia, including BNIP3 and BNIP3L, which participate in mitophagy.[175–177] Interestingly, HIF1α has been recently identified as a substrate of CMA, implying that this autophagic pathway may be important for the regulation of the cellular response to hypoxia. [178,106]

The sirtuin family of proteins are also major modulators and contributors to the balance between autophagy, metabolism and aging (for review).[179,180] Many mammalian sirtuin proteins have NAD^+-dependent protein deacetylase activity. Induction of SIRT1 deacetylation, for example, results in increased fatty acid oxidation and improved glucose homeostasis.[181] Furthermore, SIRT1 deacetylates proteins indispensable for the formation of the autophagosome.[181] Deletion of SIRT1 gene in the liver impairs fatty acid catabolism, increases susceptibility dyslipidemia, hepatic steatosis, inflammation and ER stress under high fat diet.[182] SIRT1 expression in the lung is reduced in lung aging and COPD.[183,184]

Small molecule activators of SIRT1 and AMPK such as the polyphenol resveratrol and closely related derivatives have shown promise as therapeutic agents for the treatment of age-related disease, obesity and related metabolic disorders.[185–187] Resveratrol is known to extend life span, promote autophagy, and inhibit inflammation. It also mitigates bleomycin-induced pulmonary fibrosis and ventricular remodeling in old rats with COPD.[188–190]

Substrates for SIRT1 include PPARγ and PGC-1α,[191] key regulators of the core molecular clock. Interestingly, disruption of circadian rhythm reduces lifespan. Some pathologies such as pulmonary edema, hypertensive crises, asthma and allergic attacks, peak at certain times during the circadian cycle,[192] a process that is also deregulated during aging.[193] Interestingly, it was recently found that basal autophagy is rhythmically activated in a clock-dependent manner,[194] confirming the significance of the circadian clock as a bioenergetics regulator of human physiology and pathophysiology.[195,196] The relevance of the circadian regulation of autophagy in age-related diseases and in particular in the aging lung will need to be analyzed in the future. The therapeutic targeting of these bioenergetic sensors is proposed as a way to modulate autophagy, metabolism and slow the progression of age-related diseases.

6. Conclusion

As the autophagy field continues to expand and uncover new roles for this process in cellular physiology and pathophysiology, the contribution of autophagic activity to pulmonary cellular and organ homeostasis is being elucidated. Specifically, there is much interest in understanding how autophagy regulates cellular metabolism in a tissue-specific manner. By dissecting the roles of the different types of autophagy in nutrient sensing, catabolic breakdown of macromolecules, maintenance of protein quality quality control and stress response, we will have a better understanding of how to pharmacologically manipulate this pathway to alleviate the burden of pulmonary disorders as well as to prevent or delay the deterioration in lung function that occurs with age.

Acknowledgments

Studies in Dr. Sanchez laboratory have been supported by the by the National Institute of General Medical Sciences of the National Institutes of Health under Award Number P20GM103629. The American Thoracic Society and Scleroderma Foundation award 552114G1. Dr. Schneider was supported by NIH MSTP Training Grant T32-GM007288 and NIH/NIA F30AG046109.

References

1. Lopez-Otin C, Blasco MA, Partridge L *et al.* (2013) The hallmarks of aging. *Cell* **153**: 1194–1217.
2. Rattan SI, Demirovic D. (2009) Hormesis can and does work in humans. *Dose-Response* **8**: 58–63.
3. Blagosklonny MV. (2011) Hormesis does not make sense except in the light of TOR-driven aging. *Aging* **3**: 1051–1062.
4. Salminen A, Kaarniranta K. (2009) Regulation of the aging process by autophagy. *Trends Mol Med* **15**: 217–224.
5. Hubbard VM, Valdor R, Macian F *et al.* (2012) Selective autophagy in the maintenance of cellular homeostasis in aging organisms. *Biogerontol* **13**: 21–35.

6. Bjorkoy G, Lamark T, Brech A *et al.* (2005) p62/SQSTM1 forms protein aggregates degraded by autophagy and has a protective effect on huntingtin-induced cell death. *J Cell Biol* **171**: 603–614.
7. Komatsu M, Waguri S, Chiba T *et al.* (2006) Loss of autophagy in the central nervous system causes neurodegeneration in mice. *Nature* **441**: 880–884.
8. Mathew R, Karp CM, Beaudoin B *et al.* (2009) Autophagy suppresses tumorigenesis through elimination of p62. *Cell* **137**: 1062–1075.
9. Fujiwara Y, Furuta A, Kikuchi H *et al.* (2013) Discovery of a novel type of autophagy targeting RNA. *Autophagy* **9**: 403–409.
10. Chen S, Jin YL, Yao SQ *et al.* (2013) [Autophagy in lung tissue of rats exposed to silica dust]. Zhonghua lao dong wei sheng zhi ye bing za zhi = Zhonghua laodong weisheng zhiyebing zazhi = Chinese journal of industrial hygiene and occupational diseases **31**: 607–610.
11. Dunn WA, Jr, Cregg JM, Kiel JA *et al.* (2005) Pexophagy: The selective autophagy of peroxisomes. *Autophagy* **1**: 75–83.
12. Cebollero E, Reggiori F, Kraft C. (2012) Reticulophagy and ribophagy: Regulated degradation of protein production factories. *Int J Cell Biol* **2012**: 182834.
13. Deretic V, Saitoh T, Akira S. (2013) Autophagy in infection, inflammation and immunity. *Nat Revs. Immunol* **13**: 722–737.
14. Paul S, Schaefer BC. (2012) Selective autophagy regulates T cell activation. *Autophagy* **8**: 1690–1692.
15. Hubbard VM, Valdor R, Patel B *et al.* (2010) Macroautophagy regulates energy metabolism during effector T cell activation. *J Immunol* **185**: 7349–7357.
16. Giordano S, Darley-Usmar V, Zhang J. (2014) Autophagy as an essential cellular antioxidant pathway in neurodegenerative disease. *Redox Biol* **2**: 82–90.
17. Benavides GA, Liang Q, Dodson M *et al.* (2013) Inhibition of autophagy and glycolysis by nitric oxide during hypoxia-reoxygenation impairs cellular bioenergetics and promotes cell death in primary neurons. *Free Radl Biol Med* **65**: 1215–1228.
18. Ryter SW, Cloonan SM, Choi AM. (2013) Autophagy: A critical regulator of cellular metabolism and homeostasis. *Mol Cells* **36**: 7–16.
19. Rosenfeldt MT, O'Prey J, Morton JP *et al.* (2013) p53 status determines the role of autophagy in pancreatic tumour development. *Nature* **504**: 296–300.
20. Schneider JL, Cuervo AM. (2014) Autophagy and human disease: Emerging themes. *Curr Opin Genet Dev* **26C**: 16–23.

21. Melendez A, Talloczy Z, Seaman M *et al.* (2003) Autophagy genes are essential for dauer development and life-span extension in C. elegans. *Science* **301**: 1387–1391.
22. Bjedov I, Toivonen JM, Kerr F *et al.* (2010) Mechanisms of life span extension by rapamycin in the fruit fly Drosophila melanogaster. *Cell Metabol* **11**: 35–46.
23. Juhasz G, Neufeld TP. (2008) Drosophila Atg7: Required for stress resistance, longevity and neuronal homeostasis, but not for metamorphosis. *Autophagy* **4**: 357–358.
24. Lamb CA, Dooley HC, Tooze SA. (2013) Endocytosis and autophagy: Shared machinery for degradation. *BioEssays : News Revs Mol Cell Dev Biol* **35**: 34–45.
25. Kroemer G, Marino G, Levine B. (2010) Autophagy and the integrated stress response. *Mol Cell* **40**: 280–293.
26. Mortimore GE, Lardeux BR, Adams CE. (1988) Regulation of microautophagy and basal protein turnover in rat liver. Effects of short-term starvation. *J Biol Chem* **263**: 2506–2512.
27. Cuervo AM. (2010) Chaperone-mediated autophagy: Selectivity pays off. *Trends Endocrin Met* **21**: 142–150.
28. Kelekar A. (2005) Autophagy. *Ann NY Acad Sci* **1066**: 259–271.
29. Ganley IG, Lam du H, Wang J *et al.* (2009) ULK1.ATG13.FIP200 complex mediates mTOR signaling and is essential for autophagy. *J Biol Chem* **284**: 12297–12305.
30. Kim J, Kundu M, Viollet B *et al.* (2011) AMPK and mTOR regulate autophagy through direct phosphorylation of Ulk1. *Nat Cell Biol* **13**: 132–141.
31. Ravikumar B, Sarkar S, Davies JE *et al.* (2010) Regulation of mammalian autophagy in physiology and pathophysiology. *Physiol Rev* **90**: 1383–1435.
32. Gills JJ, Lopiccolo J, Dennis PA. (2008) Nelfinavir, a new anti-cancer drug with pleiotropic effects and many paths to autophagy. *Autophagy* **4**: 107–109.
33. Richeldi L, Collard HR, du Bois RM, *et al.* (2013) Mapping the future for pulmonary fibrosis: Report from the 17th International Colloquium on Lung and Airway Fibrosis. *Euro Respir J* **42**: 230–238.
34. Koizumi R, Sasaki N, Nakamura Y *et al.* (2014) Rapamycin Attenuates Pulmonary Allergic Vasculitis in Murine Model by Reducing TGF-beta Production in the Lung. *Allergol Int* **63**: 457–466.

35. Jin X, Dai H, Ding K, Xu X *et al.* (2014) Rapamycin attenuates bleomycin-induced pulmonary fibrosis in rats and the expression of metalloproteinase-9 and tissue inhibitors of metalloproteinase-1 in lung tissue. *Chinese Med J* **127**: 1304–1309.
36. Jiang RY, Pei HL, Gu WD *et al.* (2014) Autophagic inhibitor attenuates rapamycin- induced inhibition of proliferation in cultured A549 lung cancer cells. *Euro Rev Med Pharmacol Sci* **18**: 806–810.
37. Gardner EE, Connis N, Poirier JT *et al.* (2014) Rapamycin rescues ABT-737 efficacy in small cell lung cancer. *Cancer* Res **74**: 2846–2856.
38. Klionsky DJ, Baehrecke EH, Brumell JH *et al.* (2011) A comprehensive glossary of autophagy-related molecules and processes (2nd edition). *Autophagy* **7**: 1273–1294.
39. Mizushima N, Levine B. (2010) Autophagy in mammalian development and differentiation. *Nat Cell Biol* **12**: 823–830.
40. Mizushima N, Komatsu M. (2011) Autophagy: Renovation of cells and tissues. *Cell* **147**: 728–741.
41. Zhu J, Dagda RK, Chu CT. (2011) Monitoring mitophagy in neuronal cell cultures. *Methods Mol Biol* **793**: 325–339.
42. Novak I, Kirkin V, McEwan DG*et al.* (2010) Nix is a selective autophagy receptor for mitochondrial clearance. *EMBO Reports* **11**: 45–51.
43. Lamark T, Kirkin V, Dikic I *et al.* (2009) NBR1 and p62 as cargo receptors for selective autophagy of ubiquitinated targets. *Cell cycle* **8**: 1986–1990.
44. Johansen T, Lamark T. (2011) Selective autophagy mediated by autophagic adapter proteins. *Autophagy* **7**: 279–296.
45. Pankiv S, Clausen TH, Lamark T *et al.* (2007) p62/SQSTM1 binds directly to Atg8/LC3 to facilitate degradation of ubiquitinated protein aggregates by autophagy. *J Biol Chem* **282**: 24131–24145.
46. Ichimura Y, Kominami E, Tanaka K *et al.* (2008) Selective turnover of p62/A170/SQSTM1 by autophagy. *Autophagy* **4**: 1063–1066.
47. Noda NN, Kumeta H, Nakatogawa H *et al.* (2008) Structural basis of target recognition by Atg8/LC3 during selective autophagy. *Genes Cells Mol Cell Mechan* **13**: 1211–1218.
48. Komatsu M, Waguri S, Koike M *et al.* (2007) Homeostatic levels of p62 control cytoplasmic inclusion body formation in autophagy-deficient mice. *Cell* **131**: 1149–1163.
49. Narendra D, Kane LA, Hauser DN *et al.* (2010) p62/SQSTM1 is required for Parkin-induced mitochondrial clustering but not mitophagy; VDAC1 is dispensable for both. *Autophagy* **6**: 1090–1106.

50. Dupont N, Lacas-Gervais S, Bertout J *et al.* (2009) Shigella phagocytic vacuolar membrane remnants participate in the cellular response to pathogen invasion and are regulated by autophagy. *Cell Host Microbe* **6**: 137–149.
51. Matsumoto G, Wada K, Okuno M *et al.* (2011) Serine 403 phosphorylation of p62/SQSTM1 regulates selective autophagic clearance of ubiquitinated proteins. *Mol Cell* **44**: 279–289.
52. Bitto A, Lerner CA, Nacarelli T *et al.* (2014) p62/SQSTM1 at the interface of aging, autophagy, and disease. *Age* **36**: 9626–9630.
53. Rodriguez A, Duran A, Selloum M *et al.* (2006) Mature-onset obesity and insulin resistance in mice deficient in the signaling adapter p62. *Cell Metabol* **3**: 211–222.
54. Jain A, Lamark T, Sjottem E *et al.* (2010) p62/SQSTM1 is a target gene for transcription factor NRF2 and creates a positive feedback loop by inducing antioxidant response element-driven gene transcription. *J Biol Chem* **285**: 22576–22591.
55. Hayes JD, Dinkova-Kostova AT. (2014) The Nrf2 regulatory network provides an interface between redox and intermediary metabolism. *Trends Biochem Sci* **39**: 199–218.
56. Pi J, Freeman ML, Yamamoto M. (2010) Nrf2 in toxicology and pharmacology: The good, the bad and the ugly? *Toxicol Appl Pharmacol* **244**: 1–3.
57. Chorley BN, Campbell MR, Wang X *et al.* (2012) Identification of novel NRF2-regulated genes by ChIP-Seq: Influence on retinoid X receptor alpha. *Nucleic acids Res* **40**: 7416–7429.
58. Zhan L, Zhang H, Zhang Q *et al.* (2012) Regulatory role of KEAP1 and NRF2 in PPARgamma expression and chemoresistance in human non-small-cell lung carcinoma cells. *Free Rad Biol Med* **53**: 758–768.
59. Barnes PJ, Shapiro SD, Pauwels RA. (2003) Chronic obstructive pulmonary disease: molecular and cellular mechanisms. Euro Respir J **22**: 672–688.
60. Cho HY, Kleeberger SR. (2010) Nrf2 protects against airway disorders. *Toxicol Appl Oharmacol* **244**: 43–56.
61. Makabe S, Takahashi Y, Watanabe H *et al.* (2010) Fluvastatin protects vascular smooth muscle cells against oxidative stress through the Nrf2-dependent antioxidant pathway. *Atheroscler* **213**: 377–384.
62. Singh A, Misra V, Thimmulappa RK*et al.* (2006) Dysfunctional KEAP1-NRF2 interaction in non-small-cell lung cancer. *PLoS Med* **3**: e420.

63. Mercado N, Kizawa Y, Ueda K\ *et al.* (2014) Activation of transcription factor Nrf2 signalling by the sphingosine kinase inhibitor SKI-II is mediated by the formation of Keap1 dimers. *PloS One* **9**: e88168.
64. Sosulski ML, Gongora R, Danchuck S, Dong C, Loo F, Sanchez CG, (2015) *Aging Cell.* June 9. [Epub ahead of print].
65. Artaud-Macari E, Goven D, Brayer S, *et al.* (2013) Nuclear factor erythroid 2- related factor 2 nuclear translocation induces myofibroblastic dedifferentiation in idiopathic pulmonary fibrosis. *Antioxid Redox Sign* **18**: 66–79.
66. Tracy K, Macleod KF. (2007) Regulation of mitochondrial integrity, autophagy and cell survival by BNIP3. *Autophagy* **3**: 616–619.
67. Quinsay MN, Thomas RL, Lee Y *et al.* (2010) Bnip3-mediated mitochondrial autophagy is independent of the mitochondrial permeability transition pore. *Autophagy* **6**: 855–862.
68. Hanna RA, Quinsay MN, Orogo AM *et al.* (2012) Microtubule-associated protein 1 light chain 3 (LC3) interacts with Bnip3 protein to selectively remove endoplasmic reticulum and mitochondria via autophagy. *J Biol Chem* **287**: 19094–19104.
69. Luo F, Zhuang Y, Sides MD *et al.* (2014) Arsenic trioxide inhibits transforming growth factor-beta1-induced fibroblast to myofibroblast differentiation in vitro and bleomycin induced lung fibrosis in vivo. Respir Res **15**: 51.
70. Kanzawa T, Zhang L, Xiao L *et al.* (2005) Arsenic trioxide induces autophagic cell death in malignant glioma cells by upregulation of mitochondrial cell death protein BNIP3. *Oncogene* **24**: 980–991.
71. Kirkin V, McEwan DG, Novak I *et al.* (2009) A role for ubiquitin in selective autophagy. *Mol Cell* **34**: 259–269.
72. von Muhlinen N, Thurston T, Ryzhakov G. (2010) NDP52, a novel autophagy receptor for ubiquitin-decorated cytosolic bacteria. *Autophagy* **6**: 288–289.
73. Korac J, Schaeffer V, Kovacevic I *et al.* (2013) Ubiquitin-independent function of optineurin in autophagic clearance of protein aggregates. *J Cell Sci* **126**: 580–592.
74. Wild P, Farhan H, McEwan DG *et al.* (2011) Phosphorylation of the autophagy receptor optineurin restricts Salmonella growth. *Science* **333**: 228–233.
75. Gibbings D, Mostowy S, Jay F *et al.* (2012) Selective autophagy degrades DICER and AGO2 and regulates miRNA activity. *Nat Cell Biol* **14**: 1314–1321.

76. Orvedahl A, Sumpter R, Jr., Xiao G *et al.* (2011) Image-based genome-wide siRNA screen identifies selective autophagy factors. *Nature* **480**: 113–117.
77. Kuang E, Qi J, Ronai Z. (2013) Emerging roles of E3 ubiquitin ligases in autophagy. *Trends Biochem Sci* **38**: 453–460.
78. Ashrafi G, Schwarz TL. (2013) The pathways of mitophagy for quality control and clearance of mitochondria. *Cell Death Differentiation* **20**: 31–42.
79. Owusu-Ansah E, Song W, Perrimon N. (2013) Muscle mitohormesis promotes longevity via systemic repression of insulin signaling. *Cell* **155**: 699–712.
80. Kang C, Avery L. (2008) To be or not to be, the level of autophagy is the question: Dual roles of autophagy in the survival response to starvation. *Autophagy* **4**: 82–84.
81. Marino G, Ugalde AP, Salvador-Montoliu N *et al.* (2008) Premature aging in mice activates a systemic metabolic response involving autophagy induction. *Human Mol Genet* **17**: 2196–2211.
82. Gillespie M NK, Choi AMK , Crouser ED *et al.* (2014) Mitochondria in Lung Biology and Pathology: More than just a powerhouse. *Am J Physiol. Lung Cell Mol Physiol* **306**: 962–974.
83. Geisler S, Holmstrom KM, Skujat D *et al.* (2010) PINK1/Parkin-mediated mitophagy is dependent on VDAC1 and p62/SQSTM1. *Nat Cell Biol* **12**: 119–131.
84. Manzanillo PS, Ayres JS, Watson RO *et al.* (2013) The ubiquitin ligase parkin mediates resistance to intracellular pathogens. *Nature* **501**: 512–516.
85. Cho W, Stahelin RV. (2006) Membrane binding and subcellular targeting of C2 domains. *Biochimica et biophysica acta* **1761**: 838–849.
86. Singh R, Cuervo AM. (2012) Lipophagy: connecting autophagy and lipid metabolism. *Int J Cell Biol* **2012**: 282041.
87. Cole NB, Murphy DD, Grider T *et al.* (2002) Lipid droplet binding and oligomerization properties of the Parkinson's disease protein alpha-synuclein. *J Biol Chem* **277**: 6344–6352.
88. Fujimoto T, Ohsaki Y, Cheng J *et al.* (2008) Lipid droplets: A classic organelle with new outfits. *Histochem Cell Biol* **130**: 263–279.
89. Martin S, Parton RG. (2006) Lipid droplets: A unified view of a dynamic organelle. *Nat Revs. Mol Cell Biol* **7**: 373–378.
90. Diaz G, Batetta B, Sanna F *et al.* (2008) Lipid droplet changes in proliferating and quiescent 3T3 fibroblasts. *Histochem Cell Biol* **129**: 611–621.

91. Wang H, Gilham D, Lehner R. (2007) Proteomic and lipid characterization of apolipoprotein B-free luminal lipid droplets from mouse liver microsomes: Implications for very low density lipoprotein assembly. *J Biol Chem* **282**: 33218–33226.
92. Singh R, Kaushik S, Wang Y *et al.* (2009) Autophagy regulates lipid metabolism. *Nature* **458**: 1131–1135.
93. Greenberg AS, Coleman RA, Kraemer FB *et al.* (2011) The role of lipid droplets in metabolic disease in rodents and humans. *J Clin Invest* **121**: 2102–2110.
94. Kaushik S, Rodriguez-Navarro JA, Arias E *et al.* (2011) Autophagy in hypothalamic AgRP neurons regulates food intake and energy balance. *Cell Metabol* **14**: 173–183.
95. Ouimet M, Franklin V, Mak E *et al.* (2011) Autophagy regulates cholesterol efflux from macrophage foam cells via lysosomal acid lipase. *Cell Metabol* **13**: 655–667.
96. Plantier L, Besnard V, Xu Y *et al.* (2012) Activation of sterol-response element- binding proteins (SREBP) in alveolar type II cells enhances lipogenesis causing pulmonary lipotoxicity. *J Biol Chem* **287**: 10099–10114.
97. Agarraberes F, Terlecky S, Dice J. (1997) An intralysosomal hsp70 is required for a selective pathway of lysosomal protein degradation. *J Cell Biol* **137**: 825–834.
98. Kaushik S, Cuervo AM. (2012) Chaperone-mediated autophagy: A unique way to enter the lysosome world. *Trends Cell Biol* **22**: 407–417.
99. Cuervo AM, Dice JF. (1996) A receptor for the selective uptake and degradation of proteins by lysosomes. *Science* **273**: 501–503.
100. Bandyopadhyay U, Kaushik S, Varticovski L *et al.* (2008) The chaperone-mediated autophagy receptor organizes in dynamic protein complexes at the lysosomal membrane. *Mol Cell Biol* **28**: 5747–5763.
101. Dice JF. (1990) Peptide sequences that target cytosolic proteins for lysosomal proteolysis. *Trends Biochem Sci* **15**: 305–309.
102. Aniento F, Papavassiliou AG, Knecht E *et al.* (1996) Selective uptake and degradation of c-Fos and v-Fos by rat liver lysosomes. *FEBS Lett* **390**: 47–52.
103. Cuervo AM, Palmer A, Rivett AJ *et al.* (1995) Degradation of proteasomes by lysosomes in rat liver. *Eur J Biochem* **227**: 792–800.

104. Schneider JL, Cuervo AM. (2013) Chaperone-mediated autophagy: Dedicated saviour and unfortunate victim in the neurodegeneration arena. *Biochem Soc Trans* **41**: 1483–1488.
105. Cuervo AM. (2004) Impaired degradation of mutant-synuclein by chaperone-mediated autophagy. *Science* **305**: 1292–1295.
106. Hubbi ME, Hu H, Kshitiz, Ahmed I *et al.* (2013) Chaperone-mediated autophagy targets hypoxia-inducible factor-1alpha (HIF-1alpha) for lysosomal degradation. *J Biol Chem* **288**: 10703–10714.
107. Vakifahmetoglu-Norberg H, Kim M, Xia HG *et al.* (2013) Chaperone-mediated autophagy degrades mutant p53. *Genes Dev* **27**: 1718–1730.
108. Schneider JL, Suh Y, Cuervo AM. (2014) Deficient chaperone-mediated autophagy in liver leads to metabolic dysregulation. *Cell Metabol* **20**: 417–432.
109. Franch HA, Sooparb S, Du J *et al.* (2001) A mechanism regulating proteolysis of specific proteins during renal tubular cell growth. *J Biol Chem* **276**: 19126–19131.
110. Yang Q, She H, Gearing M *et al.* (2009) Regulation of neuronal survival factor MEF2D by chaperone-mediated autophagy. *Science* **323**: 124–127.
111. Cuervo AM, Knecht E, Terlecky SR *et al.* (1995) Activation of a selective pathway of lysosomal proteolysis in rat liver by prolonged starvation. *Am J Physiol* **269**: C1200–C1208.
112. Kiffin R, Christian C, Knecht E *et al.* (2004) Activation of chaperone-mediated autophagy during oxidative stress. *Mol Biol Cell* **15**: 4829–4840.
113. Cuervo AM, Hildebrand H, Bomhard EM *et al.* (1999) Direct lysosomal uptake of alpha2-microglobulin contributes to chemically induced nephropathy. *Kidney Int* **55**: 529–545.
114. Finn PF, Dice JF. (2005) Ketone bodies stimulate chaperone-mediated autophagy. *J Biol Chem* **280**: 25864–25870.
115. Massey AC, Kaushik S, Sovak G *et al.* (2006) Consequences of the selective blockage of chaperone-mediated autophagy. *Proc Nat Acad Sci USA* **103**: 5905–5910.
116. Kon M, Kiffin R, Koga H *et al.* (2011) Chaperone-mediated autophagy is required for tumor growth. *Sci Transl Med* **3**: 109ra117.
117. Orenstein SJ, Kuo SH, Tasset I *et al.* (2013) Interplay of LRRK2 with chaperone- mediated autophagy. *Nat Neurosci* **16**: 394–406.
118. Wang Y, Martinez-Vicente M, Kruger U *et al.* (2009) Tau fragmentation, aggregation and clearance: The dual role of lysosomal processing. *Human Mol Genet* **18**: 4153–4170.

119. Rodriguez-Navarro JA, Kaushik S, Koga H *et al.* (2012) Inhibitory effect of dietary lipids on chaperone-mediated autophagy. *Proc Natl Acad Sci USA* **109**: E705–E714.
120. Pedrozo Z, Torrealba N, Fernandez C *et al.* (2013) Cardiomyocyte ryanodine receptor degradation by chaperone-mediated autophagy. *Cardiovascul Res* **98**: 277–285.
121. Martinez-Vicente M, Talloczy Z, Kaushik S *et al.* (2008) Dopamine-modified alpha-synuclein blocks chaperone-mediated autophagy. *J Clin Invest* **118**: 777–788.
122. Cuervo AM. (2000) Age-related Decline in Chaperone-mediated Autophagy. *J Biol Chem* **275**: 31505–31513.
123. Kiffin R, Kaushik S, Zeng M *et al.* (2007) Altered dynamics of the lysosomal receptor for chaperone-mediated autophagy with age. *J Cell Sci* **120**: 782–791.
124. Huang J, Xu J, Pang S *et al.* (2012) Age-related decrease of the LAMP-2 gene expression in human leukocytes. *Clin Biochem* **45**: 1229–1232.
125. Zhang C, Cuervo AM. (2008) Restoration of chaperone-mediated autophagy in aging liver improves cellular maintenance and hepatic function. *Nature Med* **14**: 959–965.
126. Ezaki J, Matsumoto N, Takeda-Ezaki M *et al.* (2011) Liver autophagy contributes to the maintenance of blood glucose and amino acid levels. *Autophagy* **7**: 727–736.
127. Lum J, Bauer D, Kong M *et al.* (2005) Growth factor regulation of autophagy and cell survival in the absence of apoptosis. *Cell* **120**: 237–248.
128. Eng CH, Yu K, Lucas J *et al.* (2010) Ammonia derived from glutaminolysis is a diffusible regulator of autophagy. *Science Signal* **3**: ra31.
129. Wing S, Chiang HL, Goldberg AL *et al.* (1991) Proteins containing peptide sequences related to KFERQ are selectively depleted in liver and heart, but not skeletal muscle, of fasted rats. *Biochem J* **275**: 165–169.
130. Cuervo AM, Dice JF, Knecht E. (1997) A population of rat liver lysosomes responsible for the selective uptake and degradation of cytosolic proteins. *J Biol Chem* **272**: 5606–5615.
131. Cuervo AM, Dice JF. (2000) Regulation of lamp2a levels in the lysosomal membrane. *Traffic* **1**: 570–583.
132. Cuervo AM, Dice JF. (2000) Unique properties of lamp2a compared to other lamp2 isoforms. *J Cell Sci* **113**: 4441–4450.

133. Kaushik S, Massey AC, Cuervo AM. (2006) Lysosome membrane lipid microdomains: Novel regulators of chaperone-mediated autophagy. *EMBO J* **25**: 3921–3933.
134. Cuervo AM, Mann L, Bonten E *et al.* (2003) Cathepsin A regulates chaperone-mediated autophagy through cleavage of the lysosomal receptor. *EMBO J* **22**: 12–19.
135. Cuervo AM, Terlecky SR, Dice JF *et al.* (1994) Selective binding and uptake of ribonuclease A and glyceraldehyde-3-phosphate dehydrogenase by isolated rat liver lysosomes. *J Biol Chem* **269**: 26374–26380.
136. Aniento F, Roche E, Cuervo AM *et al.* (1993) Uptake and degradation of glyceraldehyde-3-phosphate dehydrogenase by rat liver lysosomes. *J Biol Chem* **268**: 10463–10470.
137. Lv L, Li D, Zhao D *et al.* (2011) Acetylation targets the M2 isoform of pyruvate kinase for degradation through chaperone-mediated autophagy and promotes tumor growth. *Mol Cell* **42**: 719–730.
138. Gonzalez-Polo RA, Boya P, Pauleau AL *et al.* (2005) The apoptosis/autophagy paradox: Autophagic vacuolization before apoptotic death. *J Cell Sci* **118**: 3091–3102.
139. Sanchez CG, Penfornis P, Oskowitz AZ *et al.* (2011) Activation of autophagy in mesenchymal stem cells provides tumor stromal support. *Carcinogenesis* **32**: 964–972.
140. Fisher AB. (1984) Intermediary metabolism of the lung. *Environ Health perspect* **55**: 149–158.
141. Fisher AB, Chander A. (1984) Lung surfactant–phospholipids and apoproteins. *Exp Lung Res* **6**: 171–174.
142. Braidy N, Guillemin GJ, Mansour H *et al.* (2011) Age related changes in NAD+ metabolism oxidative stress and Sirt1 activity in wistar rats. *PloS one* **6**: e19194.
143. Krahmer N, Farese RV, Jr., Walther TC. (2013) Balancing the fat: Lipid droplets and human disease. *EMBO Mol Med* **5**: 905–915.
144. Singh M. (2009) Alteration study of lipids and phospholipids compositions of Pachysolen tannophilus membrane with aqueous ethanol media. *Nat Prod Res* **23**: 415–421.
145. Leung JK, Cases S, Vu TH. (2008) P311 functions in an alternative pathway of lipid accumulation that is induced by retinoic acid. *J Cell Science* **121**: 2751–2758.
146. Komatsu M, Waguri S, Ueno T *et al.* (2005) Impairment of starvation-induced and constitutive autophagy in Atg7-deficient mice. *J Cell Biol* **169**: 425–434.

147. Kim J W-RM. (2012) The Role of Iron Metabolism in Lung Inflammation and Injury. *J Aller Ther* **S4**:004.
148. Ghio AJ. (2009) Disruption of iron homeostasis and lung disease. *Biochimica et biophysica acta* **1790**: 731–739.
149. Philippot Q, Deslee G, Adair-Kirk TL *et al.* (2014) Increased iron sequestration in alveolar macrophages in chronic obtructive pulmonary disease. *PloS one* **9**: e96285.
150. Kurz T, Gustafsson B, Brunk UT. (2011) Cell sensitivity to oxidative stress is influenced by ferritin autophagy. *Free Rad Biol Med* **50**: 1647–1658.
151. Sirohi K, Chalasani ML, Sudhakar C *et al.* (2013) M98K-OPTN induces transferrin receptor degradation and RAB12-mediated autophagic death in retinal ganglion cells. *Autophagy* **9**: 510–527.
152. Barzilai N, Huffman DM, Muzumdar RH *et al.* (2012) The critical role of metabolic pathways in aging. *Diabetes* **61**: 1315–1322.
153. Fontana L, Klein S, Holloszy JO. (2010) Effects of long-term calorie restriction and endurance exercise on glucose tolerance, insulin action, and adipokine production. *Age* **32**: 97–108.
154. Rezzi S, Martin FP, Shanmuganayagam D *et al.* (2009) Metabolic shifts due to long-term caloric restriction revealed in nonhuman primates. *Exp Gerontol* **44**: 356–362.
155. Sonntag WE, Csiszar A, deCabo R *et al.* (2012) Diverse roles of growth hormone and insulin-like growth factor-1 in mammalian aging: Progress and controversies. *J Gerontol A Biol Sci Med Sci* **67**: 587–598.
156. Meijer AJ, Lorin S, Blommaart EF *et al.* (2014) Regulation of autophagy by amino acids and MTOR-dependent signal transduction. *Amino acids*: DOI 10.1007/s00726-014-1765-4.
157. Gouras GK. (2013) mTOR: At the crossroads of aging, chaperones, and Alzheimer's disease. *J Neurochem* **124**: 747–748.
158. Avruch J, Hara K, Lin Y *et al.* (2006) Insulin and amino-acid regulation of mTOR signaling and kinase activity through the Rheb GTPase. *Oncogene* **25**: 6361–6372.
159. Wullschleger S, Loewith R, Hall MN. (2006) TOR signaling in growth and metabolism. *Cell* **124**: 471–484.
160. Laplante M, Sabatini DM. (2012) mTOR signaling in growth control and disease. *Cell* **149**: 274–293.
161. Fuchs A, Konig K, Heukamp LC *et al.* (2014) Tuberous-sclerosis complex-related cell signaling in the pathogenesis of lung cancer. *Diagnostic Pathol* **9**: 48.

162. Yu T, Li J, Yan M *et al.* (2014) MicroRNA-193a-3p and -5p suppress the metastasis of human non-small-cell lung cancer by downregulating the ERBB4/PIK3R3/mTOR/S6K2 signaling pathway. *Oncogene* **34**: 413–423.
163. Li YC, He SM, He ZX *et al.* (2014) Plumbagin induces apoptotic and autophagic cell death through inhibition of the PI3K/Akt/mTOR pathway in human non-small cell lung cancer cells. *Cancer Letters* **344**: 239–259.
164. White E. (2012) Deconvoluting the context-dependent role for autophagy in cancer. *Nat Revs Cancer* **12**: 401–410.
165. Rao S, Tortola L, Perlot T *et al.* (2014) A dual role for autophagy in a murine model of lung cancer. *Nat Commun* **5**: 3056.
166. Araya J, Kojima J, Takasaka N *et al.* (2013) Insufficient autophagy in idiopathic pulmonary fibrosis. *Am J Physiol Lung Cell Mol Physiol* **304**: 56–69.
167. Araya J, Kojima J, Takasaka N *et al.* (2013) Insufficient autophagy in idiopathic pulmonary fibrosis. *Am J Physiol Lung Cell Mol Physiol* **304**: L56–L69.
168. Hudson ER, Pan DA, James J *et al.* (2003) A novel domain in AMP-activated protein kinase causes glycogen storage bodies similar to those seen in hereditary cardiac arrhythmias. *Curr Biol* **13**: 861–866.
169. Lamia KA, Sachdeva UM, DiTacchio L *et al.* (2009) AMPK regulates the circadian clock by cryptochrome phosphorylation and degradation. *Science* **326**: 437–440.
170. Imamura K, Ogura T, Kishimoto A *et al.* (2001) Cell cycle regulation via p53 phosphorylation by a 5'-AMP activated protein kinase activator, 5-aminoimidazole-4-carboxamide-1-beta-D-ribofuranoside, in a human hepatocellular carcinoma cell line. *Biochem Biophys Res Commun* **287**: 562–567.
171. Shackelford DB, Shaw RJ. (2009) The LKB1-AMPK pathway: metabolism and growth control in tumour suppression. *Nat Revs Cancer* **9**: 563–575.
172. Hoyer-Hansen M, Jaattela M. (2007) AMP-activated protein kinase: A universal regulator of autophagy? *Autophagy* **3**: 381–383.
173. Canto C, Auwerx J. (2010) AMP-activated protein kinase and its downstream transcriptional pathways. *Cell Mol Life Sci* **67**: 3407–3423.
174. Miloslavski R, Cohen E, Avraham A *et al.* (2014) Oxygen sufficiency controls TOP mRNA translation via the TSC-Rheb-mTOR pathway in a 4E-BP-independent manner. *J Mol Cell Biol* **6**: 255–266.

175. Liu L, Feng D, Chen G *et al.* (2012) Mitochondrial outer-membrane protein FUNDC1 mediates hypoxia-induced mitophagy in mammalian cells. *Nat Cell Biol* **14**: 177–185.
176. Band M, Joel A, Hernandez A *et al.* (2009) Hypoxia-induced BNIP3 expression and mitophagy: In vivo comparison of the rat and the hypoxia-tolerant mole rat, Spalax ehrenbergi. *FASEB J* **23**: 2327–2335.
177. Farrall AL, Whitelaw ML. (2009) The HIF1alpha-inducible pro-cell death gene BNIP3 is a novel target of SIM2s repression through cross-talk on the hypoxia response element. *Oncogene* **28**: 3671–3680.
178. Ferreira JV, Fofo H, Bejarano E *et al.* (2013) STUB1/CHIP is required for HIF1A degradation by chaperone-mediated autophagy. *Autophagy* **9**: 1349–1366.
179. Park S, Mori R, Shimokawa I. (2013) Do sirtuins promote mammalian longevity? A critical review on its relevance to the longevity effect induced by calorie restriction. *Mol Cells* **35**: 474–480.
180. Verdin E. (2014) The many faces of sirtuins: Coupling of NAD metabolism, sirtuins and lifespan. *Nat Med* **20**: 25–27.
181. Rodgers JT, Lerin C, Haas W *et al.* (2005) Nutrient control of glucose homeostasis through a complex of PGC-1alpha and SIRT1. *Nature* **434**: 113–118.
182. Purushotham A, Schug TT, Xu Q *et al.* (2009) Hepatocyte-specific deletion of SIRT1 alters fatty acid metabolism and results in hepatic steatosis and inflammation. *Cell Metabol* **9**: 327–338.
183. Luo C, Li Y, Yang L *et al.* (2013) A cigarette component acrolein induces accelerated senescence in human diploid fibroblast IMR-90 cells. *Biogerontol* **14**: 503–511.
184. Sundar IK, Yao H, Rahman I. (2013) Oxidative stress and chromatin remodeling in chronic obstructive pulmonary disease and smoking-related diseases. *Antioxid Redox Signal* **18**: 1956–1971.
185. Price NL, Gomes AP, Ling AJ *et al.* (2012) SIRT1 is required for AMPK activation and the beneficial effects of resveratrol on mitochondrial function. *Cell Metabol* **15**: 675–690.
186. Wu Y, Li X, Zhu JX *et al.* (2011) Resveratrol-activated AMPK/SIRT1/autophagy in cellular models of Parkinson's disease. *Neuro-Sign* **19**: 163–174.
187. Camins A, Sureda FX, Junyent F *et al.* (2010) Sirtuin activators: Designing molecules to extend life span. *Biochimica et biophysica acta* **1799**: 740–749.

188. Akgedik R, Akgedik S, Karamanli H *et al.* (2012) Effect of resveratrol on treatment of bleomycin-induced pulmonary fibrosis in rats. *Inflammation* **35**: 1732–1741.
189. Sener G, Topaloglu N, Sehirli AO *et al.* (2007) Resveratrol alleviates bleomycin-induced lung injury in rats. *Pulm Pharmacol Ther* **20**: 642–649.
190. Hu YX, Cui H, Fan L *et al.* (2013) Resveratrol attenuates left ventricular remodeling in old rats with COPD induced by cigarette smoke exposure and LPS instillation. *Canadian J Physiol Pharmacol* **91**: 1044–1054.
191. Canto C, Gerhart-Hines Z, Feige JN, *et al.* (2009) AMPK regulates energy expenditure by modulating NAD+ metabolism and SIRT1 activity. *Nature* **458**: 1056–1060.
192. Froy O. (2010) Metabolism and circadian rhythms–implications for obesity. *Endocrine Revs* **31**: 1–24.
193. Claustrat F, Fournier I, Geelen G *et al.* (2005) [Aging and circadian clock gene expression in peripheral tissues in rats]. *Pathologie-biologie* **53**: 257–260.
194. Ma D, Lin JD. (2012) Circadian regulation of autophagy rhythm through transcription factor C/EBPbeta. *Autophagy* **8**: 124–125.
195. Eckel-Mahan KL, Patel VR, de Mateo S *et al.* (2013) Reprogramming of the circadian clock by nutritional challenge. *Cell* **155**: 1464–1478.
196. Masri S, Patel VR, Eckel-Mahan KL *et al.* (2013) Circadian acetylome reveals regulation of mitochondrial metabolic pathways. *Proc Natl Acad Sci USA* **110**: 3339–3344.

Index